Mental Health in Public Health

AMERICAN PSYCHOPATHOLOGICAL ASSOCIATION

Volumes in the Series

Causality and Psychopathology: Finding the Determinants of Disorders and Their Cures (Shrout, Keyes, and Ornstein, eds.)

Mental Health in Public Health: The Next 100 Years (Cottler, ed.)

Trauma, Psychopathology, and Violence: Causes, Correlates, or Consequences (Widom, ed.)

Mental Health in Public Health

THE NEXT 100 YEARS

EDITED BY

LINDA B. COTTLER, PhD, MPH

Professor of Epidemiology
Department of Psychiatry
Washington University School of Medicine
St. Louis, MO

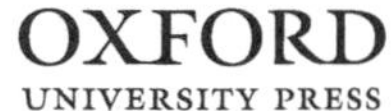

OXFORD
UNIVERSITY PRESS

Oxford University Press, Inc., publishes works that further
Oxford University's objective of excellence
in research, scholarship, and education.

Oxford New York
Auckland Cape Town Dar es Salaam Hong Kong Karachi
Kuala Lumpur Madrid Melbourne Mexico City Nairobi
New Delhi Shanghai Taipei Toronto

With offices in
Argentina Austria Brazil Chile Czech Republic France Greece
Guatemala Hungary Italy Japan Poland Portugal Singapore
South Korea Switzerland Thailand Turkey Ukraine Vietnam

Published by Oxford University Press, Inc.
198 Madison Avenue, New York, New York 10016

www.oup.com

Library of Congress Cataloging-in-Publication Data

American Psychopathological Association. Meeting (100th: 2010: New York, N.Y.)
Mental health in public health: the next 100 years/edited by Linda B. Cottler.
p.; cm.—(American Psychopathological Association series)
Includes bibliographical references and index.
ISBN 978-0-19-973594-5
1. Mental health—Congresses. 2. Public health—Congresses. I. Cottler, Linda B. II. American Psychopathological Association. III. Title. IV. Series: American Psychopathological Association series.
[DNLM: 1. Mental Disorders—epidemiology—Congresses. 2. Community Mental Health Services—Congresses. 3. Healthcare Disparities—Congresses. 4. Public Health Practice—Congresses. WM 140]
RA790.A2A44 2011
362.196'89—dc22 2010042388

This material is not intended to be, and should not be considered, a substitute for medical or other professional advice. Treatment for the conditions described in this material is highly dependent on the individual circumstances. And, while this material is designed to offer accurate information with respect to the subject matter covered and to be current as of the time it was written, research and knowledge about medical and health issues is constantly evolving and dose schedules for medications are being revised continually, with new side effects recognized and accounted for regularly. Readers must therefore always check the product information and clinical procedures with the most up-to-date published product information and data sheets provided by the manufacturers and the most recent codes of conduct and safety regulation. The publisher and the authors make no representations or warranties to readers, express or implied, as to the accuracy or completeness of this material. Without limiting the foregoing, the publisher and the authors make no representations or warranties as to the accuracy or efficacy of the drug dosages mentioned in the material. The authors and the publisher do not accept, and expressly disclaim, any responsibility for any liability, loss or risk that may be claimed or incurred as a consequence of the use and/or application of any of the contents of this material.

Printed in United States of America
on acid-free paper

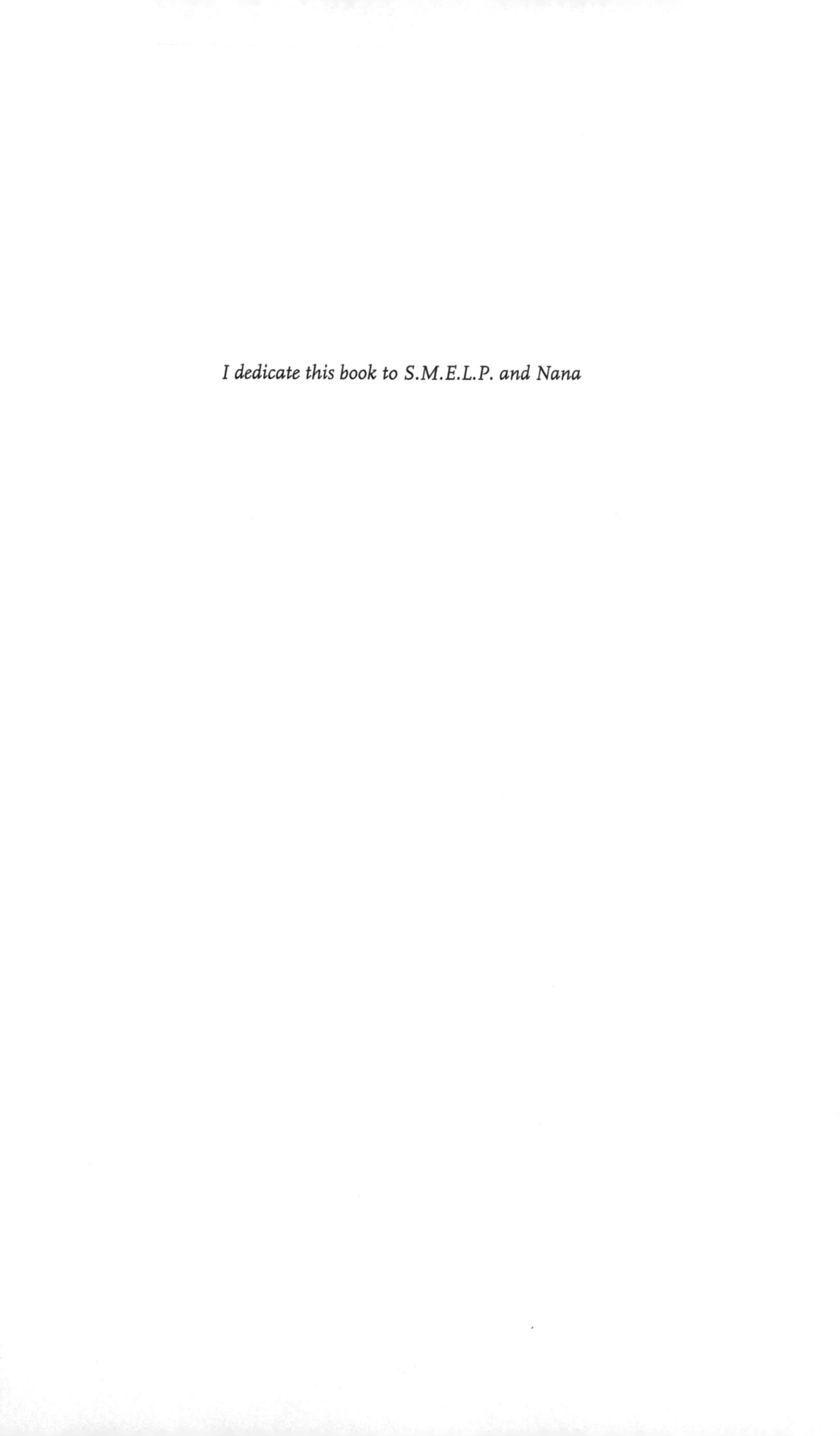

I dedicate this book to S.M.E.L.P. and Nana

Prologue

Being the President of the APPA during its Centennial year was a wonderful honor. As is customary, the President selects the topic and the speakers for the meeting with input from the Council. I am most pleased to present, in this volume, work discussed at the meeting by leaders in the field of psychiatric epidemiology. In addition, I have attached to this Prologue my opening remarks to the meeting.

Welcome to the 100th Anniversary meeting of the American Psychopathological Association! I'm honored to serve as President this year and to introduce this meeting. John Helzer, our Archivist, and I visited the APPA Archives at Cornell and have a special treat for you.

First, after 100 years, we've grown, but are still that special society to discuss the problems of psychopathology that Morton Prince and others had in mind when they started our society. There is a list of the first members of the APPA in our Archives. Sigmund Freud was a member.

The first annual meeting was held in Washington, D.C., on May 2, 1910. The papers presented were:

- Sex Symbolism in Dreams
- The Action of Suggestion in Therapeutics
- The Anxiety Neuroses
- Dreams as a Cause of Symptoms
- Mechanisms of Dreams

About 50 people attended that meeting. In the beginning, the journal was the *Journal of Abnormal Psychology*. Now, it is *Comprehensive Psychiatry*, edited by Past President David Dunner.

At 100 years, we have 457 Active Members. We started with $5 dues in 1962, $20 in 1973, $40 in 1980, $60 in 1987, $75 in 1991, and since 1996, we pay $100.

To commemorate this 100th year, we put together some things for you: a grocery bag, a nice pen, a lanyard for your name badge, a stainless steel water bottle, and an APPA commemorative booklet. The booklet has highlights including a letter from the first President, Morton Prince, the original Constitution and books we've published, as well as lists of those who have served as President, Secretary, and Treasurer.

My meeting topic, Mental Health in Public Health, is very dear to me. I believe, as you all do, that there is no public health without mental health. We've assembled a terrific group of speakers who will cover all aspects of mental health from childhood to older age. We will also focus on the most hidden populations and end with community-based strategies to give everyone a voice in health research.

I am particularly excited about the Past Presidents' Forum on Saturday where we will discuss the future of psychiatry. Living Presidents Bob Cloninger, Myrna Weissman, Alfred Freedman, and Jim Barrett send their regrets.

I cannot begin this meeting without noting those who came before me—all the Past Presidents, alive and dead, here and absent, especially Lee Robins, who died this past September. I want to thank her and John Helzer for bringing me into the world of psychiatric epidemiology. And I want to thank all of my colleagues from Washington University, and my group, EPRG, in particular.

To wrap up this introduction, I need to address a few logistics:

1. This is the first of a five-year commitment to the Grand Hyatt. It appears we are all very pleased with this new venue.
2. Nancy Newman Rice, the spouse of John Rice, donated the use of her painting for our poster and program for the Centennial meeting.
3. The NIMH R13 conference grant allowed us to support 17 travel awardees.
4. Oxford University Press will begin to publish our conference volume.
5. The number you see on the name badge below the name and affiliation is the number of years the person has been a member of the APPA.
6. A group photo will be taken.

Finally, I give thanks to our councilors—Darrel Regier, Lauren Alloy, Karestan Koenen, and Chuck Zorumski. Thanks to Mike Lyons (Membership) and John Helzer (Archivist). Thanks to officers Ezra Susser and Cathy Widom. Most of all, thanks to Kim Fader and Catina O'Leary, who do the bulk of the work for the APPA.

So, without further delay, we will begin the 2010 meeting with the striking of the gavel, which was made from Dr. Adolf Meyer's bedside table.

Linda B. Cottler, PhD, MPH
President 2010, APPA

Contents

Contributors

SERGIO AGUILAR-GAXIOLA, MD, PhD
Center for Reducing Health Disparities; and Clinical and Translational Science Center
School of Medicine
University of California, Davis
Sacramento, CA

MURRAY ALPERT, PhD
Department of Psychiatry
New York University School of Medicine
New York, NY

JAMES E. BARRETT, MD
Department of Psychiatry and Department of Community and Family Medicine
Dartmouth Medical School
Hanover, NH

O. JOSEPH BIENVENU, MD, PhD
Department of Psychiatry and Behavioral Sciences
School of Medicine
Johns Hopkins University
Baltimore, MD

MARTHA L. BRUCE, PhD, MPH
Weill Cornell Medical College
Cornell University
Ithaca, NY

ADRIE W. BRUIJNZEEL, PhD
Department of Psychiatry
University of Florida
Gainesville, FL

CATINA CALLAHAN O'LEARY, PhD, MSW
Epidemiology and Prevention Research Group
Department of Psychiatry
Washington University School of Medicine
St. Louis, MO

REDONNA K. CHANDLER, PhD
Division of Epidemiology, Services, and Prevention Research
National Institute on Drug Abuse; and Department of Health and Human Services
National Institutes of Health
Bethesda, MD

C. ROBERT CLONINGER, MD
Department of Psychiatry
Washington University School of Medicine
St. Louis, MO

WILSON M. COMPTON, MD, MPE
Division of Epidemiology, Services, and Prevention Research
National Institute on Drug Abuse; and Department of Health and Human Services
National Institutes of Health
Bethesda, MD

JOHN N. CONSTANTINO, MD
Department of Psychiatry
Washington University School of Medicine
St. Louis, MO

LINDA B. COTTLER, PhD, MPH
Epidemiology and Prevention Research Group
Department of Psychiatry
Washington University School of Medicine
St. Louis, MO

FRANCINE COURNOS, MD
Department of Psychiatry
New York State Psychiatric Institute
Columbia University
New York, NY

ROSA M. CRUM, MD, MHS
Johns Hopkins Bloomberg School of Public Health
Baltimore, MD

J. RAYMOND DEPAULO, JR., MD
Department of Psychiatry and Behavioral Sciences
Johns Hopkins University School of Medicine
Baltimore, MD

BRUCE P. DOHRENWEND, PhD
Department of Psychiatry and Mailman School of Public Health
Columbia University
New York, NY

DAVID L. DUNNER, MD, FACPsych
Center for Anxiety and Depression
Mercer Island, WA

WILLIAM W. EATON, PhD
Johns Hopkins Bloomberg School of Public Health
Baltimore, MD

MAX FINK, MD
Department of Psychiatry and Behavioral Science
Stony Brook University
Long Island, NY

ELLEN FRANK, PhD
Departments of Psychiatry and Psychology
University of Pittsburgh School of Medicine
Pittsburgh, PA

ALFRED M. FREEDMAN, MD
Department of Psychiatry and Behavioral Sciences
New York Medical College
New York, NY

SANDRO GALEA, MD, DrPH
School of Public Health
University of Michigan
Ann Arbor, MI

MARGO GENDERSON, MA
Department of Psychology
Boston University
Boston, MA

ELLIOT S. GERSHON, MD
Department of Psychiatry
University of Chicago
Chicago, IL

MARCI E. J. GLEASON, PhD
Department of Human Development and Family Sciences
University of Texas at Austin
Austin, TX

MARK S. GOLD, MD
Department of Psychiatry
McKnight Brain Institute
University of Florida
Gainesville, FL

MICHAEL D. GRANT, PhD
Department of Psychology
Boston University
Boston, MA

ALDEN L. GROSS, MHS
Johns Hopkins Bloomberg School of Public Health
Baltimore, MD

KATHERINE A. HALMI, MD
Department of Psychiatry
Weill Cornell Medical College
New York, NY

JOHN E. HELZER, MD
Department of Psychiatry
University of Vermont School of Medicine
Burlington, VT

MICHAEL HERKOV, PhD
Department of Psychiatry
University of Florida
Gainesville, FL

JAMES J. HUDZIAK, MD
Department of Psychiatry
University of Vermont College of Medicine
Burlington, VT

DAVID S. JANOWSKY, MD
Department of Psychiatry
University of North Carolina at Chapel Hill
Chapel Hill, NC

DONALD F. KLEIN, MD, DSC
Department of Child and Adolescent Psychiatry
New York University Langone Medical Center
New York, NY

MIRJA KOSCHORKE, MRCPsych
Centre for Global Mental Health
London School of Hygiene and Tropical Medicine
London, UK

MICHAEL J. LYONS, PhD
Department of Psychology
Boston University
Boston, MA

KAREN McKINNON, MA
Department of Psychiatry
New York State Psychiatric Institute
Columbia University
New York, NY

LISA J. MERLO, PhD
Department of Psychiatry
University of Florida
Gainesville, FL

CAROL S. NORTH, MD, MPE
VA North Texas Health Care System; and
Departments of Psychiatry and Surgery/ Division of Emergency Medicine
The University of Texas Southwestern Medical Center
Dallas, TX

THOMAS F. OLTMANNS, PhD
Department of Psychology
Washington University
St. Louis, MO

VIKRAM PATEL, MSC, MRCPsych, PhD, FMedsci
Centre for Global Mental Health
London School of Hygiene and Tropical Medicine
London, UK

MARTIN PRINCE, MD, MSC, FRCPsych
Centre for Global Mental Health
London School of Hygiene and Tropical Medicine
London, UK

JUDITH L. RAPOPORT, MD
Child Psychiatry Branch
National Institute of Mental Health
Bethesda, MD

DARREL A. REGIER, MD, MPH
Division of Research
American Psychiatric Association
Arlington, VA

ANNA ROYTBERG, SCB
Feinberg School of Medicine
Northwestern University
Chicago, IL

NORMAN SARTORIUS, MD, PhD
Association for the Improvement of Mental Health Programmes
Geneva, Swtizerland

PATRICK E. SHROUT, PhD
Department of Psychology
New York University
New York, NY

MARIA STEENLAND, MPH
School of Public Health
University of Michigan
Ann Arbor, MI

CATHERINE W. STRILEY, PhD, MSW, MPE
Epidemiology and Prevention Research Group
Department of Psychiatry
Washington University School of Medicine
St. Louis, MO

MING T. TSUANG, MD, PhD
Department of Psychiatry
University of California, San Diego
San Diego, CA

MILTON WAINBERG, MD
Department of Psychiatry
New York State Psychiatric Institute
Columbia University
New York, NY

MYRNA M. WEISSMAN, PhD
Departments of Epidemiology and Psychiatry
Columbia University
New York, NY

LINDA ZIEGAHN, PhD
Center for Reducing Health Disparities; and
Clinical and Translational Science Center
School of Medicine
University of California, Davis
Sacramento, CA

CHARLES F. ZORUMSKI, MD
Department of Psychiatry
Washington University School of Medicine
St. Louis, MO

PART I

Mental Health Disparities

Populations at Risk

1

Closing the Treatment Gap

A Global Health Perspective

VIKRAM PATEL, MIRJA KOSCHORKE, AND MARTIN PRINCE

The Treatment Gap

A major concern of global mental health is taking care of people with mental disorders who live in low and middle income countries (LAMIC) because they receive only a fraction of available global resources.[1] The 1990 report on the *Global Burden of Disease*[2] (GBD) highlighted the considerable burden of neuropsychiatric disorders compared with other conditions based on the health metric of the DALY (disability adjusted life years); since then there has been considerable attention to global mental health. A subsequent *World Mental Health* report emphasized a clear relationship between mental health and social factors such as violence and poverty.[3] The *World Health Report* 2001 was devoted to mental health.[4] It, and the World Health Organization's (WHO's) Commission on Social Determinants of Health, reported strong evidence demonstrating clear bi-directional relationships between social disadvantage and two mental disorders: depression in adults and ADHD in children.[5] In spite of those prior initiatives and a substantial growing evidence of the large global burden of mental disorders, mental health remains one of the least prioritised areas of global health.

In fact, mental health is not included in any major global health program, and there has been no equivalent of the Global Fund for TB, HIV, and malaria. It is exceedingly difficult to find major new donors who make mental health their priority. Recent estimates suggest that between 50 and 90% of people with severe mental disorders fail to receive even basic treatment.[6–7] While treatment gaps are evident the world over, they are particularly large in LAMIC. Moreover, an appalling neglect of human rights continues to blot the mental health care treatment landscape around the world.[8] Such a gap in services, in the face of growing evidence on cost-effective interventions for many mental disorders,[9–10] is one of the greatest public health worries.

Based on this, we review the evidence on the global burden of mental health disorders and the interaction between mental health and other health conditions to make the case that "there is no health without mental health."[11] The impact of mental illness on those who live with it, as well as their families, is the subject of this chapter, which also describes the significant burden of stigma and discrimination the world over. The chapter also reports on the barriers to scaling up services for people with mental disorders,[12] even though there is substantial evidence of the cost-effectiveness of task-shifting these treatments and new evidence on its feasibility and effectiveness in mental health care.[10] Finally, we describe new global initiatives which seek to scale up this evidence to close the treatment gap for mental disorders.

Burden and Impact of Mental Disorders

There isn't much difference in the burden of mental disorders by world regions.[2,13] Proportionately, mental disorders account for 9% of the burden in low income countries (LIC), 18% in middle income (MIC), and 27% in high income countries (HIC)[2,13] (Figures 1.1 and 1.2), resulting from the burden of other health conditions being much greater in LICs, which exaggerates the denominator. Figure 1.2 shows that the proportionate burden also varies by world region, with the lowest region Africa and the highest region the Americas.

Prince and colleagues suggest that the burden of mental disorders is underestimated in the GBD,[11] where mental disorders account for 31.7% of all years

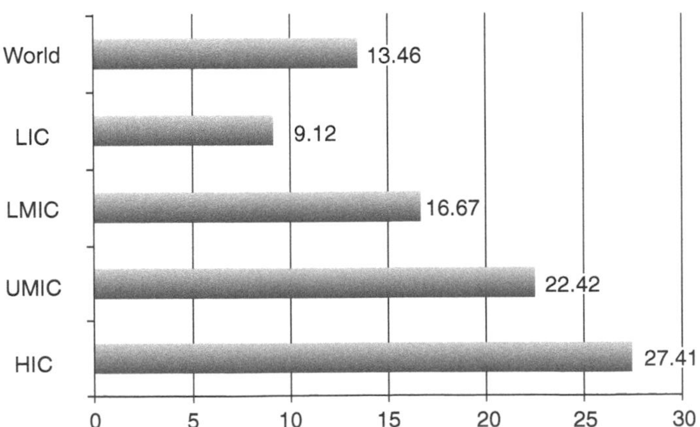

Figure 1.1 Burden of neuropsychiatric disorders by income category of countries (in proportion of total DALYs).

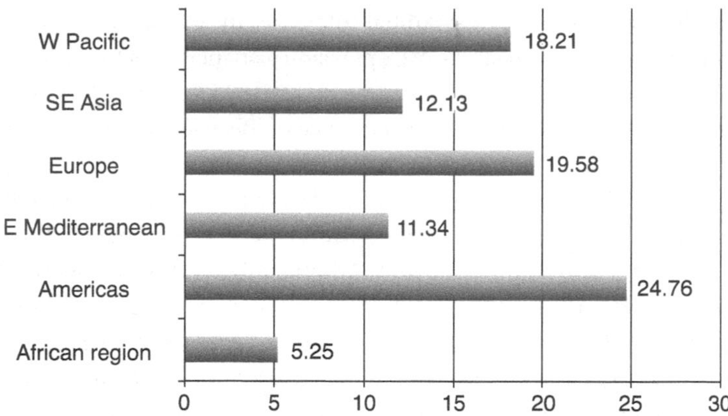

Figure 1.2 Burden of neuropsychiatric disorders by world region (in proportion of total DALYs).

lived with disability, and only 1.4% of years of life lost through premature mortality. Each year at least 800,000 people commit suicide; 86% of those who commit suicide are from LAMIC, and over half are young people.[2,13–15] Mental disorder is overwhelmingly the most important preventable factor.[16–19] Nonsuicide mortality is also elevated among persons with psychosis,[19–20] depression,[21–22] and dementia.[23] However, the poor quality of general health care received by those with mental disorders may explain some of the excess mortality.[24] Furthermore, much of the burden attributed to mental illness could be related to complex interactions with other health conditions, such as infectious diseases, reproductive health, and maternal and child health.[11]

Comorbidity with Physical Health Conditions

Comorbidity of physical and mental conditions is a major concern for people in LAMIC, especially because their symptoms are usually medically unexplained. Approximately 15% of patients seen in primary care report unexplained somatic symptoms that co-occur with psychological distress.[25–26] Those affected are chronically disabled, frequently seek health care, and account for a large proportion of health care costs.[25–27] Additionally, mental disorders are risk factors for the development of communicable and noncommunicable diseases; many physical health conditions actually increase a person's risk for mental illness. For example, in epidemiological studies, depression has been found to be a risk factor for cardiovascular disease (CVD) including angina, myocardial infarction (MI),[28–29] and stroke.[30–33] The associations are largely independent of CVD risk factors, such as hypertension,[30] obesity,[34] and smoking.[35–36]

There has also been a substantial increase in major depression after myocardial infarction[37] and stroke.[38] Depression also increases the risk for onset of type II diabetes.[39–42] We know that approximately 15% of people with schizophrenia have type II diabetes as a consequence of lifestyle factors, the metabolic effects of antipsychotic medication, and possible underlying disease-specific mechanisms.[43] Mental illness is also a risk factor for communicable diseases. For example, tuberculosis (TB) is more prevalent among people with serious mental illness[44–45] and heavy drinkers.[46] Additionally, worldwide, nearly 10% of people living with HIV/AIDS have a history of injection-drug use.[47] In the US, those with chronic severe mental illness have a high seroprevalence of HIV (5–7%),[48] and a clustering of behavioral risk factors.[49] Depression predicts seroconversion among men who have had sex with men;[50] alcohol use and depression are associated with unprotected sex among those already infected.[51]

Alternatively, persons with sexually transmitted diseases (STDs) are at higher risk for mental disorders. Persons with HIV/AIDS are more likely than those without to have affective disorder[52–54] and neurocognitive impairment.[55–56] Apart from the psychological trauma of the diagnosis, HIV infection[57] and HAART treatment[48] have direct central nervous system (CNS) effects. Multidrug-resistant TB (MDR-TB) is associated with particularly poor mental health attributed to loss of work and social roles, feelings of hopelessness, and stigma.[58] In Peru, the prevalence of mood disorders at diagnosis of TB was 52% with a further substantial incidence of mood disorders and psychosis during MDR-TB treatment.[59] In an inpatient study in Turkey, the prevalence of mood disorder was 19% for recently diagnosed TB, 22% for defaulted TB, and 26% for MDR-TB.[60]

Third, comorbidity also affects help-seeking behavior, as well as diagnosis and treatment; it affects the outcomes of treatment for physical conditions, including disease-related mortality. Comorbid depression predicts reinfarction and death after myocardial infarction.[28–29] Post-stroke depression is associated with poor functional outcomes[61–62] and a 3.4 times higher mortality over 10 years.[63] Persons with diabetes who also have depression have been found to have poor glycemic control,[64] complications,[65] and high mortality rates.[66] In the US, chronic depressive symptoms have been associated with increased AIDS-related mortality[67–68] and more rapid disease progression[67] independent of the receipt of treatment. Cognitive impairment in HIV is associated with greatly increased mortality independent of clinical stage and antiretroviral treatment.[69]

Schizophrenia complicates treatment and is associated with worse prognosis.[48] The incidence of AIDS-defining illnesses on HAART is increased among injection-drug users.[47] A common underlying mechanism may be the poor adherence to treatment for oral hypoglycemic therapy among people with schizophrenia,[70] and for diet[71–72] and exercise recommendations[72] and oral hypoglycemic medication[71–72] among diabetics with depression. There is consistent evidence from developed countries that adherence to HAART is adversely affected by depression,[73–75] cognitive impairment,[76–77] and alcohol and substance use.[47] There are fewer studies from LAMIC.[78] Alcohol use disorder has also been reported to be associated with delayed treatment-seeking, poor adherence to directly observed therapy,[79–80] and with unfavorable treatment outcomes for pulmonary TB[81] and for MDR-TB.[82]

Fourth, women are at heightened risk for mood disorders with a typical female-to-male gender ratio of 1.5 to 2.0.[83–84] Mood and substance use disorders are all robustly associated with dysmenorrhea, dyspareunia, and pelvic pain.[85] In Asian cultures, reproductive and mental health experiences may enhance these associations. Specifically, a study in south India found that a complaint of vaginal discharge was associated with mood disorder and not with reproductive tract infection.[86]

Maternal mental health may also have important implications for infant growth and survival. Maternal schizophrenia is consistently associated with preterm delivery,[87–88] low birth weight,[87–89] stillbirth, and infant mortality.[90] Postpartum depression affects 10–15% of women.[91–92] In developed countries there are adverse consequences for the early mother–infant relationship and for the child's psychological development.[93] In Asia, where physical development of infants is a particular problem, studies suggest an independent association between antenatal mood disorder and low birth weight, and associations between perinatal mood disorder and infant under-nutrition at six months.[92, 94–95] Maternal depression reduces adherence to child-health promotion and disease-prevention interventions, for example, immunization.[95] There is good evidence from developed countries[96] and LAMIC[97] that maternal depression is associated with sub-optimal breastfeeding.

Stigma and Discrimination

The stigma associated with mental illness contributes significantly to the burden of mental illness; in fact, subjective accounts of persons affected by mental illness testify that the effects of stigma and discrimination are often perceived as more burdensome and distressing than the primary condition itself.[98] The term stigma refers to "a social devaluation of a person"[99] due to an "attribute that is deeply discrediting,"[100] and can be conceptualized as consisting of "problems of ignorance, prejudice, and discrimination."[98] Discrimination, the behavioral consequence of stigma, contributes to the disability of persons with mental illness and leads to disadvantages in many aspects of life including personal relationships, education, work, housing, parenting, and childcare, as well as access to physical health care.[98,101] In addition to experiences of direct discrimination from others, persons suffering from mental illness face several forms of structural discrimination, including the lack of resources allocated to the care of mental disorders and inadequate attention to the physical health needs of people with mental illness.[102]

Paradoxically, mental health institutions and their staff are often the source of discrimination. People with mental illness frequently report feeling patronized or humiliated by contact with mental health service staff.[103] Additionally, stigmatizing views are often held by mental health staff themselves.[104–106] Human rights violations are often pervasive within the confines of mental health services.[107] Recent examples of such violations include deaths linked to malnutrition and hypothermia in a psychiatric hospital in Romania,[108] forced labor for inpatients in the Kyrgyz republic,[109] and the tragedy at Erwadi, India, where over 20 patients burned to death when a fire broke out in a healing shrine, because they had been chained to their beds.[110] In many societies where services are scarce, families resort to chaining and other inhumane practices to restrain people with mental disorders.[10,111]

Some people with mental illness accept the negative beliefs and prejudices held against them and lose self-esteem, resulting in self-stigmatization[112,119] leading to feelings of shame, hopelessness,[113] a sense of being separate from society,[114] and social withdrawal.[112,115] People with mental illness commonly anticipate discrimination and consequently try to hide their illness, become reluctant to seek help or stop themselves from applying for work,[98,115,116] thereby reinforcing the cycle of dependency and disability.

Research on stigma has been carried out in many parts of the world,[98] and findings suggest that all cultures discriminate against people with mental illness.[98] In a cross-sectional survey involving participants with schizophrenia in 27 countries, consistently high rates of experienced and anticipated discrimination were found.[116] 47% of participants said they experienced discrimination when making or keeping friends, 43% said they experienced discrimination from family members, and over 25% said it was experienced in relation to finding or keeping a job or in intimate relationships. Rates of anticipated discrimination were high; 64% reported that they had stopped themselves from applying for work, applying for training, or taking classes; over half (55%) had stopped themselves from looking for a close relationship.

High levels of ignorance and misinformation about mental disorders in the general public are a common finding. There appear to be links between popular understandings of mental illness, the perceived need to conceal the problem, and help-seeking behavior.[98]

Stigma also affects families, mental health institutions, and mental health staff.[117] In one study carried out with family caregivers of people with schizophrenia in Chennai, India, over 50% worried that other family members would not be able to marry and that other people would avoid them and treat them differently if they knew about their illness.[99] In a study from China, stigma was found to exert moderate to severe effects on the lives of over 25% of family members.[118]

Stigma and discrimination associated with mental illness are linked to the treatment gap experienced with mental illness. Stigma triggers a vicious cycle that leads to disadvantages in many aspects of life,[117] adding to increased levels of disability. Feelings of shame and low self-esteem reduce self-efficacy and produce a barrier to recovery.[112,119] Stigma lowers access to and utilization of health care because people may fear being identified and labeled, therefore delaying or avoiding seeking help for their condition.[102] Undesirable and often dehumanizing conditions in many mental health institutions further add to the barriers to treatment. The consequence of such is poor recovery rates, which further reinforce negative attitudes and discrimination.[117,120] The need to tackle this important issue has been emphasized by the World Health Organization (WHO) as a key intervention to close the treatment gap. While there are promising initiatives to combat stigma both at local and international levels,[120] much remains to be done to better understand and effectively address this complex phenomenon.

Treatment of Mental Disorders

A substantial amount of evidence is accumulating on the efficacy and cost-effectiveness of treatments for mental disorders. While much of this evidence originates from high income countries, work is now being conducted in LAMIC[9–10] and is indicating that, for most mental disorders, a combination of pharmacological and psychological treatments is the most appropriate and cost-effective treatment. Older, generic medications are just as effective as newer ones and, since they are much cheaper, they are more cost-effective. For many disorders, pharmacological treatments are indicated only for the most serious cases (for example, mood disorders). Moreover, brief structured treatments such as cognitive-behavioral or interpersonal therapies are effective. There is ample evidence that treatment of comorbid mental disorders is highly effective in improving mental health and quality of life across a range of disorders including cancer,[121] diabetes,[122] heart disease,[123–124] and HIV/AIDS.[125] In fact, structured treatment recommendations,[126–127] antidepressants,[128] and cognitive behavioral therapy (CBT)[129] have been found to reduce "medically unexplained" somatic complaints.[126]

The evidence base on whether mental health interventions can improve physical disease outcomes is mixed. Psychological interventions have been shown to improve type 1 and 2 diabetes.[130,131] Pharmacological treatments are effective for depression, but do not improve glycemic control[122] or diabetic self-care.[132–134] Antidepressants and CBT are safe and moderately effective treatments for depression post-MI,[124,135–136] but do not reduce reinfarction rates or overall mortality. The evidence base for the effectiveness of antidepressants post-stroke is weak, both for prevention and treatment.[137–138] However, one trial with a nine-year follow-up does suggest a sustained reduction in post-stroke mortality associated with antidepressant treatment.[139] In light of these findings, more intensive and tailored interventions should be advocated.[140]

In Peru, a nonrandomized evaluation of a group psychotherapy intervention coupled with recreation, symbolic celebrations, and family workshops was associated with a default rate of only 3.5% in a treatment cohort of 276 patients with MDR-TB.[141] In India, a psychotherapeutic intervention based on behavioral modification techniques was associated with significant improvements in treatment completion.[142] Similar benefits were noted for TB clubs in Ethiopia.[143] More research is needed, particularly with regard to HIV, where observational data suggests that antiretroviral adherence might be improved by antidepressant treatment.[144] As important as this seems, the number of psychosocial interventions has been surprisingly limited.[11,57] Interventions for child health and nutrition, such as infant-feeding advice, are mostly directed towards the mother, whose psychological well-being is therefore likely to be key to the success of these programs. A randomized controlled trial (RCT) of a CBT-based intervention for depressed mothers integrated into the routine work of community-based primary health workers in rural Pakistan was effective in increasing immunization rates and reducing episodes of diarrhea in their infants, while improving the mental health outcome for the mothers.[146]

Barriers to Scaling Up Evidence-Based Treatments

In spite of the evidence and many previous initiatives to highlight the crisis in global mental health care, the unmet need for care for people with mental disorders remains astonishingly large. Even where treatments are available, they tend to focus on pharmacological interventions and on care within mental hospitals (rather than primary and community care models). There are several barriers to scaling up evidence-based services,[12] and they operate in varying degrees in all countries of the world. The lack of resources is the major barrier; in Africa, for example, 80% of countries spend less than 1% of their national health budget on mental health.[147] The small overall size of health budgets makes the absolute figures even less adequate in the poorest countries. Although tax and insurance-based systems are all more appropriate than out-of-pocket payment, out-of-pocket payments are most commonly used in LAMIC.[147] Yet, a relatively modest investment of US $2–3 per capita is all that would be needed to provide a basic package of mental health services (focusing on schizophrenia, bipolar disorder, and depression) in many of the poorest LAMIC.[148]

There is an enormous scarcity of psychiatrists and other mental health specialists in most countries of the world; apart from the overall scarcity, these human resources are extremely inequitably distributed between and within countries,[1,147] which is further exacerbated by the out-migration of mental health specialists from poorer to richer countries.[149] This is further compounded within nations, when resources migrate from poorer to richer regions and from public to private services. The problem of inefficiency is also found: most mental health specialists work in very similar ways, regardless of the resource contexts in which they work. Thus, their face-to-face clinical work remains their predominant role, one which is incompatible with scaling up services to increase the pitiful coverage rates for basic mental health care.[150] Additionally, there is a concentration of scarce resources in many countries in large mental hospitals, with little or no investment in community or primary mental health care services. Other barriers include the local public health priority agenda and its impact on funding; the perceived complexity of and resistance to changing the availability of mental health services; challenges in implementing mental health care in primary care settings; and the lack of a public health perspective among leaders in mental health services sectors.[12]

Closing the Treatment Gap

One of the most important advances in mental health care in recent years has been the demonstration of the safety and effectiveness of an effort called "task-shifting" as a means to deliver efficacious treatments. Such evidence provides the key to overcoming the huge barrier posed by the scarcity of specialist mental health human resources and all of the other gaps just discussed. Task-shifting is a rational redistribution of tasks among the health workforce team: specific tasks are moved, where appropriate, from highly qualified health workers to health workers with shorter training and fewer qualifications in order to make more efficient use of the available human resources for health.[151] In recent years, a series of controlled evaluations have shown that psychological treatments or complex packages of care can be delivered by low-cost health professionals (lay people or community health workers), who are appropriately trained and supervised in the areas of depression, schizophrenia, and dementia.[145,152–155]

Mental health remains a low priority in most LAMIC. When mental disorders are seen as a distinct health domain, with separate services and budgets, investing in mental health alone is unaffordable. The ideal setting of care should be within the primary health care model using strategies which are common to all chronic diseases such as: opportunistic case finding for early detection; using a combination of pharmacological and psychosocial interventions, often in a stepped care fashion; and long-term follow up with regular monitoring and promoting adherence with treatment.[156]

Scaling Up Services: A Call to Action for Global Health

The sheer scale of unmet need for care was the key motivation for the publication, in 2007, of the landmark *Lancet* series on global mental health, a series of six articles produced independently by a group of global mental health leaders. The articles argued for scientific evidence as the basis for global advocacy[148] and ended with a call to action for the scaling up of evidence-based mental health services throughout the world and the implementation of policies protecting the rights of mentally ill people. These messages are relevant in all countries, not just in LAMIC. The principles set out in the *Lancet* global mental health series do not necessarily relate to the developed world, for example, in the nonparity in mental health care compared to general medical care in most developed countries.[157] Fortunately, local, regional, and international initiatives have begun to materialize in response to this call to action.[158] A prominent example is the World Health Organization's Mental Health Gap Action Programme (mhGAP) (http://www.who.int/mental_health/mhGAP/en/index.html),[159] which aims to identify and scale up cost-effective packages of care for eight priority conditions.

Beyond these initiatives, the call for action will also need a radical transformation in global health policy and practice whereby relevant governmental and multilateral agencies collaborate with a range of stakeholders concerned with health care and human rights. A mental health legislative framework compatible with the UN Convention on Rights of People with Disabilities is an essential requirement in every country. There is a need to overcome resistance to decentralization of resources, especially among many mental health professionals and hospital workers. Mental health investments in primary care are important but are unlikely to be sustained unless they are preceded or accompanied by the development of community mental health services. There is a need to step up mobilization and recognition of nonformal resources in the community—including community members without formal professional training, and people with mental disorders themselves and their family members—to take part in advocacy and service delivery. The voices of the mentally ill and their families—those most affected—must be listened to. Mental health professionals, primary and community health practitioners, public health experts, and policymakers must show solidarity with them. Several key questions will require systematic research in order to inform the scaling-up process.[160] The mental health community overall has to act in concert with leaders in public health to ensure the inclusion of the subject of mental health on the global public health policy agenda, and the integration of mental health care into all pertinent levels of general health care.

The Movement for Global Mental Health, born on October 10, 2008,[161] aims to build a coalition of individuals and institutions committed to improving the health care of people with mental disorders everywhere in the world. The ultimate aim of the Movement is straightforward: provision of basic, affordable care comprising generic medications, brief psychological treatments, and attention to the social needs and human rights of people with mental disorders and their families. The Movement for Global Mental Health embodies the hope that "the substantial progress in scaling up of services for people with mental disorders will take its place alongside progress in HIV/AIDS treatment and maternal and child survival as one of the great public health successes of our times" (www.globalmentalhealth.org). Only when the treatment gaps for people with mental disorders are systematically addressed on the basis of evidence derived both from biomedical disciplines and the lived experiences of people with mental disorders, will their rights and entitlements be realized at the standards which we should expect and demand.

Acknowledgment

This chapter is adapted from a chapter to be published in the *Routledge International Handbook of Global Public Health* in 2010, co-edited by Dr. Richard Parker and Dr. Marni Sommer. Vikram Patel is supported by a Wellcome Trust Senior Research Fellowship in Clinical Science. Mirja Koschorke is supported by a Wellcome Trust Clinical PhD Fellowship.

References

1. Saxena, S., Thornicroft, G., Knapp, M., & Whiteford, H. (2007). Resources for mental health: Scarcity, inequity, and inefficiency. *Lancet, 370,* 878–889.
2. Murray, C. & A. Lopez, (Eds.). (1996). *The global burden of disease.* Boston: Harvard University Press.
3. Desjarlais, R., Eisenberg, G. L., Good, B., & Kleinman, A. (1995). *World mental health: Problems and priorities in low-income countries.* Oxford: Oxford University Press.
4. World Health Organization. (2001). *The World Health Report 2001: Mental health: New understanding, new hope.* Geneva: World Health Organization.
5. Patel, V., Lund, C., Heatherill, S., Plagerson, S., Corrigal, J., Funk, M., et al. (2009). Social determinants of mental disorders. In E. Blas & A. Sivasankara Kurup, (Eds.). *Priority public health conditions: From learning to action on social determinants of health.* Geneva: World Health Organization.
6. Wang, P. S., Aguilar-Gaxiola, S., Alonso, J., Angermeyer, M. C., Borges, G., Bromet, E. J., et al. (2007). Use of mental health services for anxiety, mood, and substance disorders in 17 countries in the WHO world mental health surveys. *Lancet, 370,* 841–850.

7. Kohn, R., Saxena, S., Levav, I., & Saraceno, B. (2004). The treatment gap in mental health care. *Bull World Health Organ, 82,* 858–866.
8. Patel, V., Kleinman, A., & Saraceno, B. (in press). Protecting the human rights of people with mental disorders: A call to action for global mental health In: M. Dudley, D. Silove, & F. Gale, (Eds.). *Mental health & human rights.* Oxford: Oxford University Press.
9. Hyman, S., Chisholm, D., Kessler, R., Patel, V., & Whiteford, H. (2006). Mental disorders. In D. Jamison, J. Breman, A. Measham, G. Alleyne, D. Evans, P. Jha, A. Mills, & P. Musgrove, (Eds.). *Disease control priorities in developing countries* (*2nd edition*). New York: Oxford University Press.
10. Patel, V., Araya, R., Chatterjee, S., Chisholm, D., Cohen, A., De Silva, M., et al. (2007). Treatment and prevention of mental disorders in low-income and middle-income countries. *Lancet, 370,* 991–1005.
11. Prince, M., Patel, V., Saxena, S., Maj, M., Maselko, J., Phillips, M. R., et al. (2007). No health without mental health. *Lancet, 370,* 859–877.
12. Saraceno B, Van Ommeren M, Batniji R, Cohen A, Gureje O, Mahoney J, et al. (2007). Barriers to improvement of mental health services in low-income and middle-income countries. *Lancet, 370,* 1164–1174.
13. World Health Organization. (2006). *WHO Statistical Information System.* Working paper describing data sources, methods and results for projections of mortality and burden of disease for 2005, 2015 and 2030.
14. Aaron, R., Joseph, A., Abraham, S., Muliyil, J., George, K., Prasad, J., et al. (2004). Suicides in young people in rural southern India. *Lancet, 363,* 1117–1118.
15. Prasad, J., Abraham, V. J., Minz, S., Abraham, S., Joseph, A., Muliyil, J. P., et al. (2006). Rates and factors associated with suicide in Kaniyambadi Block, Tamil Nadu, South India, 2000–2002. *Int J Soc Psychiatry, 52,* 65–71.
16. Cavanagh, J. T., Carson, A. J., Sharpe, M., & Lawrie, S. M. (2003). Psychological autopsy studies of suicide: A systematic review. *Psychol Med, 33,* 395–405.
17. Vijayakumar, L. & Rajkumar, S. (1999). Are risk factors for suicide universal? A case-control study from India. *Acta Psychiatrica Scandinavica, 99,* 407–411.
18. Phillips, M. R., Yang, G., Zhang, Y., Wang, L., Ji, H., & Zhou, M. (2002). Risk factors for suicide in China: A national case-control psychological autopsy study. *Lancet, 360,* 1728–1736.
19. Heila, H., Haukka, J., Suvisaari, J., & Lonnqvist, J. (2005). Mortality among patients with schizophrenia and reduced psychiatric hospital care. *Psychol Med, 35,* 725–732.
20. Kebede, D., Alem, A., Shibre, T., Negash, A., Deyassa, N., Beyero, T., et al. (2005). Short-term symptomatic and functional outcomes of schizophrenia in Butajira, Ethiopia. *Schizophr Res, 78,* 171–185.
21. Saz, P. & Dewey, M. E. (2001). Depression, depressive symptoms and mortality in persons aged 65 and over living in the community: A systematic review of the literature. *Int J Geriatr Psychiatry, 16,* 622–630.
22. Mogga, S., Prince, M., Alem, A., Kebede, D., Stewart, R., Glozier, N., et al. (2006). Outcome of major depression in Ethiopia: Population-based study. *Br J Psychiatry, 189,* 241–246.
23. Dewey, M. E. & Saz, P. (2001). Dementia, cognitive impairment and mortality in persons aged 65 and over living in the community: A systematic review of the literature. *Int J Geriatr Psychiatry, 16,* 751–761.

24. Lawrence, D. M., Holman, C. D., Jablensky, A. V., & Hobbs, M. S. (2003). Death rate from ischaemic heart disease in Western Australian psychiatric patients 1980–1998. *Br J Psychiatry, 182,* 31–36.
25. Gureje, O., Simon, G. E., Ustun, T. B., & Goldberg, D. P. (1997). Somatization in cross-cultural perspective: A World Health Organization study in primary care. *Am J Psychiatry, 154,* 989–995.
26. Escobar, J. I., Waitzkin, H., Silver, R. C., Gara, M., & Holman, A. (1998). Abridged somatization: A study in primary care. *Psychosom Med, 60,* 466–472.
27. Barsky, A. J., Orav, E. J., & Bates, D. W. (2005). Somatization increases medical utilization and costs independent of psychiatric and medical comorbidity. *Arch Gen Psychiatry, 62,* 903–910.
28. Hemingway, H. & Marmot, M. (1999). Evidence-based cardiology: Psychosocial factors in the aetiology and prognosis of coronary heart disease. Systematic review of prospective cohort studies. *BMJ, 318,* 1460–1467.
29. Kuper, H., Marmot, M., & Hemingway, H. (2002). Systematic review of prospective cohort studies of psychosocial factors in the etiology and prognosis of coronary heart disease. *Semin Vasc Med, 2,* 267–314.
30. Jonas, B. S., Franks, P., & Ingram, D. D. (1997). Are symptoms of anxiety and depression risk factors for hypertension? Longitudinal evidence from the National Health and Nutrition Examination Survey I Epidemiologic Follow-up Study. *Arch Fam Med, 6,* 43–49.
31. Larson, S. L., Owens, P. L., Ford, D., & Eaton, W. (2001). Depressive disorder, dysthymia, and risk of stroke: Thirteen-year follow-up from the Baltimore epidemiologic catchment area study. *Stroke, 32,* 1979–1983.
32. Everson, S. A., Roberts, R. E., Goldberg, D. E., & Kaplan, G. A. (1998). Depressive symptoms and increased risk of stroke mortality over a 29-year period. *Arch Intern Med, 158,* 1133–1138.
33. Ohira, T., Iso, H., Satoh, S., Sankai, T., Tanigawa, T., Ogawa, Y., et al. (2001). Prospective study of depressive symptoms and risk of stroke among Japanese. *Stroke, 32,* 903–908.
34. Simon, G. E., Von, K. M., Saunders, K., Miglioretti, D. L., Crane, P. K., Van, B. G. et al. (2006). Association between obesity and psychiatric disorders in the US adult population. *Arch Gen Psychiatry, 63,* 824–830.
35. Breslau, N., Peterson, E. L., Schultz, L. R., Chilcoat, H. D., & Andreski, P. (1998). Major depression and stages of smoking. A longitudinal investigation. *Arch Gen Psychiatry, 55,* 161–166.
36. Patel, V., Kirkwood, B. R., Pednekar, S., Weiss, H., & Mabey, D. (2006). Risk factors for common mental disorders in women: Population-based longitudinal study. *Br J Psychiatry, 189,* 547–555.
37. Strik, J. J., Lousberg, R., Cheriex, E. C., & Honig, A. (2004). One year cumulative incidence of depression following myocardial infarction and impact on cardiac outcome. *J Psychosom Res, 56,* 59–66.
38. Aben, I., Lodder, J., Honig, A., Lousberg, R., Boreas, A., & Verhey, F. (2006). Focal or generalized vascular brain damage and vulnerability to depression after stroke: A 1-year prospective follow-up study. *Int Psychogeriatr, 18,* 19–35.
39. Golden, S. H., Williams, J. E., Ford, D. E., Yeh, H. C., Paton, S. C., Nieto, F. J., et al. (2004). Depressive symptoms and the risk of type 2 diabetes: The Atherosclerosis Risk in Communities study. *Diabetes Care, 27,* 429–435.

40. Eaton, W. W., Armenian, H., Gallo, J., Pratt, L., & Ford, D. E. (1996). Depression and risk for onset of type II diabetes. A prospective population-based study. *Diabetes Care, 19,* 1097–1102.
41. Anderson, R. J., Freedland, K. E., Clouse, R. E., & Lustman, P. J. (2001). The prevalence of comorbid depression in adults with diabetes: A meta-analysis. *Diabetes Care, 24,*1069–1078.
42. Grigsby, A. B., Anderson, R. J., Freedland, K. E., Clouse, R. E., & Lustman, P. J. (2002). Prevalence of anxiety in adults with diabetes: A systematic review. *J Psychosom Res, 53,* 1053–1060.
43. Holt, R. I., Bushe, C., & Citrome, L. (2005). Diabetes and schizophrenia 2005: Are we any closer to understanding the link? *J Psychopharmacol, 19,* 56–65.
44. Ohta, Y., Nakane, Y., Mine, M., Nakama, I., Michitsuji, S., Araki, K., et al. (1988). The epidemiological study of physical morbidity in schizophrenics—2. Association between schizophrenia and incidence of tuberculosis. *Jpn J Psychiatry Neurol, 42,* 41–47.
45. McQuistion, H. L., Colson, P., Yankowitz, R., & Susser, E. (1997). Tuberculosis infection among people with severe mental illness. *Psychiatr Serv, 48,* 833–835.
46. Buskin, S. E., Gale, J. L., Weiss, N. S., & Nolan, C. M. (1994). Tuberculosis risk factors in adults in King County, Washington, 1988 through 1990. *Am J Public Health, 84,*1750–1756.
47. Chander, G., Himelhoch, S., & Moore, R. D. (2006). Substance abuse and psychiatric disorders in HIV-positive patients: Epidemiology and impact on antiretroviral therapy. *Drugs, 66,* 769–789.
48. Cournos, F., McKinnon, K., & Sullivan, G. (2005). Schizophrenia and comorbid human immunodeficiency virus or hepatitis C virus. *J Clin Psychiatry, 66* Suppl 6, 27–33.
49. Kelly, J. A. (1997). HIV risk reduction interventions for persons with severe mental illness. *Clin Psychol Rev, 17,* 293–309.
50. Koblin, B. A., Husnik, M. J., Colfax, G., Huang, Y., Madison, M., Mayer, K., et al. (2006). Risk factors for HIV infection among men who have sex with men. *AIDS, 20,* 731–739.
51. Chin-Hong, P. V., Deeks, S. G., Liegler, T., Hagos, E., Krone, M. R., Grant, R. M., et al. (2005). High-risk sexual behavior in adults with genotypically proven antiretroviral-resistant HIV infection. *J Acquir Immune Defic Syndr, 40,* 463–471.
52. Bing, E. G., Burnam, M. A., Longshore, D., Fleishman, J. A., Sherbourne, C. D., London, A. S., et al. (2001). Psychiatric disorders and drug use among human immunodeficiency virus-infected adults in the United States. *Arch Gen Psychiatry, 58,* 721–728.
53. Ciesla, J. A. & Roberts, J. E. (2001). Meta-analysis of the relationship between HIV infection and risk for depressive disorders. *Am J Psychiatry, 158,* 725–730.
54. Maj, M., Janssen, R., Starace, F., Zaudig, M., Satz, P., Sughondhabirom, B., et al. (1994). WHO Neuropsychiatric AIDS study, cross-sectional phase I. Study design and psychiatric findings. *Arch Gen Psychiatry, 51,* 39–49.
55. White, D. A., Heaton, R. K., & Monsch, A. U. (1995). Neuropsychological studies of asymptomatic human immunodeficiency virus-type-1 infected individuals. The HNRC Group. HIV Neurobehavioral Research Center. *J Int Neuropsychol Soc, 1,* 304–315.
56. Maj, M., Satz, P., Janssen, R., Zaudig, M., Starace, F., D'elia, L., et al. (1994). WHO Neuropsychiatric AIDS study, cross-sectional phase II. Neuropsychological and neurological findings. *Arch Gen Psychiatry, 51,* 51–61.

57. Dube, B., Benton, T., Cruess, D. G., & Evans, D. L. (2005). Neuropsychiatric manifestations of HIV infection and AIDS. *J Psychiatry Neurosci, 30,* 237–246.
58. Sweetland, A., Acha, J., & Guerra, D. (2002). Enhancing adherence: The role of group psychotherapy in the treatment of multidrug-resistant tuberculosis in urban Peru. In A. Cohen, A. Kleinman, & B. Saraceno, eds. *The world mental health casebook: Social and mental health programmes in low-income countries* (pp. 51–79). New York: Kluwer Academic.
59. Vega, P., Sweetland, A., Acha, J., Castillo, H., Guerra, D., Smith Fawzi, M. C., et al. (2004). Psychiatric issues in the management of patients with multidrug-resistant tuberculosis. *Int J Tuberc Lung Dis, 8,* 749–759.
60. Aydin, I. O. & Ulusahin, A. (2001). Depression, anxiety comorbidity, and disability in tuberculosis and chronic obstructive pulmonary disease patients: Applicability of GHQ-12. *Gen Hosp Psychiatry, 23,* 77–83.
61. Parikh, R. M., Robinson, R. G., Lipsey, J. R., Starkstein, S. E., Fedoroff, J. P., & Price, T. R. (1990). The impact of poststroke depression on recovery in activities of daily living over a 2-year follow-up. *Arch Neurol, 47,* 785–789.
62. Chemerinski, E., Robinson, R. G., & Kosier, J. T. (2001). Improved recovery in activities of daily living associated with remission of poststroke depression. *Stroke, 32,* 113–117.
63. Morris, P. L., Robinson, R. G., Andrzejewski, P., Samuels, J., & Price, T. R. (1993). Association of depression with 10-year poststroke mortality. *Am J Psychiatry, 150,* 124–129.
64. Lustman, P. J., Anderson, R. J., Freedland, K. E., De, G. M., Carney, R. M., & Clouse, R. E. (2000). Depression and poor glycemic control: A meta-analytic review of the literature. *Diabetes Care, 23,* 934–942.
65. De Groot, M., Anderson, R., Freedland, K. E., Clouse, R. E., & Lustman, P. J. (2001). Association of depression and diabetes complications: A meta-analysis. *Psychosom Med, 63,* 619 630.
66. Katon, W. J., Rutter, C., Simon, G., Lin, E. H., Ludman, E., Ciechanowski, P., et al. (2005). The association of comorbid depression with mortality in patients with type 2 diabetes. *Diabetes Care, 28,* 2668–2672.
67. Ickovics, J. R., Hamburger, M. E., Vlahov, D., Schoenbaum, E. E., Schuman, P., Boland, R. J., et al. (2001). Mortality, CD4 cell count decline, and depressive symptoms among HIV-seropositive women: Longitudinal analysis from the HIV Epidemiology Research Study. *JAMA, 285,* 1466–1474.
68. Cook JA, Grey D, Burke J, Cohen MH, Gurtman AC, Richardson JL, et al. (2004). Depressive symptoms and AIDS-related mortality among a multisite cohort of HIV-positive women. *Am J Public Health, 94,* 1133–1140.
69. Wilkie, F. L., Goodkin, K., Eisdorfer, C., Feaster, D., Morgan, R., Fletcher, M. A., et al. (1998). Mild cognitive impairment and risk of mortality in HIV-1 infection. *J Neuropsychiatry Clin Neurosci, 10,*125–132.
70. Dolder, C. R., Lacro, J. P., & Jeste, D. V. (2003). Adherence to antipsychotic and nonpsychiatric medications in middle-aged and older patients with psychotic disorders. *Psychosom Med, 65,* 156–162.
71. Ciechanowski, P. S., Katon, W. J., & Russo, J. E. (2000). Depression and diabetes: Impact of depressive symptoms on adherence, function, and costs. *Arch Intern Med, 160,* 3278–3285.
72. Lin, E. H., Katon, W., Von, K. M., Rutter, C., Simon, G. E., Oliver, M., et al. (2004). Relationship of depression and diabetes self-care, medication adherence, and preventive care. *Diabetes Care, 27,* 2154–2160.

73. Ammassari A, Antinori A, Aloisi MS, Trotta MP, Murri R, Bartoli L, et al. (2004). Depressive symptoms, neurocognitive impairment, and adherence to highly active antiretroviral therapy among HIV-infected persons. *Psychosomatics, 45*, 394–402.
74. Gordillo,V., Del, A. J., Soriano, V., & Gonzalez-Lahoz, J. (1999). Sociodemographic and psychological variables influencing adherence to antiretroviral therapy. *AIDS, 13*, 1763–1769.
75. Paterson, D. L., Swindells, S., Mohr, J., Brester, M., Vergis, E. N., Squier, C., et al. (2000). Adherence to protease inhibitor therapy and outcomes in patients with HIV infection. *Ann Intern Med, 133*, 21–30.
76. Hinkin, C. H., Castellon, S. A., Durvasula, R. S., Hardy, D. J., Lam, M. N., Mason, K. I., et al. (2002). Medication adherence among HIV+ adults: Effects of cognitive dysfunction and regimen complexity. *Neurology, 59*, 1944–1950.
77. Hinkin, C. H., Hardy, D. J., Mason, K. I., Castellon, S. A., Durvasula, R. S., Lam, M. N., et al. (2004). Medication adherence in HIV-infected adults: Effect of patient age, cognitive status, and substance abuse. *AIDS, 18* Suppl 1, S19–S25.
78. Collins, P. Y., Holman, A. R., Freeman, M., & Patel, V. (2006). What is the relevance of mental health to HIV/AIDS care and treatment programs in developing countries? A systematic review. *AIDS, 20*, 1571–1582.
79. Davidson, H., Schluger, N. W., Feldman, P. H., Valentine, D. P., Telzak, E. E., & Laufer, F. N. (2000). The effects of increasing incentives on adherence to tuberculosis directly observed therapy. *Int J Tuberc Lung Dis, 4*, 860–865.
80. Pablos-Mendez, A., Knirsch, C. A., Barr, R. G., Lerner, B. H., & Frieden, T. R. (1997). Nonadherence in tuberculosis treatment: predictors and consequences in New York City. *Am J Med, 102*, 164–170.
81. Bumburidi, E., Ajeilat, S., Dadu, A., Aitmagambetova, I., Ershova, J., Fagan, R., et al. (2006). Progress toward tuberculosis control and determinants of treatment outcomes—Kazakhstan, 2000–2002. *MMWR Morb Mortal Wkly Rep, 55* Suppl 1, 11–15.
82. Shin SS, Pasechnikov AD, Gelmanova IY, Peremitin GG, Strelis AK, Mishustin S, et al. (2006). Treatment outcomes in an integrated civilian and prison MDR-TB treatment program in Russia. *Int J Tuberc Lung Dis, 10*, 402–408.
83. Maier, W., Gansicke, M., Gater, R., Rezaki, M., Tiemens, B., & Urzua, R. F. (1999). Gender differences in the prevalence of depression: A survey in primary care. *J Affect Disord, 53*, 241–252.
84. Kuehner, C. (2003). Gender differences in unipolar depression: an update of epidemiological findings and possible explanations. *Acta Psychiatr Scand, 108*, 163–174.
85. Latthe, P., Mignini, L., Gray, R., Hills, R., & Khan, K. (2006). Factors predisposing women to chronic pelvic pain: Systematic review. *BMJ, 332*, 749–755.
86. Patel, V., Weiss, H. A., Kirkwood, B. R., Pednekar, S., Nevrekar, P., Gupte, S., et al. (2006). Common genital complaints in women: The contribution of psychosocial and infectious factors in a population-based cohort study in Goa, India. *Int J Epidemiol, 35*, 1478–1485.
87. Nilsson, E., Lichtenstein, P., Cnattingius, S., Murray, R. M., & Hultman, C. M. (2002). Women with schizophrenia: Pregnancy outcome and infant death among their offspring. *Schizophr Res, 58*, 221–229.
88. Bennedsen, B. E., Mortensen, P. B., Olesen, A. V., & Henriksen, T. B. (1999). Preterm birth and intra-uterine growth retardation among children of women with schizophrenia. *Br J Psychiatry, 175*, 239–245.
89. Jablensky, A. V., Morgan, V., Zubrick, S. R., Bower, C., & Yellachich, L. A. (2005). Pregnancy, delivery, and neonatal complications in a population cohort of women with schizophrenia and major affective disorders. *Am J Psychiatry, 162*, 79–91.

90. Webb, R., Abel, K., Pickles, A., & Appleby, L. (2005). Mortality in offspring of parents with psychotic disorders: A critical review and meta-analysis. *Am J Psychiatry, 162,* 1045–1056.
91. O'Hara, M. (1997). The nature of postpartum depressive disorders. In L. Murray & P. J. Cooper, (Eds.). *Postpartum depression and child development* (pp. 3–31). New York: Guilford Press.
92. Patel, V., Rahman, A., Jacob, K. S., & Hughes, M. (2004). Effect of maternal mental health on infant growth in low income countries: New evidence from South Asia. *BMJ, 328,* 820–823.
93. Murray, L. & Cooper, P. J. (2003). Intergenerational transmission of affective and cognitive processes associated with depression: Infancy and the preschool years. In I. Goodyer, (Ed.). *Unipolar depression: A lifespan perspective.* Oxford: Oxford University Press.
94. Rahman, A., Bunn, J., Lovel, H., & Creed, F. (2007). Association between antenatal depression and low birthweight in a developing country. *Acta Psychiatrica Scandinavica, 115,* 481–486.
95. Rahman, A., Iqbal, Z., Bunn, J., Lovel, H., & Harrington, R. (2004). Impact of maternal depression on infant nutritional status and illness: A cohort study. *Arch Gen Psychiatry, 61,* 946–952.
96. Paulson, J. F., Dauber, S., & Leiferman, J. A. (2006). Individual and combined effects of postpartum depression in mothers and fathers on parenting behavior. *Pediatrics, 118,* 659–668.
97. Galler, J. R., Harrison, R. H., Biggs, M. A., Ramsey, F., & Forde, V. (1999). Maternal moods predict breastfeeding in Barbados. *J Dev Behav Pediatr, 20,* 80–87.
98. Thornicroft, G. (2006). *Shunned: Discrimination against people with mental illness,* Oxford: Oxford University Press.
99. Thara, R. & Srinivasan, T. (2000). How stigmatising is schizophrenia in India? *Int J Soc Psychiatry, 46,* 135–141.
100. Goffmann, E. (1963). *Stigma: Notes on the management of spoiled identity.* Englewood Cliffs: Prentice Hall.
101. Corrigan, P. (2005). *On the stigma of mental illness.* Washington, DC: American Psychological Association.
102. Link, B. G. & Phelan, J. C. (2001). On stigma and its public health implications. Paper presented at *Stigma and Global Health: Developing a Research Agenda;* September 5–7, 2001: Bethesda.
103. Thornicroft, G., Rose, D., & Kassam, A. (2007). Discrimination in health care against people with mental illness. *Int Review Psychiatry, 19,* 113–122.
104. Vibha, P., Saddichha, S., & Kumar, R. (2008). Attitudes of ward attendants towards mental illness: Comparisons and predictors. *Int J Soc Psychiatry, 54,* 469–478.
105. Lauber, C., Nordt, C., Braunschweig, C., & Rossler, W. (2006). Do mental health professionals stigmatize their patients? *Acta Psychiatr Scand Suppl,* 51–59.
106. Hugo, M. (2001). Mental health professionals' attitudes towards people who have experienced a mental health disorder. *J Psychiatr Ment Health Nurs, 8,* 419–425.
107. Hunt, P. (2006). The human right to the highest attainable standard of health: New opportunities and challenges. *Trans R Soc Trop Med Hyg, 100,* 603–607.
108. Amnesty International. (2004). Memorandum to the Romanian government concerning inpatient psychiatric treatment. London: Amnesty International.
109. Mental Disability Advocacy Center. (2004). Mental Health Law of the Kyrgyz Republic and its Implementation. Budapest: Mental Disability Advocacy Centre.

110. Patel, V., Saraceno, B., & Kleinman, A. (2006). Beyond evidence: The moral case for international mental health. *Am J Psychiatry, 163,* 1312–1315.
111. Minas, H. & Diatri, H. (2008). Pasung: Physical restraint and confinement of the mentally ill in the community. *Int J Ment Health Syst, 2,* 8.
112. Link, B. G., Struening, E. L., Neese-Todd, S., Asmussen, S., & Phelan, J. C. (2001). Stigma as a barrier to recovery: The consequences of stigma for the self-esteem of people with mental illnesses. *Psychiatric Services, 52,* 1621–1626.
113. Carroll, A., Pantelis, C., & Harvey, C. (2004). Insight and hopelessness in forensic patients with schizophrenia. *Aust N Z J Psychiatry, 38,* 169–173.
114. Ritsher, J. B. & Phelan, J. C. (2004). Internalized stigma predicts erosion of morale among psychiatric outpatients. *Psychiatry Res, 129,* 257–265.
115. Ritsher, J. B., Otilingam, P. G., & Grajales, M. (2003). Internalized stigma of mental illness: Psychometric properties of a new measure. *Psychiatry Res, 121,* 31–49.
116. Thornicroft, G., Brohan, E., Rose, D., Sartorius, N., & Leese, M. (2009). Global pattern of experienced and anticipated discrimination against people with schizophrenia: A cross-sectional survey. *Lancet, 373,* 408–415.
117. Sartorius, N. (2007). Stigma and mental health. *Lancet, 370,* 810–811.
118. Phillips, M. R., Pearson, V., Li, F., Xu, M., & Yang, L. (2002). Stigma and expressed emotion: A study of people with schizophrenia and their family members in China. *Br J Psychiatry, 181,* 488–493.
119. Vauth, R., Kleim, B., Wirtz, M., & Corrigan, P. W. (2007). Self-efficacy and empowerment as outcomes of self-stigmatizing and coping in schizophrenia. *Psychiatry Res, 150,* 71–80.
120. Sartorius, N. & Schulze, H. (2005). *Reducing the stigma of mental illness,* Cambridge: Cambridge University Press.
121. Osborn, R. L., Demoncada, A. C., & Feuerstein, M. (2006). Psychosocial interventions for depression, anxiety, and quality of life in cancer survivors: Meta-analyses. *Int J Psychiatry Med, 36,* 13–34.
122. Katon, W. J., Von, K. M., Lin, E. H., Simon, G., Ludman, E., Russo, J., et al. (2004). The Pathways Study: A randomized trial of collaborative care in patients with diabetes and depression. *Arch Gen Psychiatry, 61,* 1042–1049.
123. Rees, K., Bennett, P., West, R., Davey, S. G., & Ebrahim, S. (2004). Psychological interventions for coronary heart disease. *Cochrane Database Syst Rev, 2,* CD002902.
124. Berkman, L. F., Blumenthal, J., Burg, M., Carney, R. M., Catellier, D., Cowan, M. J., et al. (2003). Effects of treating depression and low perceived social support on clinical events after myocardial infarction: The Enhancing Recovery in Coronary Heart Disease Patients (ENRICHD) Randomized Trial. *JAMA, 289,* 3106–3116.
125. Lechner, S. C., Antoni, M. H., Lydston, D., Laperriere, A., Ishii, M., Devieux, J., et al. (2003). Cognitive-behavioral interventions improve quality of life in women with AIDS. *J Psychosom Res, 54,* 253–261.
126. Smith, G. R. Jr., Rost, K., & Kashner, T. M. (1995). A trial of the effect of a standardized psychiatric consultation on health outcomes and costs in somatizing patients. *Arch Gen Psychiatry, 52,* 238–243.
127. Dickinson, W. P., Dickinson, L. M., Degruy, F. V., Main, D. S., Candib, L. M., & Rost, K. (2003). A randomized clinical trial of a care recommendation letter intervention for somatization in primary care. *Ann Fam Med, 1,* 228–235.
128. O'Malley, P. G., Jackson, J. L., Santoro, J., Tomkins, G., Balden, E., & Kroenke, K. (1999). Antidepressant therapy for unexplained symptoms and symptom syndromes. *J Fam Pract, 48,* 980–990.

129. Kroenke, K. & Swindle, R. (2000). Cognitive-behavioral therapy for somatization and symptom syndromes: A critical review of controlled clinical trials. *Psychother Psychosom, 69,* 205–215.
130. Winkley, K., Ismail, K., Landau, S., & Eisler, I. (2006). Psychological interventions to improve glycaemic control in patients with type 1 diabetes: Systematic review and meta-analysis of randomised controlled trials. *BMJ, 333,* 65.
131. Ismail, K., Winkley, K., & Rabe-Hesketh, S. (2004). Systematic review and meta-analysis of randomised controlled trials of psychological interventions to improve glycaemic control in patients with type 2 diabetes. *Lancet, 363,* 1589–1597.
132. Lustman, P. J., Freedland, K. E., Griffith, L. S., & Clouse, R. E. (2000). Fluoxetine for depression in diabetes: A randomized double-blind placebo-controlled trial. *Diabetes Care, 23,* 618–623.
133. Lustman, P. J., Griffith, L. S., Clouse, R. E., Freedland, K. E., Eisen, S. A., Rubin, E. H., et al. (1997). Effects of nortriptyline on depression and glycemic control in diabetes: Results of a double-blind, placebo-controlled trial. *Psychosom Med, 59,* 241–250.
134. Lin, E. H., Katon, W., Rutter, C., Simon, G. E., Ludman, E. J., Von, K. M., et al. (2006). Effects of enhanced depression treatment on diabetes self-care. *Ann Fam Med, 4,* 46–53.
135. Strik, J. J., Honig, A., Lousberg, R., Lousberg, A. H., Cheriex, E. C., Tuynman-Qua, H. G., et al. (2000). Efficacy and safety of fluoxetine in the treatment of patients with major depression after first myocardial infarction: Findings from a double-blind, placebo-controlled trial. *Psychosom Med, 62,* 783–789.
136. Glassman, A. H., O'Connor, C. M., Califf, R. M., Swedberg, K., Schwartz, P., Bigger, J. T. Jr., et al. (2002). Sertraline treatment of major depression in patients with acute MI or unstable angina. *JAMA, 288,* 701–709.
137. Anderson, C. S., Hackett, M. L., & House, A. O. (2004). Interventions for preventing depression after stroke. *Cochrane Database Syst Rev, 2,* CD003689.
138. Hackett, M. L., Anderson, C. S., & House, A. O. (2005). Management of depression after stroke: A systematic review of pharmacological therapies. *Stroke, 36,* 1098–1103.
139. Jorge, R. E., Robinson, R. G., Arndt, S., & Starkstein, S. (2003). Mortality and post-stroke depression: A placebo-controlled trial of antidepressants. *Am J Psychiatry, 160,* 1823–1829.
140. Frasure-Smith, N. & Lesperance, F. (2003). Depression—a cardiac risk factor in search of a treatment. *JAMA, 289,* 3171–3173.
141. Acha, J., Sweetland, J., Guerra, D., Chalco, K., Castillo, H., & Palacios, E. (2007). Psychosocial support groups for patients with multidrug-resistant tuberculosis: Five years of experience *Glob Public Health, 2,* 404–417.
142. Janmeja, A. K., Das, S. K., Bhargava, R., & Chavan, B. S. (2005). Psychotherapy improves compliance with tuberculosis treatment. *Respiration, 72,* 375–380.
143. Demissie, M., Getahun, H., & Lindtjorn, B. (2003). Community tuberculosis care through "TB clubs" in rural North Ethiopia. *Soc Sci Med, 56,* 2009–2018.
144. Yun, L. W., Maravi, M., Kobayashi, J. S., Barton, P. L., & Davidson, A. J. (2005). Antidepressant treatment improves adherence to antiretroviral therapy among depressed HIV-infected patients. *J Acquir Immune Defic Syndr, 38,* 432–438.
145. Patel, V., Weiss, H., Chowdhary, N., Naik, S., Pednekar, S., Chatterjee, S., De Silva, M., Bhat, B., Araya, R., King, M., Simon, G., Verdeli, H. & Kirkwood, B. (2010). The effectiveness of a lay health worker led intervention for depressive and

anxiety disorders in primary care: the Manas cluster randomized controlled trial in Goa, India. *Lancet, 376*, 2086–2095
146. Rahman, A., Malik, A., Sikander, S., Roberts, C., & Creed, F. (2008). Cognitive behaviour therapy-based intervention by community health workers for mothers with depression and their infants in rural Pakistan: A cluster-randomised controlled trial. *Lancet, 372*, 902–909.
147. World Health Organization (2005). *Mental health atlas*. Geneva: World Health Organization.
148. Lancet Global Mental Health Group. (2007). Scaling up services for mental disorders—a call for action. *Lancet, 370*, 1241–1252.
149. Mullan, F. (2005). The metrics of physician brain drain. *NEJM, 353*, 1810–1818.
150. Patel, V. (2009). The future of psychiatry in low and middle income countries. *Psychological Medicine, 39*, 1759–1762.
151. Lewin, S. A., Dick, J., Pond, P., Zwarenstein, M., Aja, G., Van Wyk, B., et al. (2005). Lay health workers in primary and community health care. *Cochrane Database Syst Rev, 1*, CD004015.
152. Bolton, P., Bass, J., Betancourt, T., Speelman, L., Onyango, G., Clougherty, K. F., et al. (2007). Interventions for depression symptoms among adolescent survivors of war and displacement in northern Uganda: A randomized controlled trial. *JAMA, 298*, 519–527.
153. Bolton, P., Bass, J., Neugebauer, R., Verdeli, H., Clougherty, K., Wickramaratne, P., et al. (2003). Group Interpersonal Psychotherapy for Depression in Rural Uganda. *JAMA, 289*, 3117–3124.
154. Araya, R., Rojas, G., Fritsch, R., Gaete, J., Rojas, M., Simon, G., et al. (2003). Treating depression in primary care in low-income women in Santiago, Chile: A randomised controlled trial. *Lancet, 361*, 995–1000.
155. Rojas, G., Fritsch, R., Solis, J., Jadresic, E., Castillo, C., Gonzalez, M., et al. (2007). Treatment of postnatal depression in low-income mothers in primary-care clinics in Santiago, Chile: A randomised controlled trial. *Lancet, 370*, 1629–1637.
156. Beaglehole, R., Epping-Jordan, J., Patel, V., Chopra, M., Ebrahim, S., Kidd, M., et al. (2008). Improving the prevention and management of chronic disease in low-income and middle-income countries: A priority for primary health care. *Lancet, 372*, 940–949.
157. Patel, V. & Bloch, S. (2009). The ethical imperative to scale up health care services for people with severe mental disorders in low and middle income countries. *Postgrad Med J, 85*, 509–513.
158. Patel, V., Garrison, P., De Jesus Mari, J., Minas, H., Prince, M., & Saxena, S. (2008). The Lancet's series on global mental health: 1 year on. *Lancet, 372*, 1354–1357.
159. World Health Organization. (2008). Mental Health Gap Action Programme (mhGAP): Scaling up care for mental, neurological and substance abuse disorders. Geneva: World Health Organization.
160. Tomlinson, M., Rudan, I., Saxena, S., Swartz, L., Tsai, A., & Patel, V. (2009). Setting investment priorities for research in global mental health. *Bull World Health Organ, 87*, 438–446.
161. Editorial (2008). A movement for global mental health is launched. *Lancet, 372*, 1274.

2

Addressing Addiction and High-Risk Behaviors Using the Integrated Public Health and Public Safety Approach

WILSON M. COMPTON AND REDONNA K. CHANDLER

The number of persons under justice supervision in the United States has increased markedly over the past 30 years, driven especially by an increase in use of justice sanctions to address crimes related to drug abuse and addiction. Such a shift has led the justice system to serve as a de facto partial quarantine system. While this situation may reflect broad trends to criminalize addiction-related behavior and may also reflect deterioration of our health care system and its inability to deal with the most vulnerable in our standard facilities, it also provides an opportunity for public health strategies that reach populations which are otherwise hidden. One problem is that approaches to drug use issues that are purely justice-based are fraught with recidivism, and purely medical approaches to drug use issues are fraught with poor uptake—many persons who could benefit from treatment fail to participate. An alternative hybrid approach is the combined public health and public safety model, which may offer the most promise to address addiction, mental illness, and related health conditions within the criminal justice system. This model incorporates the strengths of health and justice systems to address the needs and weaknesses of each. Dual benefits can also encourage participation by both systems. In addition to offering promise in addressing substance use and other mental illnesses, a combined public health and public safety approach may allow rational approaches to targeting HIV/AIDS, tuberculosis, and other infectious diseases in a high-risk population.

The absolute number and the proportion of the U.S. population involved in justice settings increased tremendously during the past 30 years. Between 1980 and 2008, the number of adults incarcerated in prison or jail increased nearly five-fold from approximately 500,000 to over 2.3 million.[1] Overall, in 2008 the number of adults in prison, jail, or some other form of correctional supervision (probation, parole, work release, etc.) exceeded 7.3 million.[2] This represents

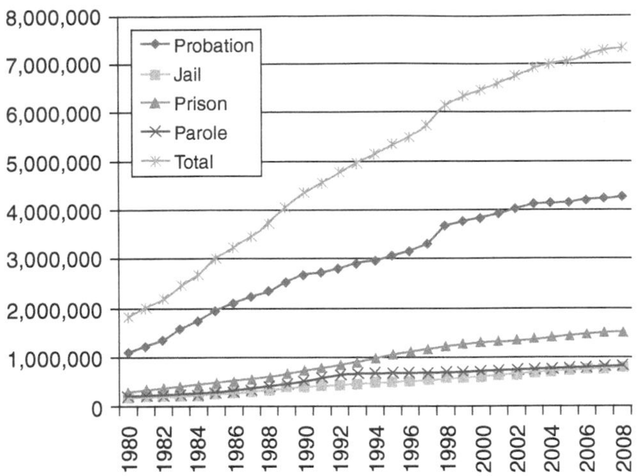

Figure 2.1 Adult United States correctional populations, 1980–2008. *Source: http://bjs.ojp.usdoj.gov/content/glance/corr2.cfm*

approximately 3.2% of the adult (age 18+) population.[3] As seen in Figure 2.1, the increases in incarceration were most dramatic during the late 1980s and early 1990s, with some leveling off in the past few years.[2] It is well known that the increases in incarceration are largely related to increases in drug-related crimes.[4] As a result, persons incarcerated exhibit very high rates of illicit drug abuse and addiction. Recent work has shown that approximately half of all those incarcerated meet the criteria for a DSM-IV (Diagnostic and Statistical Manual of Mental Disorders-IV) abuse or dependence on an illicit drug.[5,6]

One impact of high rates of incarceration is that estimates of population rates of drug use disorders are distorted if one relies solely on the major general-population surveys.[7] When data from drug use disorders collected from inmates[8–11] were combined with results from a large noninstitutionalized sample of adults (the 2001–2002 National Epidemiologic Survey on Alcohol and Related Conditions, NESARC[12]), the summed overall projected estimates of the number of persons ages 18 and older with a DSM-IV illicit drug use disorder in the U.S. were 25.1% higher than the estimates from the noninstitutionalized sample alone (increased by 1,043,000 from 4,159,000 to 5,202,000 persons). Estimates of the overall combined projected prevalence of a DSM-IV illicit drug abuse disorder increased over the base by 12.0% and DSM-IV dependence by 53.8%. Thus, high rates of DSM-IV substance use disorders among inmates combined with a large inmate population results in an incomplete picture regarding drug use disorders in major U.S. national general population surveys, such as the National Survey on Drug Use and Health,[13] because incarcerated persons are not included in the sampling frame.

Given the proportion of drug addicts that are incarcerated, it appears that prisons and jails form a pseudo-quarantine system for these disorders and associated health conditions including serious mental illness, HIV, and hepatitis C. The question is whether this system is effective in terms of improving public health and public safety or if an alternative approach could be more beneficial.

Racial Overrepresentation

Certain racial and ethnic minorities are over-represented in the U.S. criminal justice system. In 2002, approximately 43.8% of admissions to prison were African American.[14] In addition, as shown in Figure 2.2, the number of persons incarcerated since the 1980s has been disproportionately African American.[15]

Co-Occurring Mental and Physical Disorders

Psychiatric and substance use disorders frequently co-occur in the general population.[12,16–18] Psychiatric disorders are even more pronounced among those

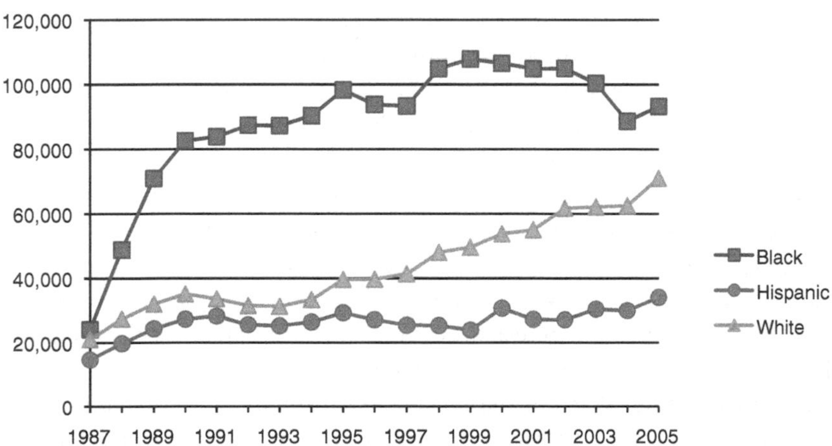

Figure 2.2 Admissions to prison for drug-related offense, by race/ethnicity (Iguchi et al., 2005),[15] based on data from Bureau of Justice Statistics, National Corrections Reporting Program, Washington, DC: US Department of Justice, 1987–2005.

in the criminal justice system. According to the Bureau of Justice Statistics, 56% of all state prisoners, 45% of federal prisoners, and 64% of jail inmates have a mental health problem.[19] These mental health problems span the full range of nonpsychotic and psychotic symptoms: 30% of jail inmates, 24% of state prisoners, and 16% of federal prisoners reported major depression and 24% of jail inmates, 15% of state prisoners, and 10% of federal prisoners reported recent hallucinations or delusions.[19] In addition, the majority of offenders with drug problems met criteria for a comorbid psychiatric disorder.[20–21] Seventy-six percent of local jail inmates as well as 74% of state prisoners and 64% of federal prisoners with a mental health problem were found to also have substance abuse or dependence.[19] High rates of mental illness among those incarcerated may relate to several factors including the increased use of jail and prison time for nonviolent drug offenses, lack of access to drug abuse treatment, and deterioration in the mental health treatment system.

Infectious diseases such as tuberculosis, HIV, and hepatitis B and C are associated with illicit drug use and occur at higher rates in offender populations than in the general population.[6] Recent research indicates that one in seven Americans living with HIV is released from a correctional facility.[22] For certain minority groups this number is even higher, with an estimated one in five African American and Hispanics living with HIV in this country being released from a prison or jail.[22] Availability of screening, treatment, and continuing care for these conditions appears to fall short of need,[23–25] despite the fact that it is feasible to implement programs in correctional settings for HIV,[26,27] hepatitis C,[28,29] and tuberculosis.[30] Programs to address these medical conditions are most available in prisons and some jails but less so in other parts of the justice system (probation, parole, etc.). This is in part due to the fact that incarcerated inmates have a constitutional right to health care.[31] Continuity of treatment for released offenders with infectious disease is difficult, but important, not just for the individual's health,[32,33] but also for the health of the community.[23,34–36] A stark example of treatment disruption for HIV was recently shown in a study of inmates who had been on anti-retroviral medications while incarcerated and then were followed after release.[36] In this study, only 5% received prescriptions for antiretroviral treatment (ART) within two weeks after release.[36] These issues have garnered the attention of public health practitioners and researchers interested in learning how to effectively address the significant treatment needs of this population.

Addressing drug addiction and related health conditions, including mental illness and infectious diseases, for individuals involved in the criminal justice system is complicated. Historically, the public health and public safety systems have used different competing models to address these vexing issues. Recent efforts have attempted to develop a new blended model combing strengths from both public health and public safety systems.

Public Health Approaches

The public health approach to drug addiction and related health conditions is built on the concept that addiction is a disease requiring treatment which is offered on a voluntary basis to patients. Advances in clinical neuroscience support the neurobiological basis of addiction as a disease that affects the brain and behavior[37] rather than a moral weakness.[38] Key findings from neuroscience research demonstrate that repeated drug use leads to longstanding changes in brain functioning.[39] These findings provide a way to understand why drug addicts have such difficulty quitting drug use despite the most severe consequences. It also presents an explanation for relapse and why punishment alone is an ineffective strategy for reducing drug use, supporting the conceptualization of addiction as a chronic condition requiring sustained treatment.[40,41] In addition, participation in drug abuse treatment provides an opportunity to screen for and treat related medical conditions including HIV and hepatitis C.

Research documents that treatment can be effective in reducing drug use and infectious disease risk behaviors as well as in improving other important outcomes.[42–44] Behavioral interventions have a strong evidence base, including cognitive therapies that teach coping skills and decision-making, contingency management interventions that shape and reinforce behaviors associated with abstinence, and motivational therapies that enhance the motivation to participate in treatment and in non-drug-related activities.[42,45] Exciting new research is exploring the use of computer technology to deliver behavioral therapies and one study has found that some components of cognitive behavioral therapy can be delivered through an automated computer platform.[46] The residential treatment approach that incorporates social learning theory in the construct of a therapeutic community has also been shown to be effective.[47] In addition, medications such as methadone, buprenorphine, and naltrexone are effective for opiate addiction, and naltrexone, acamprosate, and topiramate can be effective for alcohol addiction.[48,49] Finally, self-help support such as the 12-step Alcoholics Anonymous (and related) can be useful in supporting long-term behavior change.[50]

Cost-effectiveness studies document the potential value of public health approaches to treating drug-involved offenders.[51] In the United States, incarceration is estimated to cost about $22,000 per person per year[52] and has minimal impact on long-term drug abuse beyond the incarceration phase. One specific treatment for opiate addiction, methadone, costs about $4,000 per person per year[53,54] and has demonstrated effectiveness in reducing both drug use and criminal activity,[56] suggesting potential cost savings from this treatment approach. Overall, for every $1 spent, prison-based treatment saves between $2 and $6.[56] These economic benefits of treatment reflect in part the reduction in criminal behavior.[57,58]

A key weakness of the public health approach to drug addiction is the assumption that patients will recognize and accept their need for treatment. Large-scale epidemiological studies do not bear out this fact and in fact indicate that only 6% of those meeting the criteria of drug abuse and 31% of those meeting criteria for drug dependence actually access treatment in a given year.[12] Many individuals who enter treatment drop out prior to completion or fail to receive ongoing recovery support services. In addition, many organizations and systems serving high-risk groups (e.g., medical care settings and criminal justice system) fail to implement effective interventions for addiction. For example, it is estimated that the vast majority of prisoners (80–85%) don't participate in treatment despite clear need.[5,59]

Public Safety Approaches

The public safety approach to reducing the consequences of drug use and addiction, including illegal drug possession and sales and other drug-related crimes, is built on the concept that such drug use is primarily an issue of illegal behaviors, and so, punishment is the primary approach to changing behavior. As seen in the increases in arrests and judicial punishments (primarily probation, parole, and incarceration), this public safety approach has been a major policy and practice to address drug addiction in the United States.[15] Unfortunately, in isolation, the public safety approach to addressing drug use behaviors has significant shortcomings as seen in the high rates of recidivism.[60] Further, a strictly public safety approach to addiction also does little to impact the spread and contraction of related medical conditions including HIV.

A key assumption of the public safety approach is that incarceration will deter drug use. Yet, even in the constrained environment of incarceration, some individuals still have access to illicit drugs.[61] Further, long periods of abstinence while incarcerated fail to protect an offender from relapse when released, and rates of relapse are quite high in drug addicts released from prison or jail. This period of time after release is also fraught with excess morbidity and mortality, with drug overdose as a major contributing factor.[62] It has been suggested that the reentry process is an extremely difficult time that is filled with stressful events that contribute to both relapse and other excess morbidity and mortality. For example, reuniting with family, the need for housing and income, and the complexities of interacting with probation and parole are among the issues that offenders face after release.[63,64] In addition, returning to an environment rich in drug cues could be related to a rapid return to drug use following long periods of incarceration, and also suggests the need for ongoing treatment after release.[65]

Despite the evidence for benefits of drug treatment for offenders with addiction, a much less intense program called drug education is the most typical service provided to incarcerated addicts.[25,59] There is also some participation in self-help (i.e., Alcoholics Anonymous and other 12-step groups) with more than 20% of both federal and state inmates with addiction problems participating in these groups while incarcerated.[59] By contrast, less than 20% of inmates with drug use disorders receive formal treatment.[5,59] Taxman and colleagues, in a recent survey of U.S. programs and organizations, showed that most correctional agencies offered some type of drug abuse treatment services, but few offenders were actually able to participate.[25] The median percentage of offenders who had access to effective treatment services at any given time was generally under 10%.[25] In particular, medications, proven effective in addressing opioid and alcohol addiction, have very low availability in justice settings,[4,53] despite the fact that one recent randomized trial for heroin-dependent inmates found that those who started methadone prior to release were significantly less likely to use heroin or cocaine, or to engage in criminal activity 12 months post-release than those who received only counseling.[55,66,67] While the potential exists for immediate adoption of methadone maintenance for incarcerated opioid addicts, few U.S. prison systems have been receptive to this approach.[53,68]

Furthermore, continuity of treatment outside of prison (which is essential to recovery[69]) is frequently missing when addicts leave prison or jail and reenter the community.[35] Such lack of continuity has an impact not just on the addiction outcomes, but may also increase the risk of mortality from drug overdose and other causes.[62]

Combined Public Health/Public Safety Approaches

Given the inherent weakness of the two separate public health and public safety approaches to reducing crime and improving health outcomes, a key model has been developed that combines elements of both health and justice approaches. This "Combined Public Health/Public Safety Approach" builds on over 20 years of research documenting the effectiveness of drug treatment for addicts in the criminal justice system[69,70] by combining key elements of the health and justice systems. Such approaches include: drug court models that link drug treatment with judicial supervision,[71] prison and jail-based treatment combined with supervision and treatment during reentry,[73–75] and the use of medication-assisted treatment for addiction.[53,55,66–68] Drug court models, for instance, appear to be cost-effective in that for each dollar spent on drug courts, approximately four dollars is saved in reduced costs of incarcerations and health care.[75] In addition, therapeutic community and counseling approaches incorporated into justice settings have been shown to reduce drug use and recidivism.[76] Individuals who participated in prison-based therapeutic communities with a community-based program post-incarceration were seven times more likely to be drug-free and three times less likely to be arrested for criminal behavior than those not receiving treatment after three years post-release.[74,77] Key to the combined approaches is collaboration between drug abuse treatment and criminal justice system professionals and the use of monitoring, supervision, and potential for legal sanctions by the justice system to encourage addicts to engage in drug treatment and change their behaviors over an extended period of time.

The typical justice approach includes intermittent monitoring of behavior, including drug use, by probation/parole personnel with unpredictable but sometimes quite severe punishments for infractions, including positive testing for drug use (e.g., long-term incarceration if successfully prosecuted). By contrast, a combined public health/public safety approach, especially those promulgated under drug court models, uses an intense form of justice supervision in which offenders with particular behavioral problems are seen frequently by court personnel in a process informed by psychological science: encouragement and positive reinforcement of behavior change and careful monitoring with predictable and immediate consequences for infractions.[78]

The National Institute on Drug Abuse (NIDA) recently issued a publication entitled *Principles of Drug Abuse Treatment for Criminal Justice Population*, which synthesizes research on drug abuse treatment for criminal justice-involved drug abusers,[44] advocating for the combined public health/public safety approaches to address addiction as well as related behavioral and medical conditions and recidivism. As outlined in Table 2.1, these principles form the basis of a combined public health/public safety approach to intervention with addicts in justice settings and depend on a coordinated response by criminal justice agencies, drug abuse treatment providers, mental health and physical health care organizations, and social service agencies.

Effective integration of drug treatment and related medical interventions into criminal justice settings requires matching the intervention to the unique needs of different justice organizations (Table 2.2). For example, arrest is an entry point into the justice system and may alert an individual to the severity of their drug use. This phase can provide an opportunity for immediate evaluation of drug use and related health care needs. Since jail stays are usually brief, the interventions best suited to this environment may include screening for the various substance disorders (tobacco, drug, and alcohol abuse), other mental illnesses (i.e., co-occurring mental illnesses), and medical diseases (e.g., tuberculosis, STDs, HIV, and hepatitis B/C), the delivery of a brief intervention intended to boost motivation to seek treatment, and/or referral to community-based treatment providers. Similarly, each step in the criminal justice process (e.g., arrest, trial, sentencing, corrections, and reentry) lends itself to specific intervention opportunities, based on the specific key stakeholders who play a role in sanctioning and supervising offenders at that step in the justice process.

Table 2.1 NIDA Principles of Drug Abuse Treatment for Criminal Justice Populations[75]

	Treatment Principles
1	*Drug addiction is a chronic brain disease that affects behavior*
2	*Recovery from drug addiction requires effective treatment, followed by continued care.*
3	*Duration of treatment should be sufficiently long to produce stable behavioral changes*
4	*Assessment is the first step in treatment*
5	*Tailoring services to fit the needs of the individual is an important part of effective drug abuse treatment for criminal justice populations*
6	*Drug use during treatment should be carefully monitored*
7	*Treatment should target factors that are associated with criminal behavior*
8	*Criminal justice supervision should incorporate treatment planning for drug abusing offenders, and treatment providers should be aware of correctional supervision requirements*
9	*Continuity of care is essential for drug abusers re-entering the community*
10	*A balance of rewards and sanctions encourages prosocial behavior and treatment participation*
11	*Offenders with co-occurring drug abuse and mental health problems often require an integrated treatment approach*
12	*Medications are an important part of treatment for many drug abusing offenders*
13	*Treatment planning for drug abusing offenders who are living in or re-entering the community should include strategies to prevent and treat serious, chronic medical conditions such as HIV/AIDS, hepatitis B and C, and tuberculosis*

A key element to implementing the principles of drug abuse treatment for criminal justice populations is for the two disparate health and justice systems to coordinate as they address an addict's drug use, behavioral and health care needs, and criminal behavior. It is essential for the drug treatment staff to be aware of and tailor their approaches to the justice supervision requirements of their patients. In addition, drug abuse treatment outcomes are improved when antisocial and criminal behaviors are also targets of clinical attention.[79] Justice system staff need to be aware of and tailor their approaches based on an understanding of addiction (including the use of positive reinforcement, warning signs for mental health decompensation and relapse, and need for more intense treatment) in order to maximize their impact on reducing crime and enhancing recovery.

Next Steps

A combined public health/public safety approach to addictions, mental illness, and related health conditions has the potential to impact a wide range of

Table 2.2 Intervention Opportunities in Criminal Justice Systems[21]

STAGE	*OFFENDER EVENT*	*PARTICIPANTS*	*INTERVENTION OPPORTUNITIES*
ENTRY	Arrest	Crime Victim Police FBI	Screening/Referral
PROSECUTION	Court Pre-trial Release Jail	Crime Victim Police FBI Judge	Diversion Programs Drug Courts Community-Based Treatment TASC[a]
ADJUDICATION	Trial	Prosecutor Defense Attorney Defendant Jury Judge	N/A
SENTENCING	Fines Community Supervision Incarceration	Jury Judge	Drug Court Terms of Incarceration Release Conditions
CORRECTIONS	Probation Jail Prison	Probation Officers Correctional Personnel	Drug Treatment
COMMUNITY REENTRY	Probation Parole Release	Probation/Parole Officer Family Community-Based Providers	Drug Treatment Aftercare Housing Employment Mental Health Halfway House TASC

[a] TASC is the national Treatment Accountability for Safer Communities organization. Its interventions are based on a case management model for integrating criminal justice and drug abuse treatment services.

outcomes important to justice, behavioral health, and health care systems. This model provides a mechanism to maximize effectiveness in dealing with criminal activity and recidivism associated with drug use, which are of central importance to public safety officials. Likewise, mental illness, addiction, and infectious disease outcomes important to treatment providers are enhanced when combined approaches are applied. If this is true, why aren't these approaches used universally? Organization and management constraints, including a lack of infrastructure to support information sharing, high caseloads for criminal justice supervisors, inadequately staffed and trained drug treatment programs, and separate funding streams, create significant impediments to the implementation of these approaches. A lack of effective brief interventions may also play a role, and one approach that appears promising, especially for arrest and jail phases which generally have short time periods for intervention, is the use of screening combined with brief intervention (or linkage to treatment, depending on an individual's severity). This approach builds on established substance use Screening and Brief Intervention or Referral to Treatment (SBIRT) models in general medical settings.[80] In addition, because of their efficiency, technology-assisted implementation may make SBIRT approaches especially easy to administer.[81]

Next steps are twofold and include: First, applying principles of implementation science to build an evidence base on how to export effective principles of drug abuse treatment into criminal justice settings while simultaneously figuring out ways to create and sustain public health/public safety collaborations.[82] Second, applying effective implementation frameworks for addictions and other related health conditions. These approaches could be applied to mental illness as well as general health conditions where behavior plays a key role in disease progression and/or transmission (e.g., HIV and other STDs, tuberculosis, and hepatitis).[83]

Conclusions

There are many barriers to treatment for drug-involved offenders, including lack of resources, infrastructure, and treatment staff. Addiction remains a stigmatized disease that is often not regarded by the criminal justice system as a medical condition and as a consequence is not afforded the same guarantee of treatment like other medical conditions. In addition, the criminal justice system lacks the staff and resources needed to identify and treat frequently co-occurring mental and physical health conditions.

For behaviors that are fundamentally linked to drug addiction[4,84] punishment alone is a temporary stopgap approach. The irony is that approaches that integrate strengths of both the public health and public safety systems can be more effective than stand-alone arrest and incarceration in improving public safety outcomes. Marked increases in the number of offenders with drug addiction and other serious comorbid conditions make it imperative that we continue to respond with smarter methods. We believe a combined public safety/public health approach holds the most promise for addressing the multiple drug abuse, mental health, and health care needs of the criminal justice system.

Success in the adoption, implementation, and sustainability of this promising new approach requires a culture shift in both the public health and safety systems simultaneously. The public safety system, designed to enforce laws and punish illegal drug use, must recognize the role they can play in improving not just crime rates but community health by facilitating participation in addiction, mental health, and medical treatment. Similarly, public health officials must reach into the public safety system to establish collaborative mechanisms to deliver care. Finally, policymakers need to recognize that an integrated approach is not intended to be "soft on crime." It is often more rigorous in terms of close follow up of offenders and is designed specifically to reduce crime, in addition to addressing serious health needs. Overall, not treating the drug-abusing offender is a missed opportunity to simultaneously impact public health and public safety.

Acknowledgments

The authors acknowledge the contributions of multiple scientists supported by the National Institute on Drug Abuse whose work has informed this chapter, as well as judicial colleagues who provided essential guidance in developing the concepts. In addition, the concepts in this paper are particularly indebted to the paper by NIDA scientists, Drs. Redonna Chandler, Bennett Fletcher, and Nora Volkow.[65]

Disclaimer: The views and opinions expressed in this report are those of the authors and should not be construed to represent the views of the National Institute on Drug Abuse, the National Institutes of Health, or other parts of the U.S. government.

References

1. Bureau of Justice Statistics Prisoner Series. (2010). *Prisoners in 2008*. Web page document http://bjs.ojp.usdoj.gov/index.cfm?ty=pbdetail&iid=1763. Accessed January 31, 2010.
2. Bureau of Justice Statistics Correctional Surveys. (2010). *Total correctional population*. Available at: http://bjs.ojp.usdoj.gov/index.cfm?ty=tp&tid=11. Accessed January 31, 2010.
3. United States Census Bureau. (2010). Population estimates. Available at: http://www.census.gov/popest/states/asrh/SC-EST2005–01.html. Accessed January 20, 2010.
4. Jensen, E. L., Gerber, J., & Mosher, C. (2004). Social consequences of the War on Drugs: The legacy of failed policy. *Criminal Justice Policy Review*, *15*(1), 100–121.
5. Karberg, J. C. & James, D. J. (2005). *Substance dependence, abuse, and treatment of jail inmates, 2002*. Washington, DC: Office of Justice Programs, Bureau of Justice Statistics. DOJ publication no. NCJ 209588.
6. Weinbaum, C. A., Sabin, K. M., & Santibanez, S. S. (2005). Hepatitis B, hepatitis C, and HIV in correctional populations: A review of epidemiology and prevention. *AIDS*, *19*(Suppl3), S41–S46.

7. Compton, W. M., Dawson, D., Duffy, S. Q., & Grant, B. F. (in press). The impact of inmate populations on estimates of alcohol and drug use disorders in the United States. *Am J Psychiatry*.
8. U.S. Department of Justice, Bureau of Justice Statistics. (2003). Prison and jail inmates at midyear 2002. *Bureau of Justice Statistics Special Report*. NCJ 198877. Available at: http://www.ojp.usdoj.gov/bjs/pub/pdf/pjim02.pdf
9. U.S. Department of Justice, Bureau of Justice Statistics. (2005). Substance dependence, abuse, and treatment of jail inmates, 2002. *Bureau of Justice Statistics Special Report*. NCJ 209588. Available at: http://www.ojp.usdoj.gov/bjs/pub/pdf/sdatji02.pdf
10. U.S. Department of Justice, Bureau of Justice Statistics. (2006a). Drug use and dependence, state and federal prisoners, 2004. *Bureau of Justice Statistics Special Report*. NCJ 213530. Available at: http://www.ojp.gov/bjs/pub/pdf/dudsfp04.pdf
11. U.S. Department of Justice, Bureau of Justice Statistics. (2006b). Mental health problems of prison and jail inmates. *Bureau of Justice Statistics Special Report*. NCJ 213600. Available at: http://www.ojp.gov/bjs/pub/pdf/mhppji.pdf
12. Compton, W. M., Thomas, Y. F., Stinson, F. S., & Grant, B. F. (2007). Prevalence, correlates, disability, and comorbidity of DSM-IV drug abuse and dependence in the United States: Results from the National Epidemiologic Survey on Alcohol and Related Conditions. *Arch Gen Psychiatry, 64*, 566–576.
13. Substance Abuse and Mental Health Services Administration. (2009). *National Survey on Drug Use and Health, 2008 National Findings*. Office of Applied Studies, NSDUH Series H-36, HHS Publication No. SMA 09–4434. Rockville, MD.
14. Bureau of Justice Statistics. *National Corrections Reporting Program, 2002*. Analyzed online at: http://www.icpsr.umich.edu/cgi-bin/SDA/ICPSR/hsda?nacjd+04345–0001. Accessed January 25, 2010.
15. Iguchi, M. Y., Bell, J., Ramchand, R. N., & Fain, T. (2005). How criminal system racial disparities may translate into health disparities. *J Health Care Poor Underserved, 16*, 48–56.
16. Hasin, D. S., Stinson, F. S., Ogburn, E., & Grant, B. F. (2007). Prevalence, correlates, disability, and comorbidity of DSM-IV alcohol abuse and dependence in the United States: Results from the National Epidemiologic Survey on Alcohol and Related Conditions. *Arch Gen Psychiatry, 64*(7), 830–842.
17. Kessler, R. C., Crum, R. M., Warner, L. A., Nelson, C. B., Schulenberg, J., & Anthony, J. C. (1997). Lifetime co-occurrence of DSM-III-R alcohol abuse and dependence with other psychiatric disorders in the National Comorbidity Survey. *Arch Gen Psychiatry, 54*(4), 313–321.
18. Grant, B. F., Stinson, F. S., Dawson, D. A., Chou, S. P., Ruan, W. J., & Pickering, R. P. (2004). Co-occurrence of 12-month alcohol and drug use disorders and personality disorders in the United States. *Arch Gen Psychiatry, 61*, 361–368
19. James, D. J. & Glaze, L. E. (2006). *Mental health problems of prison and jail inmates*. Washington, DC: U.S. Department of Justice, Office of Justice Programs. NCJ Publication Number 213600. Available at: http://bjs.ojp.usdoj.gov/index.cfm?ty=pbdetail&iid=789. Accessed January 20, 2010.
20. Abram, K. M. & Teplin, L. A. (1991). Co-occurring disorders among mentally ill jail detainees: Implications for public policy. *Am Psychol, 46*(10), 1036–1045.
21. Chandler, R. K., Peters, R. H., Field, G., & Juliano-Bult, D. (2004). Challenges in implementing evidence-based treatment practices for co-occurring disorders in the criminal justice system. *Behav Sci Law, 22*(4), 431–448.

22. Spaulding, A. C., Seals, R. M., Page, M. J., Brzozowski, A. K., Rhodes, W., & Hammett, T. M. (2009). HIV\AIDS among inmates of and releases from U.S. correctional facilities, 2006: Declining share of epidemic but persistent public health opportunity. *PLoS One, 11*(4), 1–6.
23. Boutwell, A. E., Allen, S. A., & Rich, J. D. (2005). Opportunities to address the hepatitis C epidemic in the correctional setting. *Clin Infect Dis, 40*(Suppl 5), S367–S372.
24. Zaller, N., Thurmond, P., & Rich, J. D. (2007). Limited spending: An analysis of correctional expenditures on antiretrovirals for HIV-infected prisoners. *Public Health Rep, 122*(1), 49–54.
25. Taxman, F. S., Perdoni, M. L., & Harrison, L. D. (2007). Drug treatment services for adult offenders: The state of the state. *J Subst Abuse Treatment, 32*(3), 239–254.
26. Desai, A. A., Latta, E. T., Spaulding, A., Rich, J. D., & Flanigan, T. P. (2002). The importance of routine HIV testing in the incarcerated population: The Rhode Island experience. *AIDS Educ Prev, 14*(5)(Suppl), 45–52.
27. Sabin, K. M., Frey, R. L., Horsley, R., & Greby, S. M. (2001). Characteristics and trends of newly identified HIV infections among incarcerated populations: CDC HIV voluntary counseling testing and referral system 1992–1998. *J Urban Health, 78*(2), 241–255.
28. Allen, S. A., Spaulding, A. C., Osei, A. M., Taylor, L. E., Cabral, A. M., & Rich, J. D. (2003). Treatment of chronic hepatitis C in a state correctional facility. *Ann Intern Med, 138*(3), 187–190.
29. Vallabhaneni, S., Macalino, G. E., Reinert, S. E., Schwartzapfel, B., Wolf, F. A., & Rich, J. D. (2006). Prisoners favor hepatitis C testing and treatment. *Epidemiol Infect, 134*(2), 243–248.
30. Centers for Disease Control and Prevention (CDC), National Center for HIV/AIDS, Viral Hepatitis, STD, TB Prevention. (2006). Prevention and control of tuberculosis in correctional and detention facilities: Recommendations from CDC. Endorsed by Advisory Council for the Elimination of Tuberculosis, the National Commission on Correctional Health Care, and The American Correctional Association. *MMWR Recomm Rep, 55*, 1–44.
31. *Estelle* v. *Gamble*, 429 U.S. 97 (1976). U.S. Supreme Court, Number 75–929. Available at: http://supreme.justia.com/us/429/97/case.html, Accessed January 25, 2010.
32. Rich, J. D., Holmes, L., Salas, C., et al. (2001). Successful linkage of medical care and community services for HIV-positive offenders being released from prison. *J Urban Health, 78*(2), 279–289.
33. Springer, S. A., Pesanti, E., Hodges, J., Macura, T., Doros, G., & Altice, F.L. (2004). Effectiveness of antiretroviral therapy among HIV-infected prisoners: Reincarceration and the lack of sustained benefit after release to the community. *Clin Infect Dis, 38*(12), 1754–1760.
34. Freudenberg, N. (2001). Jails, prisons, and the health of urban populations: A review of the impact of the correctional system on community health. *J Urban Health, 78*(2), 214–235.
35. Hammett, T. M., Roberts, C., Kennedy, S. (2001). Health-related issues in prisoner reentry. *Crime Delinq, 47*(3), 390–409.
36. Baillargeon, J., Giordano, T. P., Rich, J. D., Wu, Z. H., Wells, K., Pollock, B. H., et al. (2009). Accessing antiretroviral therapy following release from prison. *JAMA, 301*(8), 848–857.
37. Volkow, N. & Li, T. K. (2005). The neuroscience of addiction. *Nat Neurosci*, 8, 1429–1430.
38. Kosten, T. R. (1998). Addiction as a brain disease. *Am J Psychiatry, 155*(6), 711–713.

39. Shaham, Y. & Hope, B. T. (2005). The role of neuroadaptations in relapse to drug seeking. *Nat Neurosci, 8*(11), 1437–1439.
40. Baler, R. D. & Volkow, N. D. (2006). Drug addiction: the neurobiology of disrupted self-control. *Trends Mol Med, 12*(12), 559–566.
41. McLellan, A. T., Lewis, D. C., O'Brien, C. P., & Kleber, H. D. (2000). Drug dependence, a chronic medical illness: Implications for treatment, insurance, and outcomes evaluation. *JAMA, 284*(13), 1689–1695.
42. Prendergast, M. L., Podus, D., Chang, E., & Urada, D. (2002). The effectiveness of drug abuse treatment: A meta-analysis of comparison group studies. *Drug Alcohol Depend, 67*(1), 53–72.
43. Lurigio, A. J. (2000). Drug treatment availability and effectiveness—studies of the general and criminal justice populations. *Crim Justice Behav, 27*(4), 495–528.
44. Fletcher, B. W. & Chandler, R. K. (2006). *Principles of drug abuse treatment for criminal justice populations.* Washington, DC: National Institute on Drug Abuse. NIH Publication No. 06–5316.
45. Wormith, J. S., Althouse, R., Simpson, M., Reitzel, L. R., Fagan, T. J., & Morgan, R. D. (2007). The rehabilitation and reintegration of offenders—The current landscape and some future directions for correctional psychology. *Crim Justice Behav, 34*(7), 879–892.
46. Carroll, K. M., et al. (2009). Enduring effects of a computer-assisted training program for cognitive behavior therapy: A six-month follow-up of CBT4CBT. *Drug Alcohol Depend, 100,* 178–181.
47. De Leon, G. (1997). Therapeutic communities: Is there an essential model? In G. De Leon, (Ed.). *Community as method: Therapeutic communities for special populations and special settings* (pp. 3–18). Westport, Connecticut: Praeger.
48. Volkow, N. D. & Li, T. K. (2005). Drugs and alcohol: Treating and preventing abuse, addiction and their medical consequences. *Pharmacol Ther, 108*(1), 3–17.
49. Johnson, B. A., Rosenthal, N., Capece, J. A., et al. (2007). Topiramate for treating alcohol dependence: a randomized controlled trial. *JAMA, 298*(14), 1641–1651.
50. Humphreys, K., Wing, S., McCarty, D., Chappel, J., Gallant, L., Haberle, B., et al. (2004). Self-help organizations for alcohol and drug problems: Toward evidence-based practice and policy. *J Subst Abuse Treat,* 26, 151–158.
51. McCollister, K. E., French, M. T., Prendergast, M. L., Hall, E., & Sacks, S. (2004). Long-term cost effectiveness of addiction treatment for criminal offenders. *Justice Q, 21*(3), 659–679.
52. Stephan, J. J. (2004). *State prison expenditures, 2001.* Washington, DC: Office of Justice Programs, Bureau of Justice Statistics, DOJ publication no. NCJ 202949.
53. Rich, J. D., Boutwell, A. E., Shield, D. C., Key, R. G., McKenzie, M., Clarke, J. G., et al. (2005). Attitudes and practices regarding the use of methadone in US state and federal prisons. *J Urban Health, 82,* 411–419.
54. Rich, J. D., McKenzie, M., Shield, D. C., et al. (2005). Linkage with methadone treatment upon release from incarceration: A promising opportunity. *J Addict Dis, 24*(3), 49–59.
55. Gordon, M. S., Kinlock, T. W., Schwartz, R. P., & O'Grady, K. E. (2008). A randomized clinical trial of methadone maintenance for prisoners: Findings at 6 months post-release. *Addiction, 103*(8), 1333–1342.
56. Daley, M., Love, C. T., Shepard, D. S., Petersen, C. B., White, K. L., & Hall, F. B. (2004). Cost-effectiveness of Connecticut's in-prison substance abuse treatment. *J Offender Rehab, 39*(3), 69–92.

57. Flynn, P. M., Kristiansen, P. L., Porto, J. V., & Hubbard, R. L. (1999). Costs and benefits of treatment for cocaine addiction in DATOS. *Drug Alcohol Depend, 57*(2), 167–174.
58. Zarkin, G. A., Dunlap, L. J., Hicks, K. A., & Mamo, D. (2005). Benefits and costs of methadone treatment: Results from a lifetime simulation model. *Health Econ, 14*(11), 1133–1150.
59. Mumola, C. J. & Karberg, J. C. (2006). *Drug use and dependence, state and federal prisoners, 2004.* Washington, DC: Office of Justice Programs, Bureau of Justice Statistics, DOJ publication no. NCJ 213530.
60. Langan, P. A. & Levin, D. J. (2002). *Recidivism of prisoners released in 1994.* Washington, DC: Office of Justice Programs, Bureau of Justice Statistics. DOJ publication no. NCJ 193427.
61. Simpler, A. H. & Langhinrichsen-Rohling, J. (2005). Substance use in prison: How much occurs and is it associated with psychopathology? *Addict Res Theory, 13*(5), 503–511.
62. Binswanger, I. A., Stern, M. F., Deyo, R. A., et al. (2007). Release from prison—A high risk of death for former inmates. *New Engl J Med, 356*(2), 157–165.
63. Field, G. (2004). Continuity of offender treatment: From the institution to the community. In K. Knight & D. Farabee (Eds.). *Treating addicted offenders: A continuum of effective practices.* Kingston, NJ: Civic Research Institute, 33–1–33–9.
64. Shivy, V. A., Wu, J. J., Moon, A. E., Mann, S. C., Holland, J. G., & Eacho, C. (2007). Ex-offenders reentering the workforce. *J. Couns Psychol, 54*(4), 466–473.
65. Chander, R. K., Fletcher, B. F., & Volkow, N. D. (2009). Treating drug abuse and addiction in the criminal justice system: Improving public health and safety. *JAMA,* 301, 183–190.
66. Kinlock, T. W., Gordon, M. S., Schwartz, R. P., O'Grady, K., Fitzgerald, T. T., & Wilson M. (2007). A randomized clinical trial of methadone maintenance for prisoners: results at 1-month post-release. *Drug Alcohol Depend. 91*(2–3), 220–227.
67. Kinlock, T. W., Gordon, M. S., Schwartz, R. P., & O'Grady, K. E. (2008). A study of methadone maintenance for male prisoners. *Crim Justice Behav, 35*(1), 34–47.
68. Nunn, A., Zaller, N., Dickman, S., Trimbur, C., Nijhawan, A., & Rich, J. D. (2009). Methadone and buprenorphine prescribing and referral practices in US prison systems: Results from a nationwide survey. *Drug Alcohol Depend. 105*(1–2), 83–88.
69. Inciardi, J. A., Martin, S. S., Butzin, C. A., Hooper, R. M., & Harrison, L. D. (1997). An effective model of prison-based treatment for drug-involved offenders. *J Drug Issues, 27*(2), 261–278.
70. Pearson, F. S. & Lipton, D. S. (1999). A meta-analytic review of the effectiveness of corrections-based treatments for drug abuse. *Prison J, 79*(4), 384–410.
71. Peters, R. H. & Murrin, M. R. (2000). Effectiveness of treatment-based drug courts in reducing recidivism. *Crim Justice Behav, 27*(1), 72–96.
72. Knight, K. & D. Farabee, (Eds.) (2004). *Treating addicted offenders: A continuum of effective practices.* Kingston, NJ: Civic Research Institute.
73. Leukefeld, C. G., & F. Tims, & D. Farabee, (Eds.) (2002). *Treatment of drug offenders: Policies and issues.* New York, NY: Springer.
74. Martin, S. S., Butzin, C. A., Saum, C. A., & Inciardi, J. A. (1999). Three-year outcomes of therapeutic community treatment for drug-involved offenders in Delaware: From prison to work release to aftercare. *Prison J, 79*(3), 294–320.

75. Logan, T. K., Hoyt, W. H., McCollister, K. E., French, M. T., Leukefeld, C., & Minton, L. (2004). Economic evaluation of drug court: Methodology, results, and policy implications. *Eval Program Plan, 27*(4), 381–396.
76. Mitchell, O., Wilson, D. B., & MacKenzie, D. L. (2007). Does incarceration-based drug treatment reduce recidivism? A meta-analytic synthesis of the research. *J Exp Criminol, 3*(4), 353–375.
77. Butzin, C. A., O'Connell, D. J., Martin, S. S., & Inciardi, J. A. (2006). Effect of drug treatment during work release on new arrests and incarcerations. *J Crim Justice, 34*(5), 557–565.
78. Cooper, C. S. (2003). Drug courts: Current issues and future perspectives. *Subst Use Misuse, 38*, 1671–1711.
79. Wilson, D. B., Bouffard, L. A., & Mackenzie, D. L. (2005). A quantitative review of structured, group-oriented, cognitive-behavioral programs for offenders. *Crim Justice Behav, 32*(2), 172–204.
80. Madras, B. K., Compton, W. M., Avula, D., Stegbauer, T., Stein, J. B., & Clark, H. W. (2009). Screening, brief interventions, referral to treatment (SBIRT) for illicit drug and alcohol use at multiple healthcare sites: Comparison at intake and six months. *Drug Alcohol Depend, 99*, 280–295.
81. National Institute on Drug Abuse. (2010). *NM ASSIST: Screening for drug use in general medical settings.* Available at: http://ww1.drugabuse.gov/nmassist/. Accessed January 25, 2010.
82. Wexler, H. K. & Fletcher, B. W. (2007). National criminal justice drug abuse treatment studies (CJ-DATS) overview. *Prison J, 87*(1), 9–24.
83. U.S. Department of Health and Human Services, National Institutes of Health. (2010). *Seek, test, and treat: Addressing HIV in the criminal justice system, request for applications* Number DA-10–017. 2010. Available at: http://grants.nih.gov/grants/guide/rfa-files/RFA-DA-10–017.html. Accessed January 29, 2010.
84. Dackis, C. & O'Brien, C. (2005). Neurobiology of addiction: Treatment and public policy ramifications. *Nat Neurosci, 8*(11), 1431–1436.

3

Mental Health Disparities among Latinos, the Fastest Growing Population in the US

SERGIO AGUILAR-GAXIOLA AND LINDA ZIEGAHN

Introduction

The "Latinisation" of the United States, as reported by demographer William Frey of the Brookings Institute in a January 2010 issue of *The Economist,* is one of the most important recent demographic changes in America. According to recent estimates by the U.S. Census Bureau, the Latino population will double from today's 15% to 30% by 2050.[1] Indeed, Latinos have accounted for 62% of the natural population increase of America's total population growth since 2000. From July 1, 2007, to July 1, 2008, alone, there was a 3.2% increase in the Hispanic population, making Latinos the fastest-growing minority group in the nation.[1] As of July 2008, the U.S. Latino population ranks second worldwide. Only Mexico (110 million) had a larger Latino population than the United States (46.9 million). However, knowledge of general statistics on Latino growth tells us little about the many vibrant cultures which are subsumed under the "Latino" rubric. Furthermore, without knowing the nuances of how mental illness affects different Latino populations, we cannot know how to ultimately improve access to care and specific treatment options for mental health conditions affecting Latinos.

Relevant questions include, first, who are the Latinos, and which subgroups represent the largest populations within the US? Second, what is the nature of disparities in mental health status in Latinos and for the major Latino subgroups? Third, what is the pattern of mental health utilization among the various Latino subgroups? The preliminary research reported on these questions in this chapter provides researchers with an important baseline for further investigation of the context of Latino mental health disparities, as well as perceived barriers to receiving care and potential opportunities for improving mental health service utilization among Latinos.

The Latino Population in the United States

With a U.S. population of 46.8 million on July 1, 2008, Latinos are the largest and fastest growing minority group, comprising15% of the nation's total population.[1] Between 2000 and 2006, Latinos accounted for one-half of the nation's growth, and the growth rate of Latinos was more than three times the growth rate of the total population (24.3% vs. 6.1%, respectively).[1]

The 50% growth rate is driven primarily by Latino births in the US, and secondarily by immigration. The dominant Hispanic subgroups are from Mexico (64%); Central and South America (14%), most notably El Salvador, Guatemala and Colombia; Puerto Rico (9%); Cuba (3.5%); and the Dominican Republic (2.7%). Foreign-born Latinos comprise 6% of the total U.S. population.[2] Nearly half of all foreign-born in the United States are Hispanic, and the United States has the fifth largest Spanish-speaking population in the world, exceeded only by Mexico, Colombia, Spain, and Argentina. These subgroups have differing life experiences, natural histories, and risks of psychiatric disorders. Of special significance to the field of mental health are the different immigration experiences, which include war experiences and traumas. Another significant feature of the Latino population in the US is its youth. Compared with the total U.S. population, a higher percentage of the Hispanic population is under 18 years (34% compared with 26%); over one-third (36.8%) of all Latinos are under the age of 18.[1]

Hispanic and Latino are adjectives used to describe people who come from different countries, with different cultures and sociopolitical histories, including Mexico, Puerto Rico, Cuba, Argentina, Colombia, the Dominican Republic, Brazil, Guatemala, Costa Rica, Nicaragua, El Salvador, and people from all other countries in Central and South America, and most of the Caribbean islands. The term Hispanic, which dates back to the 1970s and the U.S. Department of Education, refers to the influence of the Spanish culture and language on a group of people who suffered years of colonization. The term Latino, on the other hand, refers to people who came from Mexico, Central and South America, and territories in the United States that were taken from Mexico, and some of the Caribbean islands. It considers the influences of indigenous cultures and African ancestry on people who share a history of colonization by Spain. Except for Brazilians, who speak Portuguese, Latinos are bonded together in the United States by the Spanish language. Most first generation Latinos (68%) identify themselves with their native land or country of origin. In contrast, most third or higher generation Latinos (57%) identify themselves as Americans.[3]

Latinos: A Heterogeneous Population

Despite a tendency to lump "Hispanics or Latinos" together, Latinos are heterogeneous in several factors that may influence the prevalence, incidence, presentation, course, and treatment of mental disorders. These factors include birthplace, acculturation, genetics, race, health care access, service utilization, and language. While epidemiological studies tend to aggregate Latino subgroups into a homogenous category, there are significant differences in mental health status, access to care, and service utilization across subgroups. Just looking at key socio-demographic variables, we see significant differences among the three largest Latino subgroups—Mexicans, Puerto Ricans, and Cubans:

Mexicans. Mexicans comprise the largest group of Latinos (approximately 29 million or 64.2%) in the United States. They have been in the US the longest, having arrived in the 1600s and 1700s when they worked with the Spaniards to establish missions and communities that later became important cities. Large numbers of Mexicans began to immigrate into the United States during the early 1900s, when they attempted to escape Mexico's economic depression and the Mexican Revolution of 1910. They settled primarily in Texas, California, New Mexico, and Arizona, where the largest number remains. However, traditional migration problems have changed in recent times, and new patterns of settlement are being created in rural communities in the Midwest, Southeast, and Northeast. Although some Mexican-Americans have achieved financial success, the majority of this population subgroup continues to have incomes below the poverty line.

Puerto Ricans. At about 4.1 million (or 9.1% of the Latino population), Puerto Ricans are the second largest group of Latinos living in the United States. They began to arrive in large numbers after the Depression and World War II. While most live in the Northeast, especially in New York City, there also are Puerto Rican communities in Texas, Florida, and Illinois. Because they are U. S. citizens, Puerto Ricans are able to go back and forth between the island and the U.S. mainland. Puerto Ricans have the highest unemployment rate of all Latinos; one-third live in poverty, making them the poorest of the Latino groups. However, they are eligible for public assistance and benefits such as Medicare and Medicaid.

Cubans. Cubans are the third largest subgroup of Latinos in the United States, comprising 1.6 million or 3.5% of the Latino population. Their primary places of residence are Florida, New York, and New Jersey. The first wave of immigrants arrived in the 1960s, after Fidel Castro's revolution and establishment of a socialist government. Most were upper class Whites with educational resources, business acumen, and financial backing. The majority settled in Miami and viewed themselves as exiles waiting to return to Cuba when the revolution was over. Their situation was greatly aided by the Cuban Adjustment

Act of 1966, which helped to legalize their status in the US, and the Cuban Refugee Program. The second wave of Cuban immigrants, known as the *Marielitos*, a term applied to exiles who fled to the United States from the port of Mariel, arrived in 1980.[4] Most members of that group were of lower socioeconomic status and more racially mixed.

Another important group in the US includes Dominicans, who came to the US primarily via Puerto Rico. Most of the estimated 1.2 million Dominicans reside in New York and New Jersey, with the majority living in Washington Heights in New York City.[5] Those who migrate to the US tend to be of lower socioeconomic status. Other large Central American groups such as Salvadorans (1.5 million), who settled primarily in Los Angeles area, and Nicaraguans, many of whom live in Florida, add to the increasing Latino diversity of the US.

Despite great diversity among Latino subgroups, research studies have traditionally treated them as a monolithic population group.

Disparities in Mental Health Status: The Immigrant Paradox

In the aggregate, Latinos have equal or better mental health than Whites, despite having lower socioeconomic status and greater social problems, and yet they suffer from disparities in mental health care access and service utilization.[6] Latinos report lower prevalence rates for all psychiatric disorders except agoraphobia without panic disorder.[7] For example, Latinos report a lifetime rate of any psychiatric disorder of 29.7% compared to 43.2% in Whites. However, this overall difference in mental health becomes more complex and nuances are revealed when Latinos are disaggregated into subgroups. Indeed, when the unitary category of Latinos is disaggregated by subgroup, significant differences are found by nativity,[i] by time of residence in the United States, and by age of migration.

Specifically, Puerto Ricans have the highest lifetime prevalence rates of mental disorders (37.4%), followed by Mexicans (29.5%), Cubans (28.2%), and other Latinos (27.0%).[7] Additionally, U.S.-born Latinos have higher rates (37.1%) of mental disorders compared to immigrants (24.9%). For Mexican immigrants, as an example, rates of mental disorders increase according to time in the United

i. "Nativity refers to whether a person is native or foreign born. The native-born population includes anyone who was a U.S. citizen or U.S. national at birth. Respondents who were born in the United States, Puerto Rico, a U.S. Island Area (U.S. Virgin Islands, Guam, American Samoa, or the Commonwealth of the Northern Mariana Islands), or abroad of a U.S. citizen parent or parents, are defined as native. The foreign-born population includes anyone who was not a U.S. citizen or U.S. national at birth. Respondents who are not U.S. citizens as well as those who have become U.S. citizens through naturalization are considered foreign born."

States, with individuals living in the United States longer than 13 years having higher prevalence rates than those who lived in the US less than 13 years.[8] Similar patterns are repeated, to varying degrees, in other major Latino subgroups, leading to what has been termed the "immigrant paradox," wherein protective effects of Latino culture from countries of origin pre-immigration lessen as immigrants establish residency in the United States. Further, mental health declines over time in the host country, as acculturation in the US leads to changes in lifestyle, cultural practices, and social norms.[7–9] However, the relative impact of these various factors on mental health pre- and post-immigration varies considerably by some Latino sub-ethnic populations.

Mental Health Status in Latinos

Earlier studies: 1980s and 1990s. Before 1980 there were no large scale psychiatric epidemiological studies that ascertained the rates of mental disorders for any population, much less the Hispanic population. Prior to the 1980s, the data available for Latinos from existing studies were limited to relatively small studies of limited circulation and generalizability. Further, these studies lacked the scientific rigor to have an impact in the development of mental health policy and services. Starting in the 1980s, researchers trying to unravel the correlates of mental health status for the different subgroups conducted psychiatric epidemiological studies that revealed increasingly nuanced interpretations of differences emerging from Latino subgroups.[7,8,10–13]

The Epidemiological Catchment Area (ECA) study, conducted from 1981 to 1984, was the first of several large studies that ascertained prevalence rates of mental disorders in the US. Using the Diagnostic Interview Schedule (DIS)[10] and DSM-III criteria,[14] the ECA included nearly 20,000 participants from five major U.S. cities (New Haven, CT; Baltimore, MD; St Louis, MO; Raleigh-Durham, NC; and Los Angeles, CA). Los Angeles was the only city and ECA site that included an oversample of Hispanics. The findings presented below are based on the LA-ECA.[11]

The LA-ECA sample of 1,243 adult Latinos reported a lifetime rate of any psychiatric disorder of 34.6%; 7.8% met criteria for any affective disorders, 14.5% for any anxiety disorders, and 18.4% for any substance use disorders. In general, it was found that Latinos had similar rates to the rest of the ECA sample, and that overall, Latinos had similar rates of psychiatric disorders as compared to the general sample that included other ECA study sites.[11,12] However, when the Latino sample was analyzed by birthplace, the rates for each of the disorders studied were higher for the U.S.-born Latinos than the immigrant sample. Specifically, the rate of major depression among the immigrant sample ranged from 3% to 3.7% according to their level of acculturation to the United States.

The rates for the U.S.-born Hispanic sample were nearly double, at 5.5% to 6.9%. One of the lasting legacies of the ECA study was not only that it was the first study to systematically outline the psychiatric status of a population by using a fully structured diagnostic interview based on the DSM criteria in the US, but also that it identified subgroups that were at increased risk for developing psychiatric disorders, and thus opened the door for future research on Hispanic populations.

The National Comorbidity Survey (NCS) was the first large psychiatric epidemiological study that included a national representative sample of the general U.S. population. It included a national probability sample of 8,098 participants aged 15 to 54 and used the University of Michigan CIDI (Composite International Diagnostic Interview) based on DSM-III-R criteria. Close to 10% of the total NCS sample identified itself as Hispanic. One of the limitations of the NCS was that it only included English-speaking Latinos. Compared with Whites, Latinos were found to have a lower risk of having a psychiatric disorder in their lifetime. Similar to the findings of the LA-ECA sample, the NCS reported that, compared to Whites, Latinos had similar lifetime rates for any anxiety disorders (28%) and any substance use disorders (24.7%), but significantly higher rates of affective disorders (20.4% vs. 19.5%).[8,13] Latinos with mood disorders were nearly twice as likely to be persistently ill as Whites.[15] Immigrant Latinos were also found to have the lowest prevalence rates across all psychiatric disorders.[8]

Given the results of the ECA-LA and the NCS that documented differing rates by place of birth among Latinos, Vega and colleagues (1998)[8] initiated the regional Mexican American Prevalence and Services Survey (MAPSS) of 3,011 randomly selected participants aged 18 to 54 years of age. Launched in Fresno County, CA, the MAPSS study, which used the Fresno CIDI, remains one of the largest epidemiological mental health surveys conducted with the Latino (specifically, Mexican origin) population in the US.

Overall, MAPSS/DSM-III-R lifetime prevalence rates for any psychiatric disorder were reported to be 33.8%. Among the specific diagnostic categories, substance use disorders had the highest lifetime prevalence rates (17.1%), followed by any anxiety disorder (16.8%), and affective disorders (12.1%). Given the earlier findings of differences by place of birth, the MAPSS study analyzed its sample by nativity and found immigrants to have a 24.9% lifetime rate for any psychiatric disorder compared to a 48.1% rate for U.S.-born Mexican Americans. Further comparisons across the immigrant and the U.S.-born Mexican origin adults found that immigrants had significantly lower lifetime rates for any substance use (10.5% vs. 27.7%), any affective (8% vs. 18.7%), and any anxiety disorders (13% vs. 23.2%) than the U.S.-born. Researchers further reported that the Mexican U.S.-born sample had prevalence rates (48.7%) that were very similar to the general U.S. population (48.6%). Thus, Mexican immigrants were found to have about one-half the lifetime prevalence rates of any psychiatric disorder and any major diagnostic categories of either native-born Mexican Americans or other Americans and had similar rates of psychiatric disorders (24.9%) to residents of Mexico City (23.4%).

The Mexican immigrant sample was further analyzed to determine whether length of stay in the US had any impact on lifetime prevalence rates. In fact, individuals who had lived in the US less than 13 years had lower prevalence rates of mental illness than those immigrants who had lived in the US equal to or longer than 13 years.[8] Consistent with previous studies, MAPSS researchers concluded that there are protective factors within the Hispanic culture that may become eroded with length of stay in the US. In other words, there are risk factors associated with living in the US that lead to an increased risk for the development of psychiatric disorders.

Recent studies: 2000s. From 2000 to 2009, there have been three large, national probabilistic studies that included Latino samples. A brief description of each, along with the main findings, follows.

The National Comorbidity Survey Replication (NCSR) is a national probabilistic household study representative of the U.S. general population conducted by Kessler and colleagues between 2001 and 2003.[9] With a sample of 9,282 English-speaking adults, the NCSR was fielded a decade later than the original NCS. Using an expanded survey, with DSM-IV diagnostic criteria, the NCSR found that Latinos had lower rates than Whites of mood and anxiety disorders but not substance use disorders.

The National Epidemiologic Survey on Alcohol and Related Conditions (NESARC) conducted by Grant and colleagues is a national probabilistic study representative of the U.S. general population of 43,093 adults 18 years and older.[16] The NESARC included a Hispanic sample of 7,995; 4,558 were of Mexican origin. The participants were interviewed with the Alcohol Use Disorder and Associated Disabilities Interview Schedule (AUDADIS)–DSM-IV version.[17] This study was the first to compare four groups regarding nativity (U.S.-born vs. immigrants and Mexican origin vs. Whites). Consistent with previous studies that have demonstrated the important protective role of culture in immigrants' mental health, this study found that both U.S.-born Mexicans and U.S.-born Whites had higher lifetime rates of any disorder (47.6% and 52.5%, respectively) than their immigrant counterparts born either in Mexico or other countries (28.5% and 32.3%). This pattern was consistently found for any mood disorder, anxiety disorder, alcohol use disorder, and drug use disorder with ratios ranging from 2:1 to 8.3:1 for the U.S.-born Mexicans and Whites than for foreign-born Mexicans and Whites.

The National Latino and Asian American Study (NLAAS) was the first large national probability study of English and Spanish-speaking Latinos to compare lifetime and past-year prevalence rates of psychiatric disorders across Latino subgroups using the World Health Organization Composite International

Diagnostic Interview (WHO-CIDI).[18] This study of 2,554 Latinos—Mexican, Puerto Rican, Cuban, and "other"—revealed overall lifetime psychiatric disorder prevalence estimates of 28.1% for men and 30.2% for women. Rates among Latino subgroups varied depending upon the specific psychiatric disorders: for major depressive episode (MDE), U.S.-born Puerto Ricans revealed a 20.2% lifetime rate, Mexicans 19.2%, Cubans 17.9%, and other Latino, 16.2%; whereas for immigrant Latinos, the prevalence rates were highest for Cubans (18.5%), 17.6% for Puerto Ricans, 14.1% for other Latinos, and 11.8% for Mexicans. U.S.-born Puerto Ricans, Cubans, Mexicans and other Latinos had similar rates of substance use disorders (20.4 to 21.4%); whereas for immigrant Latinos, the rates were 11.1% for Puerto Ricans, 6.4% for Cubans, 7.0% for Mexicans, and 5.7% for other Latinos. Based on these findings, Alegria and her colleagues[7] concluded that the immigrant paradox appeared to hold true for Mexicans—foreign-born Mexicans had consistently lower rates of disorders than U.S.-born across mood, anxiety, and substance disorders. However, for Cubans and other Latinos, this paradox seemed evident only for substance disorders; and for Puerto Ricans, no differences were found in lifetime prevalence rates across the three diagnostic categories between immigrants and the U.S.-born.

The NLAAS findings further revealed that, in the immigrant sample, a longer stay in the US was associated with higher lifetime and 12-month rates of psychiatric disorders than those with a shorter stay. However, once age was controlled it was found that the difference of years of residence in the US disappeared. A further breakdown revealed the importance of age of arrival and risk of disorder. There was basically no difference in risk between U.S.-born and Latino immigrants arriving between the ages of 0–6. However, the longer immigrants remain in their country of origin before migrating, the less the risk of onset for psychiatric disorders such as MDE, anxiety, and substance use. For example, 17.2% of immigrants arriving between the ages of 0–6 were at risk for MDE, versus 14.9% aged 7–17, and 13.5% arriving at 18 and older. Thus, the age of immigration to the US emerged as a strong predictor of risk for psychiatric disorders, and the protective function played by native Latino culture was reinforced, particularly for individuals in their teens and early twenties for depressive and substance use disorders, and childhood and early teens for anxiety disorders.

Disparities in Mental Health Care

Racial, ethnic, and socioeconomic disparities in access to and quality of health care are a major public health problem that challenges the U.S. health systems. The Institute of Medicine's landmark report on *Unequal Treatment: Confronting Racial and Ethnic Disparities in Health Care* provides extensive evidence that racial and ethnic minorities are more likely to receive lower quality health services than White Americans.[19] In the past 3 years, the Agency for Healthcare Research and Quality (AHRQ) *National Healthcare Disparities Reports*[20–22] have consistently documented that, while health care disparities appear to be narrowing overall for many ethnic minority populations, disparities have *worsened* for Latinos in both access to and quality-of-care measures. Efforts to counteract these troubling trends are sorely needed given the fact that Latinos are the fastest growing population in the US. The previous section focused on disparities in mental health status in Latinos in comparison to other ethnic groups and within Latino subgroups. This section focuses on disparities in access to care, patterns of service utilization for Latinos, and factors that influence seeking and receiving services.

Disparities in Access to Care

Current disparities in health care for Latinos are severe, persistent, and well documented.[18,23–27] Latinos have less access to mental health services than do Whites, are less likely to receive needed care, and are more likely to receive poor quality care when treated. Further, there is little indication of progress toward eliminating disparities in mental health care provided in primary care settings, the settings where ethnic minorities (including Latinos) are mostly likely to get their care for common mental disorders. The reasons range from poor access and quality of care, limited insurance coverage, ineffective communication between provider and patient, patients' lack of trust, doctors' assumptions about the distribution of disease and their inability to perceive severity among minorities, and low minority representation in the workforce (with implications for health insurance coverage).

Recently, Alegria and colleagues[28] reported differences in use of mental health services by Latino subgroups as follows: Puerto Ricans had higher use patterns of the general medical sector as well as the mental health specialty sector than the other Latino subgroups. Specifically, one in five Puerto Ricans (19.9%) reported using mental health services in the past year, compared with only 10.1% of Mexicans, and approximately 11% for Cubans and other Latino groups. Individuals who spoke primarily Spanish reported less use of total services and mental health services than those who spoke primarily English. No differences were found in use of general medical services between English and Spanish speakers. Immigrants who had resided in the US less than 5 years had lower use of services than those who had 20 years or more residing in the US. Once again, the age of immigration played an important difference: A higher percentage of individuals immigrating to the US at age 12 or younger (13.4%)

or 35 years or older (14.5%) reported using more mental health services within the past year than those who immigrated between the ages of 18 to 34. Perhaps not surprisingly, mental health service use rates were all significantly lower among individuals with no insurance coverage than among those who were insured.

For Mexicans and Mexican-Americans: While Mexican-Americans are by far the largest and fastest growing Latino subgroup, research findings from the MAPSS study[8] indicated that dramatic disparities in utilization of mental health care services exist for Mexican-Americans compared to other ethnic minorities. According to MAPSS, only about one in four (27%) Mexican-origin adults who had one or more psychiatric disorders in the last year received any kind of service provided by mental health providers, general medical providers, or other professionals or informal providers. This means that approximately three out of four Latinos (73%) with a diagnosable mental disorder who are in need of services remain untreated, compared to the national rate of one out of two people receiving mental health services.

For Migrant Agricultural Workers: The problem of underutilization is even more pronounced in Mexican immigrants working in the agricultural sector in the US. Again, according to the MAPSS study, 85% of Mexican immigrants who needed services remained untreated.[26] Research has repeatedly shown that this population receives no care unless they are extremely dysfunctional or a danger to themselves or others.[26] Often this is a result of barriers that can best be understood as problems related to accessibility, availability, appropriateness, affordability, and advocacy.

Factors That Influence Seeking and Receiving Mental Health Care

Factors that may influence access to and acceptance of professional help by Latinos can be organized into two broad categories: patient variables and organizational/structural variables.[29] Patient variables include demographic characteristics and cultural factors; organizational/structural variables encompass issues related to the appropriateness, accessibility, and affordability of mental health services. Patient variables related to demographics (i.e., age, gender, educational status, and legal status in the US) and culture factors (i.e., cultural beliefs, beliefs about mental illness and treatment, provider preference, language, and acculturation) have been extensively investigated in the mental health literature. An abridged review of the previous research on the aforementioned variables follows.

Patient Factors

Demographic Characteristics

Extensive research has examined the influence of demographic characteristics, such as age, gender, educational level, and legal status in the US, on mental health care for Mexican-Americans.

Age: Differential availability of services based on age constitutes a barrier to mental health care for Latinos. In contrast to other ethnic groups, the Latino population is relatively young[1,30] compared to a significantly aging White population. Although the aged may have special problems related to dementia, depression, poverty, general health, and substance abuse,[31] the needs of children, youth, young adults, and young families—developmental, family, peer, health, vocational, academic, and behavioral problems—may be the most critical in the Latino population. However, the availability of mental health services is typically based on the needs of the majority group; thus, age-appropriate mental health services for Latinos may not be as available.

Gender: Previous research has shown that men and women differ in their rates and patterns of mental health service utilization.[32–38] Gender differences are especially notable in the Latino population;[29] however, differential rates of psychiatric disorders do not explain these differences.[39] According to previous research, women tend to recognize mental health disorders and take action earlier than men,[33,37] while men, particularly Latinos, may view help-seeking as emasculating.[29]

Educational Level: Aguilar-Gaxiola and colleagues (2000) found that 58% of Mexican-Americans in the California Central Valley did not know where to obtain help or treatment for a mental health problem; low levels of education may explain these findings.[40] Notably, Latinos have the lowest level of education in the nation[29] with only 51% of Latinos graduating from high school, and fewer than half entering college.[41,42] College retention rates for Latinos are strikingly low; some estimate rates are as low as 20%.[43] These data imply that educational status is positively correlated with having some knowledge about mental health services.

Legal Status in the US: Immigration to the United States increases the likelihood of the development of psychological problems.[40] However, immigrants may not have knowledge about service eligibility or know where to receive mental health services. Further, immigrants may not be aware that mental health services are available to all who need them at adjustable rates or no cost.[44] Fear may also underlie mental health service underutilization, especially among undocumented immigrants. Although most mental health clinics do not inquire about legal status, immigrants may fear being reported to the

US Department of Homeland Security (formerly the Immigration and Naturalization Service or INS) and consequent deportation. Thus, because of its implications on perceived eligibility and service availability, legal status in the US may be the most important barrier to mental health treatment for Mexican-Americans.

Cultural Factors

Research shows that while culture mediates seeking and receiving mental health services,[45] research on how to provide culturally sensitive mental health care for Mexican-Americans is limited.[46] The most noted cultural barriers in the service literature are cultural beliefs about mental illness and treatment, provider preference, language, and acculturation.

In Latino culture, mental and emotional problems are often believed to be a sign of weakness, lack of strength, bad luck, the result of a spell or supernatural event, or the will of God. For example, illness caused by a frightening experience or exposure to upsetting situations, which results in periods of languor, listlessness, and anorexia is called "susto." Culture also determines the path in which help is sought. A case study which exemplified the influence of culture on help-seeking pathways found that Latinos, especially first generation low socioeconomic groups, tend to be more fatalistic.[45] Thus, for those who embrace fatalism, human actions are perceived to be ineffective; therefore, help-seeking is suppressed.[47]

Latino clients often find mental health services strange, foreign, and unhelpful.[48] When help is sought in this culture, it is typically within the nuclear or extended family.[45] Because Latino families have a strong sense of supporting one another and family obligation, Mexican-Americans may primarily rely on the protective effects of the family to deal with mental illness.[49] Positive family attitudes may lead to strengthened social support abating the need for professional help; however, negative family attitudes may lead to greater stigma about mental illness and treatment, which may attenuate help-seeking in the professional domain.

Most mental health services are provided in English; however, Aguilar-Gaxiola, et al.[50] found that 50% of Mexican-Americans reported that if they went for mental health treatment they would prefer to speak in Spanish, even if they speak English in daily life. The situation is far more serious for those Spanish-monolingual individuals in need of mental health care, given the predominance of English-speaking care providers.[51,52] Consequently, the patient is likely to give less information, thereby increasing the potential for misdiagnosis and inappropriate treatment.[53]

Organizational/Structural Factors

Organizational/structural factors also play a role in mental health care for Mexican-Americans. To understand the appropriateness of mental health services for ethnic minorities, special concerns must be considered with regard to compatibility between the patient and therapist, mutual trust, health literacy, and therapeutic efficacy. Speaking the language of a client is a key feature in mental health treatment; yet, often there is an assumption that speaking the language equates to cultural competence.[46] In a case study of miscommunication between two Spanish speakers in a mental health setting, a paranoid Hispanic client described delusions about people she thought were following her as "*estaban trabajando commigo*," which translated means "they were working with me." The therapist, who spoke Spanish but lacked cultural competence, missed the double meaning of *trabajo*, which translated can mean work/occupation or work/spirits. He responded "*En que trabajabas?*" which translated means "What was your work?".[46]

Credibility refers to the "client's perception of the therapist as an effective and trustworthy helper."[48] Individuals who believed in their therapist's credibility had more positive outcomes.[54] Some researchers assert that lack of ascribed credibility, or the position that one is assigned by others, may be the primary reason for underutilization in mental health care by ethnic minorities.[48]

Conclusion

Extensive research has examined the importance of age of immigration in explaining a seeming "immigrant paradox" wherein the later the age at which persons immigrate to the US, the less likely they are to suffer from a range of mental disorders because they are protected by years of living in their native cultures.[7] However, when Latinos do suffer from mental illness, they are not as likely to access professional care and services, particularly Mexican-Americans. Several steps must be taken to further understand the nature of the gaps in mental health service utilization by Latinos. Although rates of mental health service use among Latinos appear to have increased over the past decade compared to rates reported in the 1990s, there are still significant gaps in access to and utilization of services. Cultural and immigration factors should be considered in providing mental health services to Latinos who need services.

First, limited research has been conducted on certain Latino subgroups (e.g., Mexican-Americans) most in need of mental health services, the severely mentally ill and functionally impaired. Second, few studies have comparatively assessed the effect of barriers on mental health service utilization. Third, insufficient research has qualitatively examined barriers and predictors of mental health care for Mexican-Americans and other Latinos. Furthermore, insufficient research has analyzed the relative effect of these barriers on service underutilization. Future research has been recommended to identify the social determinants of disparities in mental health services, and to assess the relative importance of these determinants.[26]

Disclaimer: The views and opinions expressed in this report are those of the authors and should not be construed to represent the views of any of the sponsoring organizations, agencies, or the University of California.

References

1. U.S. Census Bureau. (2009). Hispanic Heritage Month 2009: Sept. 15–Oct. 15. *Census Bureau News*. Available at: *www.census.gov/PressRelease/www/releases/pdf/cb09ff-17_hispmonth09eng.pdf*. Accessed March 14, 2010.
2. Grieco, E. M. (2010). *Race and Hispanic origin of the foreign-born population in the United States; 2007*. Washington, DC: U.S. Census Bureau.
3. Pew Hispanic Center. Hispanics: A people in motion. In: *Trends 2005*. Washington, DC: Pew Research Center; 2005. Available at *http://pewresearch.org/assets/files/trends2005-hispanic.pdf*. Accessed on January 14, 2011.
4. Aguirre, B. R., Sáenz, R., & James, B. S. (1997). Marielitos ten years later: The Scarface legacy. *Soc Sci Q, 78*(2), 487–507.
5. U.S. Census Bureau (2007). *American community survey reports*. The American community- Hispanics: 2004. Available at *http://www.census.gov/prod/2007pubs/acs-03.pdf*. Accessed on January 14, 2011.
6. McGuire, T. G. & Miranda, J. (2008). New evidence regarding racial and ethnic disparities in mental health: Policy implications. *Health Affairs, 27*, 393–403
7. Alegria, M., Canino, G., & Shrout, P. E., et al. (2008). Prevalence of mental illness in immigrant and non-immigrant U.S. Latino groups. *Am J Psychiatry, 165*, 359–369.
8. Vega, W. A., Kolody, B., Aguilar-Gaxiola, S., Alderete, E., Catalano, R., & Caraveo-Anduaga, J. (1998). Lifetime prevalence of DSM-III-R psychiatric disorders among urban and rural Mexican Americans in California. *Arch Gen Psychiatry, 55*, 771–778.
9. Kessler, R. C., Berglund, P., Demler, O., Jin, R., Merikangas, K. R., & Walters, E. E. (2005). Lifetime prevalence and age-of-onset distributions of DSM-IV disorders in the national comorbidity survey replication. *Arch Gen Psychiatry, 62*, 593–768.
10. Robins, L. N. & Regier, D. A. (1991). *Psychiatric disorders in America: The epidemiologic catchment area study*. New York: The Free Press.
11. Karno, M., Hough, R. L., & Burnam, M. A., et al. (1987). Lifetime prevalence of specific psychiatric disorders among Mexican Americans and non-Hispanic whites in Los Angeles. *Arch Gen Psychiatry, 44*, 695–701.
12. Burnam, M. A., Hough, R. L., Karno, M., Escobar, J. I., & Telles, C. A. (1987). Acculturation and lifetime prevalence of psychiatric disorders among Mexican Americans in Los Angeles. *J Health Soc Behav, 28*, 89–102.
13. Kessler, R. C., McGonagle, K. A., Zhao, S., et al. (1991). Lifetime and 12-month prevalence of DSM-III-R psychiatric disorders in the United States: Results from the National Comorbidity Survey. *Arch Gen Psychiatry, 51*, 8–19.

14. American Psychiatric Association. (1980). *Diagnostic and Statistical Manual of Mental Disorders.* 3rd ed. Washington, DC: American Psychiatric Association.
15. Breslau, J., Aguilar-Gaxiola, S., Kendler, K. S., Su, M., Williams, D., & Kessler, R. C. (2006). Specifying race-ethnic differences in risk for psychiatric disorder in a USA national sample. *Psychol Med, 36*(1), 57–68
16. Grant, B. F., Dawson, D. A., Stinson, F. S., Chou, P. S., Kay, W., & Pickering, R. (2003). The Alcohol Use Disorder and Associated Disabilities Interview Schedule-IV (AUDADIS-IV): Reliability of alcohol consumption, tobacco use, family history of depression and psychiatric diagnostic modules in a general population sample. *Drug Alcohol Depend, 71,* 7–16.
17. Grant, B. F., Stinson, F. S., Dawson, D. A., et al. (2004). Prevalence and co-occurrence of substance use disorders and independent mood and anxiety disorders: results from the National Epidemiologic Survey on Alcohol and Related Conditions. *Arch Gen Psychiatry, 61,* 807–816.
18. Alegria, M., Mulvaney-Day, N., Torres, M., Polo, A., Cao, Z., & Canino, G. (2007). Prevalence of psychiatric disorders across Latino subgroups in the United States. *Am J Public Health, 97*(1), 68–75.
19. Smedley, B. D., Stith, A. Y., & Nelson, A. R. (Eds.). (2003). *Unequal treatment: Confronting racial and ethical disparities in health care.* Washington, DC: National Academy Press.
20. Agency for Healthcare Research and Quality. (2006). *National healthcare disparities report, 2006.* Rockville, MD: Author.
21. Agency for Healthcare Research and Quality. (2007). *National healthcare disparities report, 2007.* Rockville, MD: Author.
22. Agency for Healthcare Research and Quality. (2008). *National healthcare disparities report, 2008.* Rockville, MD: Author.
23. Padgett, D., Patrick, C., Burns, B., & Schlesinger, H. (1994). Women and outpatient mental health services: Use by Black, Hispanic, and White women in national insured populations. *J Ment Health Adm, 21,* 347–360.
24. Alderete, E., Vega, W. A., Kolody, B., & Aguilar-Gaxiola S. (2000). Lifetime prevalence of and risk factors for psychiatric disorders among Mexican migrant farmworkers in California. *Am J Public Health, 90*(4), 608–614.
25. Ruiz, P. (1995). Assessing, diagnosing and treating culturally diverse individuals: A Hispanic perspective. *Psychiatr Q, 66,* 329–341.
26. Vega, W. A., Kolody, B., Aguilar-Gaxiola, S., & Catalano, R. (1999). Gaps in service utilization by Mexican Americans with mental health problems. *Am J Psychiatry, 156,* 928–934.
27. Woodward, A. M., Dwinell, A. D., & Arons, B. S. (1995). Barriers to mental health care for Hispanic Americans: A literature review and discussion. *J Ment Health Adm, 19,* 224–236.
28. Alegria, M., Mulvaney-Day, N., Woo, M., Torres, M., Gao, S., & Oddo, V. (2007). Correlates of past-year mental health service use among Latinos: Results from the National Latino and Asian American Study. *Am J Public Health, 97*(1), 1–8.
29. Echeverry, J. J. (1997). Treatment barriers: Accessing and accepting professional help. In: J. G. Garcia & M. C. Zea, (Eds.). *Psychological interventions and research with Latino populations* (pp. 94–107). Boston: Allyn & Bacon.
30. Espino, D. V., Neufeld, R. R., Mulvihill, M., & Libow, L. S. (1988). Hispanic and non-Hispanic elderly on admission to the nursing home: A pilot study. *Gerontologist, 28,* 821–824.

31. Baker, F. M. & Lightfoot, O. B. (1993). Psychiatric care of ethnic elders. In: A. C. Gaw AC, (Ed.). *Culture, ethnicity, and mental illness* (pp. 516–552). Arlington, VA: American Psychiatric Publishing, Inc.
32. Veroff, J., Hulka, R. A., & Douvan, E. (1981). *Mental health in America: Patterns of help-seeking from 1957–1976.* New York: Basic Books.
33. Kessler, R. C., Brown, R. L., & Broman, C. L. (1981). Sex differences in psychiatric help-seeking: Evidence from four large-scale surveys. *J Health Soc Behav, 22,* 29–64.
34. Gove, W. R. & Tudor, J. F. (1973). Adult sex roles and mental illness. *Am J Sociol, 98,* 812–835.
35. Mechanic, D. (1982). The epidemiology of illness behavior and relationship to physical and psychological distress. In D. Mechanic, (Ed.). *Symptoms, illness behavior and help-seeking* (pp. 1–24). New Brunswick, NJ: Rutgers University Press.
36. Gurwitz, P. M. (1981). Paths of psychotherapy in the middle years: A longitudinal study. *Soc Sci Med, 15E,* 67–76.
37. Horowitz, A. V. (1977). The pathways in to psychiatric treatment: Some differences between men and women. *J Health Soc Behav, 18,* 169–178.
38. Greenley, J. R. (1984). Social factors, mental illness, and psychiatric care: Recent advances from a sociological perspective. *Hosp Community Psychiatry, 35,* 813–820.
39. Myers, J. K., Weissman, M. M., Tischler, G. L., et al. (1984). Six-month prevalence of psychiatric disorders in three communities: 1980–1982. *Arch Gen Psychiatry, 41,* 959–970.
40. Aponte, J. F. & Barnes, J. M. (1995). Impact of acculturation and moderator variables on the intervention and treatment of ethnic groups. In: J. F. Aponte, R. Young Rivers, J. Wohl, (Eds.). *Psychological interventions and cultural diversity* (pp. 19–39). Boston, MA: Allyn and Bacon; 1995.
41. O' Brien, E. M. (1993). Latinos in higher education. *Research Briefs, 4*(4), 1–15.
42. Zea, M. C., Jarama, S. L., & Trotta Bianchi, F. (1995). Social support and psychosocial competence: Explaining the adaptation to college of ethnically diverse students. *Am J Community Psychol, 23,* 509–531.
43. Solberg, V. S., Valdez, J., &Villarreal, P. (1994). Social support, stress, and Hispanic college adjustment: Test of a diathesis-stress model. *Hispanic Journal of Behavioral Sciences, 16,* 230–239.
44. Stefl, M. E. & Prosperi, D. C. (1985). Barriers to mental health service utilization. *Community Ment Health J, 21*(3), 167–178.
45. Rogler, L. H. & Cortes, D. E. (1993). Help seeking pathways: A unifying concept in mental health care. *Am J Psychiatry, 150*(4), 554–561.
46. Guarnaccia, P. J. & Rodriguez, O. (1996). Concepts of culture and their role in the development of culturally competent mental health services. *Hisp J Behav Sci, 18,* 419–443.
47. Smart, J. F. & Smart, D. W. (1991). Acceptance of disability and the Mexican American culture. *Rehabil Couns Bull, 34*(4), 357–367.
48. Sue, S. & Zane, N. (1987). The role of culture and cultural techniques in psychotherapy: A critique and reformulation. *Am Psychol, 42*(1), 37–45.
49. Marin, G. & Marin, B. (1991). *Research with Hispanic populations.* Newbury Park, CA: Sage Publications.
50. Aguilar-Gaxiola, S. A., Zelezny, L., Garcia, B., Edmonson, C., Alejo-Garcia, C., & Vega, W. A. (2000). Translating research into action: Reducing disparities in mental health care for Mexican Americans. *Psychiatr Serv, 53*(12), 1563–1568.

51. Bamford, K. W. (1991). Bilingual issues in mental health assessment and treatment. *Hisp J Behav Sci, 13*(4), 377–390.
52. Malgady, R. G., Rogler, L. H., & Constantino, G. (1987). Ethnocultural and linguistic bias in mental health evaluation of Hispanics. *Am Psychol, 42*(3), 228–234.
53. Gomez, R., Ruiz, P., & Rumbaut, R. D. (1985). Hispanic patients: A linguo-cultural minority. *Hisp J Behav Sci, 7*(2), 177–186.
54. Phares, E. J. (1984). *Clinical psychology*. Homewood, IL: Dorsey.

4

Global Initiatives for HIV/AIDS and Programs Promoting Global Access to Mental Health Care

Putting Mental Health into Public Health

FRANCINE COURNOS, KAREN MCKINNON, AND MILTON WAINBERG

Introduction

The global response to the growing number of people infected with HIV has included unrivaled international donor funding for a medical illness that has particularly strong associations with psychiatric comorbidities. This paper examines how the struggle to contain the devastating effects of the HIV epidemic has created an unprecedented opportunity to test out models for the integration of mental health care and health care.

The past two decades have seen the publication of multiple studies demonstrating that at a population level, good physical health cannot be achieved without good mental health.[1] These studies demonstrate that mental illnesses can be as disabling as physical illnesses, and that major depression, the most common disabling mental illness, is strongly associated with increased morbidity and mortality both by itself and in association with other medical disorders.

Translating this awareness into successful models of integrated care has been slow and difficult in developed and developing countries. Barriers have included the profound stigma of mental illnesses, the lack of education about mental illnesses among lay people and health care workers, and discriminatory funding for psychiatric disorders. Global efforts associated with the HIV epidemic could provide new impetus to address those barriers and make progress toward integrating mental health care into health care.

Funding

Unprecedented donor funding for HIV/AIDS has made the health systems response to this epidemic an area of rapid new program development unlike that ever seen for a specific disease.[2] Using data from multiple sources, Lieberman et al. estimated that between 1998 and 2007 international donor funding commitments for health care in constant U.S. dollars nearly tripled from $5.5 billion to $15.6 billion.[3] During this same period of time, the percentage of funding targeted to HIV/AIDS grew from 5.5% of the total donor health care commitment to 47.2%, nearly half of the total funding.[4]

The Joint United Nations Program on HIV/AIDS (UNAIDS) and Kaiser Family Foundation estimate that global donor funding specifically intended to combat HIV/AIDS has increased from US $2.1 billion in 2001 to US $10 billion in 2007.[5] Much of this money targets countries with severe HIV epidemics, most notably those in sub-Saharan Africa, which is the epicenter of the HIV epidemic, as well as countries in the Caribbean.[3]

Concentrating so much health care spending on HIV/AIDS in low-income countries most affected by the epidemic raises concern about how this might impact the treatment of other illnesses.[3,5] Negative consequences could include a shift of health care workers, structural support, and other resources from existing health programs to AIDS programs, undermining the care of other diseases. Positive outcomes could occur if the influx of new money into AIDS programs contributed to general health systems strengthening. Thus far there is relatively little data to clarify these potential outcomes.[2] Moreover, the outcomes are interrelated: It is difficult to deliver comprehensive HIV/AIDS care if health systems are generally weak.

The enormous global investment in HIV prevention and care initiatives is creating a window of opportunity to test out innovative approaches for integrating mental health care into HIV/AIDS care, with the hope that the lessons learned might eventually benefit health care systems more generally.

Mental Health Conditions among People at Risk for HIV Infection

HIV infection has always been comorbid with substance use disorders and other mental illnesses in part because throughout the world, HIV begins its spread among three vulnerable populations with high rates of these disorders: injection drug users (IDUs), men who have sex with men (MSM), and sex workers. The literature on rates of mental disorders in these three populations is limited but growing.

Injection Drug Users (IDU) and Opioid Users

The prevalence of substance use disorders among IDUs is the most obvious link between psychiatric illness and injection drug use. Most studies of mental disorders among IDUs focus on opioid use.

Brooner et al. studied 716 opioid abusers seeking methadone maintenance treatment in Baltimore, MD.[6] Using the Structured Clinical Interview for DSM-III-R (SCID) to establish diagnoses, the authors found that 100% of subjects met criteria for current opioid dependence. In addition, lifetime rates of drug dependence with other substances were as follows: cocaine, 65%; cannabis, 51%; alcohol, 50%; sedatives, 45%; stimulants, 19%; and hallucinogens, 18%. In another U.S. study of 158 people who had a lifetime history of injection drug use, 99.4% met criteria for a lifetime substance abuse or dependence diagnosis when assessed with the Diagnostic Interview Schedule (DIS).[7] In a study of 55 young adult incarcerated heroin users in Taiwan, of whom 46 were injectors, 87% had a current diagnosis of substance dependence as assessed by the Mini International Neuropsychiatric Interview (MINI).[8]

Comorbidity between substance use disorders and other mental illnesses has been another focus of research in this population. Between 1980 and 1985, a series of U.S.-based studies found that up to 80% of opioid users met criteria for at least one non-substance use psychiatric disorder, with rates of mood disorder and antisocial personality disorder far exceeding general population estimates.[6] In an attempt to distinguish between psychiatric syndromes induced by drug intoxication/withdrawal from those that are independent of drug use, Brooner et al. assessed 716 opioid abusers after they had been stabilized on methadone maintenance.[6] Using the SCID, the authors found that 24% of subjects met lifetime criteria for an Axis I non-substance psychiatric disorder, most commonly major depression. On Axis II, 35% had a personality disorder, most commonly antisocial personality disorder.

Unfortunately, there are significant barriers to treating both substance use and comorbid psychiatric diagnoses because in many countries alcohol and other drug use disorders are not addressed with effective treatment but instead are neglected or criminalized.[9]

Men Who Have Sex with Men (MSM)

MSM is a term that describes men of various identities and social contexts who engage in sexual behavior with other men. In many parts of the world, HIV surveillance, prevention, and treatment are impeded by the stigma, secrecy, and even criminal penalties that surround same-sex behavior. Stigma and discrimination probably both contribute to elevated rates of certain psychiatric disorders that have been documented among MSM in some countries.[10]

King et al. conducted a systematic review of mental disorders, suicide, and deliberate self harm among lesbian, gay, and bi-sexual people.[11] Twenty-five studies were considered to be of sufficient quality to be included in a meta-analysis. Using data drawn from this group of studies the authors concluded that MSM had elevated rates of depression, anxiety disorders, alcohol and other substance dependence, and suicide attempts when compared to their heterosexual counterparts. It is not clear the extent to which prevalent HIV infection explains some of this mental illness comorbidity.[12]

Using data from a comprehensive health survey conducted among 571 gay men in Geneva, Switzerland, Wang et al. found the following 12-month rates of the five disorders studied: major depression, 19%; specific and social phobia, 22%; and alcohol and drug dependence, 17%.[13] These rates contrasted with the European Study of the Epidemiology of Mental Disorders which provided population prevalence for ten psychiatric disorders among Western European men, and found the following 12-month prevalences: any mood disorder, 2.8%; any anxiety disorder, 3.8%; and any alcohol disorder, 1.7%.[14]

Sex Workers

Commercial sex work, whether legal or illegal, is an economic exchange in which specific sexual activities are purchased or traded for other goods. Many social and economic factors are associated with prostitution, including extreme poverty, illiteracy, and unaddressed (or even sanctioned) violence against women and MSM. Childhood sexual abuse histories are common among male and female sex workers. Most female sex workers report being raped and physically assaulted during the course of their work. These childhood and adult traumas are associated with significant suicide risk and high rates of mental disorders.[15]

Using a variety of outreach techniques, Farley et al. interviewed 475 people engaged in prostitution in five countries: South Africa, Thailand, Turkey, the US, and Zambia.[16] The sample included women, men, and transgendered people who were primarily working on the street. Histories of abuse and violence were pervasive: 54% of interviewees reported physical abuse in childhood, and 58% reported childhood sexual abuse. In the context of prostitution, 73% had been physically assaulted, 68% had been threatened with a weapon, and 62% had been raped. The US had some of the highest rates of these violent events and offered some of the poorest support services. Using the Posttraumatic Stress Disorder Checklist (PCL), a 17-item scale which assesses DSM-IV (Diagnostic and Statistical Manual of Mental Disorders) symptoms for this disorder, 67% of respondents met the criteria for PTSD. On average, 92% stated that they wanted to leave prostitution. The authors argue that prostitution, whether legal or not, primarily exploits the poorest people with the fewest choices and should be seen as a human rights violation.

Farley and Kelly's review of the literature on prostitution published in 2000 cited many other studies that found similar rates of abuse and violence: sexual abuse in childhood, 50–90%; physical abuse in childhood, 60–90%; rape during prostitution, 40–85%; and physical assault during prostitution, 60–87%.[17] The authors conclude that women in prostitution are socially invisible battered women and that focusing on them as simply vectors of HIV transmission overlooks their many vulnerabilities and needs.

Increasingly, studies on prostitution have included data on psychiatric symptoms and disorders. The Roxburgh et al. study of 72 female street-based sex workers in Australia found that 75% of these sex workers experienced sexual abuse in childhood with the mean age of the first episode being seven years of age.[18] Among these women, 47% met a lifetime DSM-IV diagnosis of post-traumatic stress disorder (PTSD).

A study of suicidal behavior among 326 female sex workers in Goa, India, found that in the previous three months, 35% of the women had suicidal ideation and 19% had attempted suicide. This compared with a 0.8% annual incidence of attempted suicide in the general population of women in Goa.[19]

A study of 310 female sex workers in China found that 30% had elevated depressive symptoms, 18% had suicidal ideation, and 9% had made a suicide attempt in the past six months.[20] Greater perceived stigma on the part of sex workers was associated with poorer mental health.

Interviews were conducted with 193 female sex workers in Zurich, Switzerland using the Composite International Diagnostic Interview (CIDI) to determine rates of mental disorders. One-year prevalence data showed that 50% of the women had a mental disorder: 24% had major depression, 12% had dysthymia, 13% had PTSD, and 34% had other anxiety disorders.[21]

Two studies found that both male and female sex workers had elevated rates of psychopathology when compared to matched controls.[22,23] Matched controls in the study of male prostitutes were two normative samples of adults (nonpatient normals and psychiatric outpatients) for the Symptom Checklist-90-R (SCL-90-R);[22] matched controls in the study of female prostitutes were women without prostitution histories attending the same three methadone maintenance clinics.[23]

Some studies suggest that mental illness is associated with higher HIV prevalence and lower rates of condom use among sex workers. In one study conducted in Puerto Rico,[24] sex workers with high levels of depressive symptoms had a 70% HIV infection rate, whereas those with low depressive symptoms had a 30% infection rate. This did not appear to be a consequence of HIV infection, since depressive symptoms were independent of HIV status.

Vanwesenbeck conducted an exhaustive review of the research literature on prostitution from 1990 through 2000 and analyzed it from a "pro-sex work feminist frame of reference," meaning that sex work is on principal considered legitimate work.[25] Vanwesenbeck emphasized that the tendency of researchers to focus on street prostitutes and those recruited in jails or through social service agencies paints a much bleaker picture than would studies focused on indoor sex workers. She further concludes that in the Western world, IDU and non-commercial sexual activity are the most important risk factors for HIV infection in female sex workers. Vanwesenbeeck agrees that in Africa, the current epicenter of the HIV epidemic, prostitution does have a role in the spread of HIV. Documented rates of HIV among sex workers in Africa include: 58% among female sex workers in Burkina Faso;[26] and 61% and 43%, respectively, among female sex workers recruited from truck stops who did or did not have anal sex with their clients.[27] Extensive social networking of commercial sex workers has been documented in Nigeria and Uganda.[28,29]

Overlap among Vulnerable Populations

Vulnerable groups are not mutually exclusive. An individual simultaneously or over time may belong to more than one vulnerable group. Addiction to drugs can lead to sex work in exchange for drugs or for money to purchase drugs.

Vaddiparti et al. developed a model to evaluate the association between childhood victimization, perpetration of violence, and later cocaine dependence and adult sex trading among drug-using women.[30] A cohort of 594 women (362 sex traders) was recruited using community outreach strategies for HIV prevention studies in St. Louis. Rates of cocaine dependence were higher among traders (85% vs. 56%). Path analysis confirmed that childhood victimization had a significant and direct association with both adult cocaine dependence and sex trading. However, the association between childhood perpetration and adult sex trading was mediated by cocaine dependence.

A study of 1,606 women and 3,001 men entering substance use treatment in the US found high rates of prostitution.[15] In the past year, 41% of women and 11% of men reported having engaged in prostitution; lifetime rates were 51% among women and 19% among men. In both men and women, prostitution was associated with more mental health symptoms, injection drug use, and HIV infection.

Rates of injection drug use are high among sex workers.[9] In Roxburgh et al.'s study of sex workers in Australia, more than 80% were heroin dependent and injecting drugs.[18] About half of these sex workers had begun injecting drugs prior to sex work and used sex work to pay for their drugs. Half of the woman reported using drugs to facilitate their sex work largely through their numbing effects. What emerges is a complex intertwinement of childhood abuse and neglect, PTSD, symptoms of depression, injection drug use, and engaging in sex work.

An example is St. Petersburg (Russia), where 81% of surveyed sex workers said they injected drugs at least once a day (65% had used nonsterile injecting equipment) and 48% of sex workers were HIV-positive.[9] Similar rates of HIV infection were reported among female sex workers who inject drugs in Ho Chi Minh City in Vietnam.[9] A study in Puerto Rico found that 47% of female sex workers injected drugs.[24] In Farley's studies of 475 people who engaged in prostitution in five countries, 38% self-reported the need for alcohol or drug-addiction treatment.[16]

Mental Health Conditions Seen Following HIV Infection

Mental illness not only precedes HIV infection, but also follows it. HIV is a neurotropic virus that enters the central nervous system at the time of initial infection and persists there. It remains unclear the degree to which the presence of HIV in the brain in and of it itself is a risk factor for the onset or worsening of mental illness. What is certain is that HIV-related illnesses and their treatments are associated with mental disorders and that HIV in the brain can impair cognition and actually manifest in neurological and behavioral symptoms.

Neurocognitive Complications of HIV Infection

Neurocognitive complications of the direct effects of HIV in the brain become more frequent as illness advances.[31] Common problems include decreased attention and concentration, psychomotor slowing, reduced speed of information processing, executive dysfunction, and, in more advanced cases, verbal memory impairment.[31] Neurocognitive manifestations occur with a range of severity varying from subclinical manifestations to specific disorders. There have been multiple shifts in the nomenclature used to describe HIV-associated neurocognitive disorders. The most recent proposed system suggests three categories: asymptomatic neurocognitive impairment (ANI), mild neurocognitive disorder (MND), and HIV-associated dementia (HAD).[32] However, the diagnoses of ANI and MND require neuropsychological testing that is more likely to be available in research settings as opposed to clinical settings.

Psychiatric disturbances are commonly seen in HAD, where symptoms can range from apathy and depression to mania and psychosis, mimicking functional psychiatric disorders and thus requiring a thorough differential diagnosis.[33] Neurocognitive manifestations of HIV are diagnoses of exclusion after eliminating all other possible medical causes, including opportunistic infections, metabolic problems, side effects of antiretrovirals, and substance use syndromes (including intoxication, withdrawal, and the long-term deleterious impact of chronic use).[33]

Overview of Psychiatric Disorders among HIV-Infected People

Psychiatric illness can exist premorbidly or result from the progression and treatment of HIV infection, influencing the course of the illness both through behavior and putative biological factors.[34] Epidemiological studies indicate that a high percentage of HIV-infected individuals will suffer from psychiatric disorders, most commonly anxiety, depression, or psychosis.[35] Mental health disorders are associated with poor medical outcomes and the secondary transmission of HIV infection. This is particularly well demonstrated among people suffering from substance use disorders and/or depression. Both are associated with poor adherence to antiretroviral regimens, secondary transmission of HIV, and increased morbidity and mortality from HIV-related diseases and co-morbidities.[36,37] Findings from the following studies combined suggest that behaviors associated with untreated mental health symptoms increase the chances for HIV transmission, and that routine HIV care should include assessment and treatment of mental health issues to enhance access to needed care and reduce morbidity and mortality. Therefore, ensuring that these conditions are detected and treated is an essential component of both early and ongoing HIV disease management.

Accuracy of available prevalence estimates of rates of psychiatric disorders among people living with HIV infection is unclear because most studies of prevalence used convenience samples, often of the historic risk groups, had small sample sizes, or were confined to specific geographical areas. Population-based estimates of psychiatric disorders among HIV-positive people are scarce but necessary.

The landmark HIV Cost and Services Utilization Study (HCSUS) found that a large, nationally representative probability sample of adults receiving medical care for HIV in the United States in early 1996 (N = 2,864: 2,017 men, 847 women) reported major depression (36%), dysthymia (27%), generalized anxiety disorder (16%), panic attack (11%), and drug dependence (12%), as well as heavy drinking at a rate (8%) almost twice that found in the general population and high rates of drug use (50%).[38,39] In this sample, 48% of patients met criteria for at least one psychiatric disorder.

The HCSUS study remains the most comprehensive view we have of the prevalence of psychiatric disorders among people living with HIV/AIDS, even though the study was not designed as a diagnostic assessment of psychiatric disorders in this population. Thus, rates of psychosis, bipolar disorder, alcohol abuse or dependence, and drug abuse, among others, were not obtained. Another important aspect of the HCSUS study is that people with HIV who are receiving medical care may be different from those not receiving medical care in terms of underlying comorbidities and their impact on illness progression.

Hospital admissions for AIDS-related illnesses decreased soon after the introduction of highly active antiretroviral therapy (HAART) in 1996, but a study of hospitalizations of 8,376 patients in six U.S. HIV care sites showed that among patients hospitalized at least once, the third most common admission diagnosis after AIDS-defining illnesses (21%) and gastrointestinal disorders (9.5%) was a mental illness (9%).[40] This study also found that compared with Caucasians, African Americans had higher admission rates for mental illnesses but not for AIDS-defining illnesses. Overall, the majority of these patients were hospitalized for reasons other than AIDS-defining illnesses, and the relatively large number of mental illness admissions highlights the need for co-management of psychiatric disease, substance abuse, and HIV.

PTSD and depression have been shown to be significant predictors of health care utilization, whereas symptoms and indices of HIV disease progression were not.[41] Among 210 patients attending two HIV primary care clinics who were screened for depression, PTSD, and acute stress disorder (ASD),[42] 38% met criteria for depression, 34% for PTSD, and 43% for ASD; 38% screened positive for two or more disorders. Of the 118 patients with at least one of these disorders, 43% reported receiving no concurrent mental health treatment.

One probability sample study was conducted using South Carolina Hospital Discharge Data from all of the state's 68 hospitals. Among 378,710 adult cases of discharge from all hospitalizations and emergency room visits during 1995, 422 had a diagnosis of HIV/AIDS and mental illness (using ICD-9 [International Classification of Diseases] criteria), 1,353 had a diagnosis of HIV/AIDS alone, and 67,092 had a diagnosis of mental illness alone. People with a mental illness, regardless of race, gender, or age, were 1.44 times as likely to have HIV/AIDS than people without a mental illness.[43] In this study, two categories of mental illness—alcohol/drug abuse and depressive disorders—were found to have relative risks significantly associated with HIV infection.

The prevalence of HIV infection in the general psychiatric population is unknown, but one retrospective review of all psychiatric outpatients at one medical center in North Carolina from 2001 to 2004 found that HIV infection was present in 1.2% of patients and that the diagnostic categories with the highest prevalence of HIV infection were substance use disorders (5%), personality disorders (3.1%), bipolar disorders (2.6%), and PTSD (2.1%).[44]

Recent studies of psychiatric disorders have expanded the knowledge base to focus on women, youth, acute or early HIV infection, epidemiology of psychiatric disorders among those living with HIV/AIDS in low-income countries, the persistence over time of psychiatric disorders among HIV/AIDS patients, and benefits of mental health service utilization and specific screening tools. Using U.S. hospital discharge data from the 1994–2004 Nationwide Inpatient Sample, Bansil et al. found that, after adjusting for demographic factors and alcohol/substance abuse, HIV-infected women were more likely to be hospitalized for mood, anxiety disorders, or psychotic disorders in 2004 than in 1994.[45] The authors concluded that the number of hospitalizations with a psychiatric diagnosis among HIV-infected women in the US has increased substantially as HIV-infected women live longer. This highlights the need for targeted public health interventions to address mental health issues.

Among 174 inner-city HIV-positive youth in Chicago, screened during primary care appointments between 1998 and 2006, 31% had substance use disorders, 28% had PTSD, 19% had alcohol abuse, 17% had generalized anxiety disorder, and 15% had major depressive disorders.[46]

The psychiatric context of acute/early HIV infection was the focus of one part of The NIMH Multisite Acute HIV Infection Study.[47] Thirty-four participants with acute/early HIV infection from six U.S. cities were assessed with the MINI International Diagnostic Interview, Beck Depression Inventory II, State-Trait Anxiety Inventory, Brief COPE, and an in-depth interview. Most had a pre-HIV history of alcohol or a substance use disorder (85%); a majority (53%) had a history of major depressive or bipolar disorder.

Although mood disorders encompass the range of unipolar and bipolar conditions, mania secondary to HIV infection is rare, generally occurring in late stages of AIDS. By contrast, depression and anxiety disorders are seen throughout the course of HIV infection; these conditions commonly coexist.[48] There is an increased likelihood of the emergence of symptoms during pivotal disease points such as with HIV antibody testing, declines in immune status, and the occurrence of opportunistic infections. Mkanta et al.[49] demonstrated that survival after AIDS is associated with mental health service use.

Research on mental health is scarce in low-income countries such as those in sub-Saharan Africa where HIV-infection levels are highest, but recent studies support the need to continue aggressive assessment and treatment of mental health disorders in these settings.

Current diagnoses of DSM-IV psychiatric disorders were obtained using the MINI among 88 HIV-positive and 87 HIV-negative healthy controls in Nigeria. The HIV group had significantly higher rates of affective disorders (OR=3.58, 95% CI=1.44–8.94), anxiety disorders (OR=3.57, 95% CI=1.65–7.72), and psychotic disorders (OR=1.10, 95% CI=1.01–1.12) than healthy controls.[50]

A sample of 900 HIV-positive individuals in South Africa was administered the Composite International Diagnostic Interview (CIDI) to determine the presence of selected mental disorders; 43.7% were found to have a mental disorder, mainly depression (11.1% major depression and 29.1% minor depression), alcohol abuse disorder (12.9%), posttraumatic stress disorder (event HIV) (4.2%), intermittent explosive disorder (3.9%), and alcohol dependence (2.9%). For all other disorders measured, the prevalence was below 2%. Prevalence was highest in stages 3 (49.7%) and 4 (68%) of the disease (using World Health Organization staging criteria).[51]

Few prospective studies on the rates of psychiatric disorders in HIV/AIDS have been done, particularly in the developing world. Among 65 patients with recently diagnosed HIV in a hospital-based HIV clinic in South Africa, 56% had at least one psychiatric disorder at baseline, and 48% had at least one at six-month follow-up, demonstrating that the rate of psychiatric disorders in HIV/AIDS patients was consistent over time and that regular evaluation for psychiatric disorders is important.[52]

A cross-sectional study of 220 HIV-positive outpatients at a dedicated Tanzanian HIV/AIDS care center examined prevalence of ICD-10 common mental health diagnoses using a standardized psychiatric questionnaire (the Clinical Interview Schedule - Revised).[53] Depression or mixed anxiety and depression was identified in 15.5% of subjects, with 4.5% suffering from other anxiety disorders. Finally, newly validated screening tools such as the K-10 for common conditions seen in HIV/AIDS are making assessment a more streamlined process.[54]

Depression among People with HIV Infection

Depression associated with HIV/AIDS has been linked in high-income countries with faster disease progression and reduced drug adherence. Mortality also has been linked to depression in one recent study. The Women's Interagency HIV Study examined its representative U.S. cohort, focusing on HIV deaths over a 10-year period among participants. Although HIV-associated factors predicted AIDS and non-AIDS deaths, other treatable conditions predicted mortality, most strongly depressive symptoms.[55]

Depression is the most common reason for psychiatric referral among people with HIV-infection.[56] Overall, rates of depression among people with HIV infection are nearly 50%.[38,57,58] Among HIV-infected patients referred for psychiatric evaluation, rates of major depression range from 8% to 67%,[59] with up to 85% of HIV-seropositive individuals reporting some depressive symptoms.[60] A meta-analysis of published studies[61] found that people with HIV were almost twice as likely as those who were seronegative to be diagnosed with major depression, and that depression was equally prevalent in people with both symptomatic and asymptomatic HIV.

Depression is frequently underdiagnosed and when recognized is often poorly treated, particularly in primary medical settings where HIV/AIDS patients receive care. Clinicians working with HIV/AIDS patients must consider underlying medical causes for depression (for example, medication side effects, central nervous system infections, and endocrine disorders). Rates are generally lower among community-based HIV-positive samples and are highest among IDUs and women engaging in high-risk behaviors.[62] Elevated rates of depression are also seen among patients with more advanced HIV disease, particularly those hospitalized for medical illness.[62] Other risk factors for depression include prior history of depression, substance abuse, unemployment, lack of social support, use of avoidance coping strategies, HIV-related physical symptoms, and multiple losses.[63]

International studies suggest that 20–37% of HIV-positive patients have diagnosable depression though this may be an underestimate.[64] Among 205 HIV-positive patients in an outpatient clinic in Denmark, 38% had Beck Depression Inventory II (BDI-II) symptoms of depression greater than 14 and 26% had scores of 20 or more, indicating major depression.

Several studies published in the last two years show high prevalence of depression among those living with HIV/AIDS. For example, 81% of 850 Rwandan HIV-positive women in the prospective observational cohort study assessed with the Epidemiologic Studies Depression Scale (CES-D) showed depressive symptoms (CES-D > or = 16);[65] 78% of 127 pregnant women in Thailand reported depressive symptoms;[66] 40.8% of 82 HIV-seropositive adolescents at a specialized HIV/AIDS Health Care Centre in Kampala, Uganda met ICD-10 criteria for depression;[67] and 18.7% of 584 men living with HIV in Vietnam self-reported depression over a 1-month period.[68] Among 214 HIV-positive people in eastern China and 200 controls, Symptom Check List 90 (SCL-90) mean subscale scores in the HIV-positive group were all higher than those of the control group ($P<0.001$), especially for depression.[69]

Anxiety Disorders among People with HIV Infection

Estimates of the prevalence of anxiety disorders in HIV/AIDS patients range from almost negligible to as high as 40%.[70,71,72] The rates vary for numerous reasons, including a host of psychosocial correlates and because anxiety frequently coexists with depression and substance use problems. Higher rates generally are seen as HIV illness progresses. Despite the wide range of prevalence estimates, a pattern emerged in the late 1990s when several studies found that anxiety disorders did not differ between HIV-seropositive patients and HIV-seronegative clinical comparison groups. Still, lifetime rates are higher in the HIV clinical population than in the general population.[70,71,73]

Among 82 HIV seropositive adolescents who were consecutively enrolled in a study at a specialized HIV/AIDS Health Care Centre in Kampala, Uganda, anxiety disorder was the most common psychiatric disorder, with 45.6% meeting ICD-10 criteria.[67]

Substance Use Disorders among People with HIV Infection

The prevalence of current alcohol use disorders among people with HIV infection has been estimated to range from 3% to 12%.[70,71,74–76] In the HCSUS study, participants were screened for heavy drinking in the previous

12 months; 8% of participants met this criterion.[38] In the general population, the 12-month prevalence of current alcohol use disorders was estimated to be between 7% and 10%.[77,78]

The HCSUS study screened participants for drug dependence in the previous 12 months, and 12% were found to meet criteria for this disorder.[38] Specific drugs for which dependence had developed were not reported. Earlier studies had provided estimates of 2% to 19% for current drug use disorders in HIV-positive people.[70,71,75,76] The general population 12-month prevalence for drug use disorders was estimated to be just under 4%.[77,78]

Lifetime prevalence for both alcohol and other drug use disorders appears to be higher among people with HIV infection than in the general population. Across studies, the lifetime prevalence of alcohol use disorders for people with HIV was 26% to 60%[70,75,76] compared with a general population prevalence of 14%[77] to 24%.[78] Similarly, the lifetime prevalence of drug use disorders for people with HIV has been found to be between 23% and 56%,[70,75,76] whereas for the general population it is between 6%[77] and 12%.[78]

To screen and assess for mental health disorders, HIV-positive youth in Chicago, IL, between the ages of 13 to 24 consecutively enrolled in an adolescent and young adult HIV clinic between 1998–2006 (n = 174), were screened for mental health disorders using the Client Diagnostic Questionnaire (CDQ). The most prevalent disorder was substance abuse disorder (31%), followed by posttraumatic stress disorder (28%), alcohol abuse disorder (19%), generalized anxiety disorder (17%), and major depressive disorder (15%).[46]

PTSD among People with HIV Infection

In addition to PTSD studies already described, several cross-sectional studies have shown strong associations between PTSD and HIV; many of these focused on HIV-related risk behaviors. Rates of PTSD among those with HIV/AIDS have not been established in population-based studies.

Traumatic childhood experiences and other psychosocial stressors can contribute to the acquisition of HIV and further exacerbate mental health problems. Sexual abuse, for instance, whether in childhood or as an adult, has been shown to increase the risk of HIV infection in adolescent girls, commercial sex workers, gay men, people with severe mental illness, and other groups.[79]

One recent study sought to determine the percentage of individuals who met criteria for lifetime PTSD and HIV-related PTSD among 85 recently diagnosed HIV-positive patients attending public health clinics in the Western Cape, South Africa. The PTSD module of the Composite International Diagnostic Interview (CIDI) was used to determine the percentage of those who met criteria for lifetime PTSD and HIV-related PTSD. The rate of lifetime PTSD was 54.1% and the incidence of HIV-related PTSD was 40%.[80]

Among adolescents and young adults with HIV, 13% met criteria for PTSD in response to their HIV diagnosis; the rate was 47% among those with other trauma such as being a victim of a personal attack, sexual abuse, or being abandoned by a caregiver.[81] In a U.S. study of medication adherence in HIV/AIDS care settings, 164 individuals provided data at five time points, with participants screening positive for PTSD at 20% of visits.[82]

Compared to HIV-infected people without PTSD, those with PTSD were found to have lower levels of medication adherence; however, those with HIV-related PTSD were more adherent to HIV medications than those with non-HIV-related PTSD.[83]

Psychosis among People with HIV Infection

An overview of the literature suggests that the pathophysiology of psychosis in HIV infection is complex, and a multifactorial etiology of psychotic symptoms is likely in many cases. There are many reports of psychotic symptoms in HIV-infected persons in the absence of concurrent substance abuse, iatrogenic causes, evidence of opportunistic infection or neoplasm, or detectable cognitive impairment. A common clinical feature of new-onset psychosis in HIV-infected patients is the acute onset of HIV symptoms. Estimates of the prevalence of new-onset psychosis in HIV-infected patients vary widely, from less than 0.5% to 15%.[84–88]

Suicide Risk among People with HIV Infection

Suicide risk is classified as a psychiatric disorder in the ICD-10 although not in the DSM-IV. Risk for suicide has been a long-standing concern among people with HIV infection and classifying it as a disorder has the advantage of bringing greater attention to this problem.

Before the introduction of highly active antiretroviral treatment (HAART), rates of suicide in the US were shown to be considerably higher among HIV-positive patients than among the HIV-negative.[89] In Switzerland, rates of suicide were tracked among 15,275 HIV-positive patients from 1988 to 2008.[89] Suicide rates decreased significantly with the introduction of HAART, but remained above the rate observed for the general population.

Conclusion

A small but growing body of international literature suggests that substance use disorder and other mental illnesses precede and follow HIV infection at rates substantially higher than those seen in the general population, creating a strong need to integrate mental health care into health care provided to people with

HIV/AIDS. Such integration would diminish the likelihood of HIV transmission, and reduce disability and improve medical outcomes of those already infected. Donor global health funding is currently disproportionately targeted to HIV/AIDS programs. The intersection between need and funding has created an unprecedented opportunity for developing and studying models for integrating mental health and health care in HIV/AIDS programs. These models could pave the way for similar integration in the treatment of other disorders as funding for global mental health care becomes more available.

References

1. Prince, M., Patel, V., & Saxena, S., et al. (2007). Global Mental Health 1: No health without mental health. *Lancet, 370,* 859–877.
2. Rabkin, M., El-Sadr, W. M., & De Cock, K. M. for the Bellogio HIV/Health Systems Working Group 1. (2009). The impact of HIV scale-up on health systems: A priority research agenda. *J Acquir Immune Defic Syndr, 52,* S6–11.
3. Lieberman, S., Gottret, P., Yeh, E., de Beyer, J., Oelrichs, R., & Zewdie, D. (2009). International health financing and the response to AIDS. *J Acquir Immune Defic Syndr, 52,* S38–44.
4. Shiffman, J., Berlan, D., & Hafner, T. (2009). Has aid for AIDS raised all health funding boats? *J Acquir Immune Defic Syndr, 52,* S45–48.
5. Levine, R. & Oomman, N. (2009). Global HIV/AIDS funding and health systems: Searching for the Win-Win. *J Acquir Immune Defic Syndr, 52,* S3–5.
6. Brooner, R., King, V., Kidorf, M., Schmidt, C., & Bigelow, G. (1997). Psychiatric and substance use comorbidity among treatment-seeking opioid abusers. *Arch Gen Psychiatry, 54,* 71–80.
7. Dinwiddie, S. H. (1997). Characteristics of injection drug users derived from a large family study of alcoholism. *Compr Psychiatry, 38,* 218–229.
8. Chiang, S-C., Chen, S-J., Sun, H-J., Chan, H-Y., & Chen, W-J. (2006). Heroin use among youths incarcerated for illicit drug use: Psychosocial environment, substance use history, psychiatric comorbidity, and route of administration. *Am J Addiction, 15,* 233–241.
9. Joint United Nations Programme on HIV/AIDS. Available at: http://www.unaids.org/en/default.asp (last accessed on 25 February, 2010).
10. McKirnan, D. J. & Peterson, P. L. (1989). Alcohol and drug use among homosexual men and women: Epidemiology and population characteristics. *Addict Behav, 14,* 545–553.
11. King, M., Semlyen, J., Tai, S. S., et al. (2008). A systematic review of mental disorder, suicide, and deliberate self harm in lesbian, gay and bisexual people. *BMC Psychiatry, 8,* 70–97.
12. Cochran, S. D. & Mays, V. M. (2009). Burden of psychiatric morbidity among lesbian, gay, and bisexual individuals in the California quality of life survey. *J Abnorm Psychol, 118,* 647–658.
13. Wang, J., Hausermann, M., Ajdacis-Gross, V., Aggleton, P., & Weiss, M. G. (2007). High prevalence of mental disorders and comorbidity in the Genera Gay Men's Health Study. *Soc Psychiatry Psychiat Epidemiol, 42,* 414–420.

14. The ESEMeD/MHEDEA 2000 Investigators. (2004). 12-month co-morbidity patterns and associated factors in Europe: Results from the European Study of the Epidemiology of Mental Disorders (ESEMeD) project. *Acta Psychiatr Scand, 109,* 21–27.
15. Burnette, M. L., Lucas, E., Ilgen, M., et al. (2008). Prevalence and health correlates of prostitution among patients entering treatment for substance use disorders. *Arch Gen Psychiatry, 65,* 337–344.
16. Farley, M., Baral, I., Kiremire, M., & Sezgin, U. (1998). Prostitution in five countries: Violence and post-traumatic stress disorders. *Fem Psychol, 8,* 405–426.
17. Farley, M. & Kelly, V. (2000). Prostitution: A critical review of the medical and social sciences literature. *Women and Criminal Justice, 11,* 29–64.
18. Roxburgh, A., Degenhardt, L., & Copeland, J. (2006). Posttraumatic stress disorder among female street-based sex workers in the greater Sydney area, Australia. *BMC Psychiatry, 6,* 24–36.
19. Shahmanesh, M., Wayal, S., Cowan, F., Mabey, D., Copas, A., & Patel, V. (2009). Suicidal behavior among female sex workers in Goa, India: The silent epidemic. *Am J Public Health, 99,* 1239–1246.
20. Hong, Y., Li, X., Liu, Y., Li, M., & Tai-Seale, T. (2010). Self-perceived stigma, depressive symptoms, and suicidal behaviors among female sex workers in China. *J Transcult Nursing, 21,* 29–34
21. Rössler, W., Koch, U., & Lauber, C., et al. (2010). The mental health of female sex workers. *Acta Psychiatr Scand, 25* (Epub ahead of print).
22. Simon, P. M., Morse, E. V., & Osofsky, H. J., et al. (1992). Psychological characteristics of a sample of male street prostitutes. *Arch Sexual Behav, 21,* 33–44.
23. El-Bassel, N., Schilling, R. F., & Irwin, K. L., et al. (1997). Sex trading and psychological distress among women recruited from the streets of Harlem. *Am J Publ Health, 87,* 66–70.
24. Alegría, M., Vera, M., Freeman, D. H., et al. (1994). HIV infection, risk behaviors and depressive symptoms among Puerto Rican sex workers. *Am J Publ Health, 84,* 2000–2002.
25. Vanwesenbeeck, I. (2001). Another decade of social scientific work on sex work: A review of the research 1990–2000. *Annu Rev Sex Res, 12,* 242–289.
26. Lankoande, S., Meda, N., Sangare, L., et al. (1998). Prevalence and risk of HIV infection among female sex workers in Burkina Faso. *Int J STD AIDS, 9,* 146–150.
27. Karim, S. S. A. & Ramjee, G. (1998). Anal sex and HIV transmission in women. *Am J Publ Health, 88,* 165–166.
28. Asowa Omorodian, F. I. (2000). Sexual and health behaviour of commercial sex workers in Benin City, Edo State, Nigeria. *Health Care Women Int, 21,* 335–345.
29. Pickering, H., Okongo, M., Nnalusiba, B., Bwanika, K., & Whitworth, J. (1997). Sexual networks in Uganda: Casual and commercial sex in a trading town. *AIDS Care, 9,* 199–207.
30. Vaddiparti, K., Bogetto, J., Callahan, C., Abdallah, A. B., Spitznagel, E., & Cottler, L. B. (2006). The effects of childhood trauma on sex trading in substance using women. *Arch Sex Behav, 35,* 451–459.
31. Boissé, L., Gill, M. J., & Power, C. (2008). HIV infection of the central nervous system: Clinical features and neuropathogenesis. *Neurol Clin, 26,* 799–819.
32. Antinori, A., Arendt, G., Becker, J. T., et al. . (2007). Updated research nosology for HIV-associated neurocognitive disorders. *Neurology, 69,* 1789–1799.
33. Bartlett, J. A. & Ferrando, S. J. Identification and management of neurologic and psychiatric side effects associated with HIV and HAART. Available at: http://www.medscape.com/viewprogram/2960_pnt. (last accessed on 26 February, 2010)

34. Brogan, K. & Lux, J. (2009). Management of common psychiatric conditions in the HIV-positive population. *Curr HIV/AIDS Rep, 6,* 108–115.
35. Stoff, D. M., Mitnick, L., & Kalichman, S. (2004). Research issues in the multiple diagnoses of HIV/AIDS, mental illness and substance abuse. *AIDS Care, 16,* S1–5.
36. Williams, C. T. & Latkin, C. A. (2005). The role of depressive symptoms in predicting sex with multiple and high-risk partners. *J Acquir Immune Defic Syndr, 38,* 69–73.
37. Yun, L. W., Maravi, M., Kobayashi, J. S., et al. (2005). Antidepressant treatment improves adherence to antiretroviral therapy among depressed HIV-infected patients. *J Acquir Immune Defic Syndr, 38,* 432–438.
38. Bing, E. G., Burnam, A., Longshore, D., et al. (2001). Psychiatric disorders and drug use among human immunodeficiency virus–infected adults in the United States. *Arch Gen Psychiatry, 58,* 721–728.
39. Galvan, F. H., Bing, E. G., Fleishman, J. A., et al. (2002). The prevalence of alcohol consumption and heavy drinking among people with HIV in the United States: results from the HIV Cost and Services Utilization Study. *J Stud Alcohol, 63,* 179–186.
40. Betz, M. E., Gebo, K. A., Barber, E., et al., for the HIV Research Network. (2005). Patterns of diagnoses in hospital admissions in a multistate cohort of HIV-positive adults. *Med Care, 43,* 3–14.
41. O'Cleirigh, C., Skeer, M., Mayer, K. H., & Safren, S. A. (2009). Functional impairment and health care utilization among HIV-infected men who have sex with men: The relationship with depression and post-traumatic stress. *J Behav Med, 32,* 466–477.
42. Israelski, D. M., Prentiss, D. E., Lugega, S., et al. (2007). Psychiatric co-morbidity in vulnerable populations receiving primary care for HIV/AIDS. *AIDS Care, 19,* 220–225.
43. Stoskopf, C. H., Kim, Y. K., & Glover, S. H. (2001). Dual diagnosis: HIV and mental illness, a population-based study. *Community Ment Health J, 37,* 469–479.
44. Beyer, J. L., Taylor, L., Gersing, K. R., Krishnan, K. R. (2007). Prevalence of HIV infection in a general psychiatric outpatient population. *Psychosomatics, 48,* 31–37.
45. Bansil, P., Jamieson, D. J., Posner, S. F., & Kourtis, A. P. (2009). Trends in hospitalizations with psychiatric diagnoses among HIV-infected women in the USA, 1994–2004. *AIDS Care, 21,* 1432–1438.
46. Martinez, J., Hosek, S. G., & Carleton, R. A. (2009). Screening and assessing violence and mental health disorders in a cohort of inner city HIV-positive youth between 1998–2006. *AIDS Patient Care STDs, 23,* 469–475.
47. Atkinson, J. H., Higgins, J. A., Vigil, O., et al. (2009). Psychiatric context of acute/early HIV infection. The NIMH Multisite Acute HIV Infection Study: IV. *AIDS Behav, 13,* 1061–1067.
48. McDaniel, J. S. & Blalock, A. C. (2000). Mood and anxiety disorders. *New Dir Ment Health Serv,* 87, 51–56.
49. Mkanta, W. N., Mejia, M. C., & Duncan, R. P. (2010). Race, outpatient mental health service use, and survival after an AIDS diagnosis in the highly active antiretroviral therapy era. *AIDS Patient Care STDs, 24,* 31–37.
50. Adewuya, A. O., Afolabi, M. O., Ola, B. A., Ogundele, O. A., Ajibare, A. O., & Oladipo, B. F. (2007). Psychiatric disorders among the HIV-positive population in Nigeria: A control study. *J Psychosom Res, 63,* 203–206.
51. Freeman, M., Nkomo, N., Kafaar, Z., & Kelly, K. (2007). Factors associated with prevalence of mental disorder in people living with HIV/AIDS in South Africa. *AIDS Care, 19,* 1201–1209.

52. Olley, B. O., Seedat, S., & Stein, D. J. (2006). Persistence of psychiatric disorders in a cohort of HIV/AIDS patients in South Africa: A 6-month follow-up study. *J Psychsom Res, 61,* 479–484.
53. Marwick, K. F. & Kaaya, S. F. (2010). Prevalence of depression and anxiety disorders in HIV-positive outpatients in rural Tanzania. *AIDS Care, 22,* 415–419.
54. Spies, G., Kader, K., Kidd, M., et al. (2009). Validity of the K-10 in detecting DSM-IV-defined depression and anxiety disorders among HIV-infected individuals. *AIDS Care, 21,* 1163–1168.
55. French, A. L., Gawel, S. H., Hershow, R., et al. (2009). Trends in mortality and causes of death among women with HIV in the United States: A 10-year study. *J Acquir Immune Defic Syndr, 51,* 399–406.
56. Strober, D. R., Schwartz, J. A. J., McDaniel, J. S., & Abrams, R. F. (1997). Depression and HIV disease: Prevalence, correlates and treatment. *Psychiatr Ann, 27,* 372–377.
57. Ickovics, J. R., Hamburger, M. E., Vlahov, D., et al. for the HIV Epidemiology Research Study Group. (2001). Mortality, CD4 cell count decline, and depressive symptoms among HIV-seropositive women: Longitudinal analysis from the HIV Epidemiology Research Study. *JAMA, 285,* 1466–1474.
58. Morrison, M. F., Petitto, J. M., Ten Have, T., et al. (2002). Depressive and anxiety disorders in women with HIV infection. *Am J Psychiatry, 159,* 789–796.
59. Acuff, C., Archambeault, J., Greenberg, B., et al. (1999). *Mental health care for people living with or affected by HIV/AIDS: A practical guide.* Substance Abuse and Mental Health Services Administration monograph. Rockville, MD: Research Triangle Institute.
60. Stolar, A., Catalano, G., Hakala, S., Bright, R. P., & Fernandez, F. (2005). Mood disorders and psychosis in HIV. In K. Citron, M-J. Brouillette, & A. Beckett, (Eds.). *HIV and psychiatry: A training and resource manual,* 2nd ed. Cambridge, UK: Cambridge University Press.
61. Ciesla, J. A. & Roberts, J. S. (2001). Meta-analysis of the relationship between HIV-1 infection and risk for depressive disorders. *Am J Psychiatry, 158,* 725–730.
62. Cournos, F. & McKinnon, K. (2008). Epidemiology and prevalence of psychiatric disorders associated with HIV/AIDS. In M. A. Cohen & J. A. Gorman, (Eds.). *Comprehensive textbook of AIDS psychiatry.* Oxford, UK: Oxford University Press.
63. Goodkin, K., Wilkie, F. L., Concha, J., et al. (1997). Subtle neuropsychological impairment and minor cognitive-motor disorder in HIV-1 infection. Neuroradiological, neurophysiological, neuroimmunological, and virological correlates. *Neuroimaging Clin N Am, 3,* 561–579.
64. Rodkjaer, L., Laursen, T., Balle, N., & Sodemann, M. (2010). Depression in patients with HIV is under-diagnosed: A cross-sectional study in Denmark. *HIV Med, 11,* 46–53.
65. Cohen, M. H., Fabri, M., Cai, X., et al. (2009). Prevalence and predictors of posttraumatic stress disorder and depression in HIV-infected and at-risk Rwandan women. *J Womens Health (Larchmt), 18,* 1783–1791.
66. Ross, R., Sawatphanit, W., & Zeller, R. (2009). Depressive symptoms among HIV-positive pregnant women in Thailand. *J Nurs Scholarsh, 41,* 344–350.
67. Musisi, S. & Kinyanda, E. (2009). Emotional and behavioural disorders in HIV seropositive adolescents in urban Uganda. *East Afr Med J, 86,* 16–24.
68. Esposito, C. A., Steel, Z., Gioi, T. M., Huyen, T. T., & Tarantola, D. (2009). The prevalence of depression among men living with HIV infection in Vietnam. *Am J Public Health,* 99 Suppl 2:S439–444.

69. Jin, C., Zhao, G., Zhang, F., Feng, L., & Wu, N. (2010). The psychological status of HIV-positive people and their psychosocial experiences in eastern China. *HIV Med, 11*,253–259.
70. Dew, M. A., Becker, J. T., Sanchez, J., et al. (1997). Prevalence and predictors of depressive, anxiety and substance use disorders in HIV-infected and uninfected men: A longitudinal evaluation. *Psychol Med, 27*, 395–409.
71. Rabkin, J. G., Ferrando, S. J., Jacobsberg, L. B., & Fishman, B. (1997). Prevalence of axis I disorders in an AIDS cohort: A cross-sectional, controlled study. *Compr Psychiatry, 38*, 146–154.
72. Blalock, A. C., Sharma, S. M., & McDaniel, J. S. (2005). Anxiety disorders and HIV disease. In K. Citron, M-J Brouillette, & A. Beckett, (Eds.). *HIV and psychiatry: A training and resource manual*, 2nd ed. Cambridge, UK: Cambridge University Press.
73. Sewell, M. C., Goggin, K. J., Rabkin, J. G., Ferrando, S. J., McElhiney, M. C., & Evans, S. (2000). Anxiety syndromes and symptoms among men with AIDS: A longitudinal controlled study. *Psychosomatics, 41*, 294–300.
74. Brown, G. R., Rundell, J. R., McManis, S. E., Kendall, S. N., Zachary, R., & Temoshok, L. (1992). Prevalence of psychiatric disorders in early stages of HIV infection. *Psychosom Med, 54*, 588–601.
75. Rabkin, J. G. (1996). Prevalence of psychiatric disorders in HIV illness. *Int Rev Psychiatry, 8*, 157–166.
76. Ferrando, S. J., & Batki, S. L. (2000). Substance abuse and HIV infection. *New Dir Ment Health Serv, 87*, 57–67.
77. Regier, D. A., Farmer, M. E., Rae, S., et al. (1990). Comorbidity of mental disorders with alcohol and other drug abuse. *JAMA, 264*, 2511–2518.
78. Kessler, R. C., McGonagle, K. A., Zhao, S., et al. (1994). Lifetime and 12-month prevalence of DSM III-R psychiatric disorders in the United States: Results from the National Comorbidity Study. *Arch Gen Psychiatry, 51*, 8–19.
79. Goodman, L. A., Koss, M. P., Fitzgerald, L. F., et al. (1993). Male violence against women. Current research and future directions. *Am Psychol, 48*, 1054–1058.
80. Martin, L. & Kagee, A. (2008). Lifetime and HIV-related PTSD among persons recently diagnosed with HIV. *AIDS Behav, 12* (Epub ahead of print).
81. Radcliffe, J., Fleisher, C. L., Hawkins, L. A., et al. (2007). Posttraumatic stress and trauma history in adolescents and young adults with HIV. *AIDS Patient Care STDs, 21*, 501–508.
82. Vranceanu, A. M., Safren, S. A., Lu, M., et al. (2008). The relationship of post-traumatic stress disorder and depression to antiretroviral medication adherence in persons with HIV. *AIDS Patient Care STDs, 22*, 313–321.
83. Boarts, J. M., Buckley-Fischer, B. A., Armelie, A. P., Bogart, L. M., & Delahanty, D. L. (2009). The impact of HIV diagnosis-related vs. non-diagnosis-related trauma on PTSD, depression, medication adherence, and HIV disease markers. *Evid Based Soc Work, 6*, 4–16.
84. Navia, B. A., Jordan, B. D., & Price, R. W. (1986). The AIDS dementia complex: I. Clinical features. *Ann Neurol, 19*, 517–524.
85. Halstead, S., Riccio, M., Harlow, P., Oretti, R., & Thompson, C. (1988). Psychosis associated with HIV infection. *Br J Psychiatry, 153*, 618–623.
86. Harris, M. J., Jeste, D. V., Gleghorn, A., & Sewell, D. D. (1991). New-onset psychosis in HIV-infected patients. *J Clin Psychiatry, 52*, 369–376.
87. Prier, R. E., McNeil, J. G., & Burge, J. R. (1991). Inpatient psychiatric morbidity of HIV-infected soldiers. *Hosp Community Psychiatry, 42*, 619–623.

88. Boccellari, A. A. & Dilley, J. W. (1992). Management and residential placement problems of patients with HIV-related cognitive impairment. *Hosp Community Psychiatry*, *43*, 32–37.
89. Keiser, O., Spoerri, A., Brinkhof, M., et al. (2010). Suicide in HIV-infected individuals and the general population in Switzerland, 1988–2008. *Am J Psychiatry*, *167*:2.

PART II

Conditional Disorders and the Public's Mental Health

5

Veterans' Mental Health

The Effects of War

MICHAEL J. LYONS, MARGO R. GENDERSON, AND MICHAEL D. GRANT

Introduction

The psychological, medical, and social effects of stress and trauma have been an important focus for a number of disciplines. Accounts of the painful and tragic consequence of war have appeared throughout recorded history in writings as far back as Homer and Sophocles. Books such as Remarque's *All Quiet on the Western Front,* Crane's *The Red Badge of Courage,* Trumbo's *Johnny Got His Gun,* Solzhenitsyn's *August 1914,* and O'Brien's *Going After Cacciato* have provided brilliant and compelling literary accounts. More recently there have been a number of systematic and sophisticated empirical investigations of the effects of combat. Certainly, posttraumatic stress disorder (PTSD), the clinical definition of which is based on psychological sequelae among combat veterans, has received a great deal of attention, but the pervasive and multifarious nature of combat influences numerous domains. In this chapter we consider the consequences of combat primarily reviewing results from previous research along with findings from our work with a sample of twins who served in the military during the Vietnam Era.

The Vietnam Era Twin Registry (VETR) consists of over 8,000 male-male twin pairs in which both siblings served on active military duty during the Vietnam era (May 1965 to August 1975). Twins were identified in the late 1980s from Department of Defense computer files.[1,2] From a list of approximately 5.5 million veterans, 15,711 potential twin pairs were identified. In 1992, information about lifetime history of psychiatric disorders was collected by telephone interview in the Harvard Drug Study.[3] Of 10,300 eligible individuals, data were successfully collected from 8,169. VETR members are representative of all twins who served in the military during the Vietnam War on a variety of sociodemographic and other variables.[4] Data were also available from military records and several questionnaire-based studies of the VETR. This chapter includes some preliminary findings from the ongoing Vietnam Era Twin Study of Aging (VETSA), a comprehensive follow-up study of a subsample of VETR members.[5]

Because individuals are not randomly assigned to a combat role, it is important to consider factors that make it more likely that an individual will be exposed to combat. Among Operation Iraqi Freedom (OIF) veterans, traumatic experiences such as exposure to violent combat and killing another person were associated with increased risk-taking propensity, including alcohol use and increased verbal and physical aggression towards others.[6] Although prior research has suggested that combat veterans have heightened aggressive behavior, one study demonstrated that combat exposure was indirectly associated with aggression primarily through its relationship with PTSD symptoms.[7] VETR analyses demonstrated significant genetic influences on volunteering for service in Southeast Asia and for actually serving in Southeast Asia.[8] Using the Combat Experiences Scale (CES), in which individuals indicate which of 18 different combat situations (e.g., being in a fire-fight, being a prisoner of war) they experienced, we found a significant genetic influence on level of combat exposure. Because of concerns about the validity of self-reported combat exposure, we correlated CES scores with the number of medals that were awarded to the individual based on military records and found a substantial correlation. We also found that genetic factors significantly affected being awarded combat decorations. Among members of the VETR, higher scores on the personality traits of social potency, alienation, and aggression and lower scores on social closeness and harm avoidance were associated with volunteering for service in Vietnam. Higher scores on the personality traits of social potency and aggression and lower scores on social closeness, control, and harm avoidance were associated with higher levels of combat exposure among those who served in Vietnam.

When suggesting that preexisting characteristics of an individual, such as genetic endowment, may influence the likelihood of being exposed to trauma in combat, it is important to be sensitive to concerns about the possibility of "blaming the victim," that is, the suggestion that there is something about the individual that caused the trauma to happen to him—that he "brought it on himself." Of course, the fact that genetic factors can increase the probability of experiencing trauma no more warrants blame for the victim than do genetic factors that influence the risk of cancer. However, this point may be less obvious when dealing with behavioral rather than purely biological characteristics.

Psychiatric Effects of War

War veterans have an increased risk for developing numerous psychiatric illnesses, such as PTSD, substance dependence, major depression, and anxiety disorders,[9] and symptoms including anger/irritation, hopelessness, and suicidal ideation/attempts.[10] Understanding the effects of war on mental health is particularly timely, as this knowledge may inform prevention and intervention strategies for soldiers currently returning from Iraq and Afghanistan. Veteran health is of great public health concern; in fact, of 289,328 Operation Iraqi Freedom/Operation Enduring Freedom (OIF/OEF) veterans, 36.9% were diagnosed with a mental illness.[11] Over half of OIF/OEF veterans diagnosed with one mental disorder received two or more diagnoses.[12] The prevalence of mental illness among OIF/OEF veterans nearly doubles from predeployment to post-deployment assessment.[13]

While it is difficult to compare prevalence rates across studies due to varying diagnostic assessments, subject characteristics, and other methodological factors, a series of studies from the Veterans Administration (VA) have directly examined mental health among OIF/OEF, WWII, Korean War, and Persian Gulf War veterans, controlling for age and other factors. Compared to the Vietnam War, veterans of Iraq/Afghanistan were less likely to report witnessing and participating in atrocities in the military, were less likely to be diagnosed with substance abuse disorders, had lower rates of VA disability compensation because of PTSD, and displayed more violent behavior. Persian Gulf veterans were less often diagnosed with PTSD compared to Vietnam and Iraq/Afghanistan war veterans.[14] Even after controlling for severity of traumatic exposure and other variables, WWII veterans demonstrated significantly less severe symptomatology compared with Korean and Vietnam veterans.[15] The authors suggested that differences among wars in terms of public support may explain these findings. The positive reception upon returning from WWII may have mitigated the effects of trauma on psychiatric symptoms, consistent with research findings demonstrating that the quality of social support that Vietnam veterans received upon returning from war was significantly related to the development of psychiatric symptoms.[16] On the other hand, it is possible that WWII veterans under-reported their symptoms, reflecting a greater stigma attached to mental illness for that generation.

To achieve a more comprehensive understanding of the effects of war on mental health, researchers have explored the effects of varying levels of combat exposure, pointing to a dose-response relationship, in which the risk of mental illness increases as combat severity increases. This relationship has been demonstrated across wars; a positive linear relationship between the severity of traumatic experiences and psychiatric outcomes (general psychiatric symptoms,

PTSD, guilt, suicidality) has been reported among WWII, Korean, and Vietnam War veterans.[15] Such a relationship has also been demonstrated with the current wars in Iraq and Afghanistan, in which psychiatric symptoms of Army and Marine combatants were significantly associated with combat experiences.[17] An association between the severity of physical injury experienced during battle and mental health symptoms among OIF veterans has also been reported.[18] Younger veterans (age 18–24) of OIF/OEF have been found to be at a significantly greater risk for developing mental disorders compared to older veterans (40 years and older), possibly because younger veterans experienced more combat.[12] The association between combat severity and psychiatric symptoms is long lasting, with one study reporting a significant dose response relationship on numerous outcomes of mental health almost 30 years after combat exposure.[10]

Exposure to combat is a well-known and robust risk factor for PTSD. Results from the National Comorbidity Survey (NCS) indicated that after adjusting for potential confounding influences, individuals who experienced combat were 6.4 times more likely to have PTSD.[19] This is similar to reports of Australia's Korean War veteran population, indicating that veterans were 6.4 times more likely to have PTSD. The most recent results from the National Vietnam Veterans Readjustment Study (NVVRS) indicated the prevalence of lifetime war-related PTSD to be 18.7% among veterans, with 9.1% prevalence up to 12 years after the Vietnam War.[20] Among military personnel in the Gulf War, the prevalence of PTSD was 1.9% for deployed individuals versus 0.8% among nondeployed personnel.[21] In the largest study of OEF/OIF veterans with a sample of 289,328, the rate of PTSD was reported to be 21.8%,[11] compared to 3.5% in the general population.[22] However, prevalence rates of PTSD vary from 11.5%[13] to 37%[23] among OEF/OIF studies depending on subject characteristics, assessment measures, and other methodological inconsistencies.

Numerous factors influence the risk of developing combat-related PTSD, including longer and multiple deployments[11,24] and branch of service, with members of the Army (OR= 2.81) and Marine Corps (OR=2.13) more likely to screen positive for PTSD compared with Navy veterans.[23] These findings likely reflect difference in level of combat exposure, which has been found to be significantly higher among Army, Marine Corps, and National Guard veterans compared to Navy veterans.[23] Similarly, being of enlisted rank as opposed to officer rank is associated with increased risk for PTSD.[11] Those who were injured during combat were three times more likely to screen positive for PTSD.[13,23]

The severity of the experienced trauma is directly related to PTSD symptom severity or increased risk,[11,20,25,26] and this association has been found to be significant up to 25 years after combat exposure.[27] According to the NVVRS, veterans who experienced high combat were four times more likely to develop PTSD compared to veterans with moderate or low combat.[28] One study examined identical twin pairs from the VETR who were discordant for military service in southeast Asia and found that the rate of PTSD among twins who served in southeast Asia was 16.8% compared to 5.0% among twins who did not serve in southeast Asia; twins who served in southeast Asia who experienced high levels of combat were nine times more likely to develop PTSD compared to their co-twins.[25] The twin method controls for possible genetic and shared environmental effects that might influence the development of PTSD.

The relationship between combat exposure and PTSD is complex, and other factors may interact with levels of combat exposure to influence risk for developing PTSD. In a sample from the VETR, we found a significant dose-response relationship between cognitive ability assessed by the Armed Forces Qualification Test (AFQT) prior to combat and risk for PTSD.[29] After controlling for confounders, the highest cognitive ability quartile had a 48% lower risk than the lowest ability quartile ($P < 0.001$). Lower cognitive ability may be a marker of less adaptive coping against adverse mental health consequences of exposure to traumatic events. Thompson, Gottesman, and colleagues[21] also examined the relationship between AFQT scores and the risk of developing PTSD during the Vietnam War.[30] They found an interaction between AFQT score and combat exposure, in which veterans with higher AFQT scores had a decreased risk of PTSD in the low-combat exposure group, but AFQT score was not associated with risk for PTSD in veterans with high exposure to combat. Results suggest the possibility that high combat exposure may overwhelm cognitive resources available for coping with stressful events.

Other factors may moderate the relationship between combat and PTSD. The personality dimension Stress Reactivity from the Multidimensional Personality Questionnaire (MPQ),[31] which reflects the tendency to experience negative emotions such as anxiety and guilt, interacted with level of combat exposure to predict risk of PTSD. Individuals who were high on stress reactivity responded to combat stress differently from individuals low in stress reactivity. Specifically, individuals high in stress reactivity were more likely to develop PTSD when exposed to high levels of combat. Individuals with low stress reactivity were less affected by combat exposure. Another variable that interacted with combat exposure in the VETR to influence the development of PTSD was whether the individual had volunteered to serve in Vietnam. The effect of combat exposure on the risk of developing PTSD was stronger among those who had not volunteered for Vietnam. This might reflect personality and other relevant differences among volunteers versus nonvolunteers, or it might reflect the benefit of experiencing some sense of control over exposure to stressors.

Although PTSD is the most salient mental health consequence of combat exposure, combat and PTSD have been linked to numerous other psychiatric outcomes; rates of depression are elevated among military personnel and based on findings from the National Comorbidity Survey, individuals who experience combat are 2.12 times more likely to develop major depressive disorder.[19]

The risk of developing depression among Korean War veterans has been reported to be 5.45 times higher than a comparison group.[32] The prevalence of having major depression among veterans deployed during the Gulf War was two times greater than among veterans who were not deployed,[33] and other findings show that 17% of military personnel deployed had major depression versus 10.9% of nondeployed personnel.[21] Among OIF/OEF veterans, the prevalence of having major depressive disorder (MDD) was reported to be up to 17.4%, with women at a higher risk than men.[11] Risk for depression is also strongly associated with lower military rank.[32,33] Several studies have found that as combat intensity increases, the severity of depression, dysthymia, and physical symptoms of depression increase, and life happiness and general life satisfaction decrease.[10,34,35]

Not all studies, however, have found a significant association between combat and depression.[36] Results from studies of Vietnam veterans indicated that combat exposure was only related to continuous measures of depression but not significantly associated with being diagnosed with major depression.[34,37] Sher[38] suggested that many individuals who are diagnosed with both PTSD and MDD have a psychobiological condition that is distinct from either disorder by itself. He asserted that individuals with "posttraumatic mood disorder" are different clinically and neurobiologically and demonstrate greater symptom severity, increased suicidality, and greater social and occupational impairment.

An associated feature of combat-related depression includes survivor guilt,[39] characterized by dreams of friends dying in battle and avoidance of interpersonal intimacy due to a fear of abandonment or death of loved ones.[39] Survivor guilt is common among veterans with depression as well as PTSD[40,41] and is associated with avoidance of trauma-related stimuli and with the re-experiencing symptoms of PTSD.[41,42] Survivor guilt has also been found to be related to risk of suicide.[43] A study of Nigerian army veterans who served as peace keepers in the Liberian and Sierra-Leonean wars found that 38% of respondents struggled with survivor guilt.[42]

Substance use disorders are also elevated in war veterans. In a study from the National Comorbidity Survey, Part II,[19] individuals who experienced combat were 2.22 times more likely to abuse substances. The prevalence of drug use disorders in a large sample of OIF/OEF veterans was 3%, with men having over twice the risk for developing drug use disorders compared to women,[11] and younger veterans having five times the risk for developing drug disorders compared to those older than 40 years.[11] Some studies, however, have not found an association between war stressors and drug abuse.[26]

Although some early studies suggested that increased alcohol consumption among veterans is a function of demographic differences between veterans and nonveterans,[44,45] there is a clear consensus in more recent literature that combat exposure influences alcohol use. One study assessed OIF/OEF personnel before and after deployment and found that individuals who experienced combat were significantly more likely to develop new-onset heavy weekly drinking (OR=1.63), binge drinking (OR= 1.46), and alcohol-related problems (OR = 1.61) compared with nondeployed personnel.[46] Prevalence rates of alcohol use disorders among veterans have been reported to be 7.1% among OIF/OEF personnel,[11] and according to the NVVRS, 11.2% of veterans suffered from alcohol-related disorders up to 20 years after discharge from the military. Younger veterans are more likely to develop drinking problems compared to veterans older than 40 years.[11] Numerous studies have also reported that alcohol abuse and dependence increases as combat severity increases.[10,28,37,47] Goldberg and colleagues[48] examined identical (MZ) twin pairs discordant for combat exposure from the VETR and reported that 4% of veterans who were not exposed to combat were heavy drinkers compared to 6.7% of their co-twins who experienced high combat. These results indicated that combat exposure has a modest long-term effect on drinking.[48]

Findings on the effects of combat on tobacco use are equivocal. While some studies found no association between smoking and combat,[47] other findings have demonstrated that smoking increases with combat severity.[10] One study measured smoking before and after deployment to Iraq and Afghanistan and found that the percentage of new smokers and of smoking recidivism was greater in deployed versus nondeployed individuals. Among individuals who were deployed, combat exposure and length and number of deployments were related to smoking.[49] Furthermore, military personnel who smoke to reduce stress report significantly higher stress levels than those who do not use tobacco, and tobacco users engaged more frequently in negative coping behaviors.[50,51]

Experiencing combat has been associated with an increased risk of numerous anxiety disorders, including generalized anxiety disorder (GAD), panic disorder, social phobia, simple phobia, and obsessive compulsive disorder.[36] Compared to a comparison group, Korean War veterans were 5.7 times more likely to demonstrate high levels of anxiety.[32] The prevalence of anxiety disorders among veterans deployed during the Gulf War was 2 times greater than among veterans who were not deployed,[33] and 4.3% of Gulf War veterans who were deployed had nonPTSD anxiety disorders compared to 1.4% of veterans who were not deployed.[21] Although the prevalence of nonPTSD anxiety disorders among all veterans declined after 10 years, the prevalence remained higher in the deployed group.[21] Studies have reported that as combat intensity increases, anxiety symptoms also increase,[10,32,35] and risk for anxiety disorders is associated with lower rank.[32,33] Findings from the NVVRS indicated that veterans who experienced high war-zone stress had significantly elevated rates of GAD and panic disorder compared to veterans who experienced low war-zone stress.[35] Not all studies, however, have found a significant association between combat and anxiety. Results from one study indicated that combat exposure was only related to continuous measures of anxiety but not significantly associated with being diagnosed with GAD.[34,37] Other studies have reported similar findings that GAD is not related to war stressors.[52]

The prevalence of pathological gambling is higher among PTSD treatment-seeking veterans[51] compared to a representative sample of the U.S. population,[53] with prevalence rates of 17% and 0.6%, respectively. Studies have also found that having a history of trauma and specific traumatic events—such as witnessing someone being badly hurt or killed and physical attacks—are significantly related to gambling severity and pathological gambling.[54–56] Trauma in these studies, however, was not exclusively combat related. While several studies have reported that combat and PTSD are not significantly associated with gambling,[36,51] other studies have demonstrated a strong association.[53,57] Findings from the National Comorbidity Survey Replication indicate that the onset of pathological gambling was predicted by DSM-IV anxiety, mood, impulse control, and substance use disorders, and pathological gambling predicted the subsequent onset of GAD, PTSD, and substance dependence.[53] A study from the VETR examined twin pairs discordant for gambling behavior and reported that the association between trauma and gambling was partially accounted for by genetic and family environmental influences.[55]

Suicide is a very serious concern among veterans since psychiatric disorders and psychosocial problems upon returning from war increase risk for suicide. Suicide rates among OIF/OEF veterans are startling, and rates have increased since 2004. There were 64 deaths by suicide in 2004; this number doubled in 2008, with 128 confirmed deaths and 15 pending investigation. Rates of suicide among Army personnel were 12.7 per 100,000 in 2005, 15.3 in 2006, 16.8 in 2007, and 20.2 in 2008.[58] These rates are the highest since the Army started keeping track about 30 years ago.[59] While suicide rates among Army personnel are historically 20% lower than that of the U.S. general population,[60] the 2008 suicide rate among active-duty Army personnel exceeded that of demographically matched civilians.[59] Research indicates that OIF/OEF veterans diagnosed with a mental disorder have a 77% increased risk of suicide compared to civilians.[61] Other studies have shown that male veterans were twice as likely to die by suicide compared to male nonveterans, controlling for other factors.[62] Risk of suicide has been found to vary little by military service branches (Army, Marines, Navy, and Air Force).[61] Firearms are the most common method used in military suicide fatalities, with 72% of Army suicides involving firearms, compared to 52% of those in the general population.[63] The widespread availability of firearms in the military undoubtedly increases the degree of lethality of suicide attempts.[64]

A comparison of suicidality among World War II, Korean War, and Vietnam War veterans seeking treatment at VA facilities found differences in suicidality across wars.[15] Though suicidality did not differ for Korean and Vietnam veterans, veterans from those wars were more suicidal than WWII veterans. This study also found a significant relationship between trauma severity and suicidality among Vietnam veterans but not WWII or Korean War veterans. While some studies of Vietnam veterans have supported these findings,[65,66] others do not.[67] In a previous study of the VETR, we asked a series of questions from the Diagnostic Interview Schedule for DSM-III-R[68] about thoughts of death and suicide. VETR members with high levels of combat exposure compared to those veterans without combat exposure were significantly more likely to report having had a two-week period during which they often thought about death, a two-week period during which they wanted to die, suicidal ideation, and previous suicide attempts.

Comorbidity

The relationship between combat exposure and development of other psychopathologies is challenging since combat-related PTSD is highly comorbid with other mood, anxiety, and substance use disorders. One study found that Vietnam veterans without PTSD had a mean of 1.1 psychiatric diagnoses, while those with PTSD had a mean of 3.6 diagnoses.[36] A longitudinal study of war veterans from the 1982 Lebanon War found that almost half of veterans endorsed a lifetime triple comorbidity of PTSD, depression, and anxiety and that PTSD predicted the development of depression, anxiety, and other comorbid disorders, but not vice versa.[69] It is possible, therefore, that combat does not directly increase the risk of developing psychiatric disorders other than PTSD and that the observed relationship between combat and psychopathology exists due to the presence of PTSD.

Earlier studies have attempted to control for the effects of PTSD when examining the relationship between combat and psychiatric illnesses. Two studies of Vietnam veterans found that *before* controlling for PTSD, combat was significantly related to numerous disorders, such as panic disorder, obsessive compulsive disorder, alcohol abuse and dependence, social phobia, simple phobia, and somatoform pain disorder.[26,36,52] Findings were mixed regarding the association between combat and depression, dysthymia, and GAD. Both studies found that drug abuse or dependence was not related to combat, although other research has demonstrated that veterans are at an increased risk for developing substance use disorders. However, after controlling for PTSD, no association was found between war experiences and other psychiatric diagnoses. In addition, although prior research has suggested that combat veterans have heightened aggressive behavior,[6] one study demonstrated that combat exposure was indirectly associated with aggression primarily through its relationship with PTSD symptoms.[7] These findings suggest that it may not be the traumatic event itself, but the development of PTSD after the trauma that increases risk for developing comorbid psychopathologies.

On the other hand, an association between combat exposure and having any mental health diagnosis after controlling for PTSD has been reported.[34] A strong association between alcohol abuse and dependence and combat exposure in the absence of PTSD has also been reported,[70] which is inconsistent with reports described above of no direct relationship. Nicotine dependence has also been found to be associated with experiencing trauma after controlling for PTSD, although the prevalence of nicotine dependence was significantly lower in individuals without PTSD.[71] The association between combat and antisocial personality disorder also remained significant after controlling for PTSD.[36] Taken together, these studies demonstrate that "any psychiatric diagnosis," is directly related to combat and other disorders after controlling for PTSD. However, when examining specific disorders individually, PTSD seems to mediate the relationship between trauma and most psychiatric disorders. Nicotine dependence and antisocial personality disorder are two exceptions, and findings are mixed regarding alcohol use and dependence.

Several hypotheses explain the association between PTSD and comorbid disorders. Preexisting psychiatric disorders may increase the risk for developing PTSD, either by influencing the risk of exposure to a traumatic event or by influencing one's response to trauma.[72–75] This is supported by studies demonstrating that depression, dysthymia, and substance use disorders precede PTSD onset, reflecting vulnerability to PTSD.[36,52,76] Another hypothesis suggests that PTSD directly influences the development of comorbid disorders, thereby mediating the relationship between combat and other disorders. For example, PTSD may cause substance use onset since specific substances may alleviate specific PTSD symptoms, and the course of substance abuse has been found to parallel the course of PTSD,[77] which is consistent with a self-medication model of comorbidity.[78] Other studies have also reported that depression and anxiety tend to develop after PTSD onset.[79,80] Alternatively, a shared vulnerability reflecting genetic or environmental risk factors may influence the development of PTSD and other disorders and explain the high co-occurrence, and this hypothesis has been tested through twin modeling.

VETR studies have investigated the relationship between combat and psychiatric illnesses and familial vulnerability common to PTSD. Koenen and colleagues[81] utilized a co-twin control design to examine the effects of combat on major depression, dysthymia, generalized anxiety disorder, and panic disorder and found that PTSD probands had more psychopathology than their MZ non-combat exposed co-twins. These co-twins also had significantly more psychiatric illness compared to MZ co-twins of combat controls or dizygotic (DZ) co-twins of veterans with PTSD. These findings suggest that major depression, GAD, and panic disorder encompass a psychological response to combat and that the association between PTSD and depression and dysthymia in part reflects a shared familial vulnerability mediated by genetic factors.

Koenen and colleagues[82] also examined the level of combat exposure and prevalence of combat-related PTSD in MZ twin pairs discordant for five psychiatric outcomes and found that MZ twins with MDD, alcohol, drug, tobacco, or cannabis dependence had higher levels of combat exposure (unadjusted for combat-related PTSD) compared to their co-twins. After controlling for PTSD, the association between combat exposure with alcohol and cannabis dependence remained significant, suggesting a direct relationship between combat and these disorders. However, combat exposure was not significantly related to major depression and tobacco dependence after adjusting for PTSD. Results indicated that PTSD mediated the relationship between combat exposure and MDD and tobacco dependence, suggesting that the observed relationship between combat and these two disorders is attributable to the presence of combat-related PTSD and not to the direct effects of combat. These results are supported by other findings from VETR studies suggesting that much of the association between PTSD and nicotine dependence[83] and between PTSD and MDD[84,85] is explained by shared genetic effects. However, these findings challenge previous studies indicating a direct relationship between nicotine dependence and combat, as described above,[71] although that study did not utilize twin subjects and therefore cannot control for genetic or shared environmental factors.

In a study by Scherrer and colleagues[86] that built upon Koenen and colleagues'[82] study, twin structural equation models indicated that among individuals exposed to combat, the prevalence of nicotine and alcohol dependence and MDD was higher in individuals with PTSD compared to those without PTSD. Further, the association between combat exposure and MDD, and alcohol and nicotine dependence was due to genetic and unique environmental contributions in common with PTSD. These results support findings from Koenen and colleagues[82] suggesting that combat exposure is not independently associated with MDD and nicotine dependence.

The relationship between combat and alcohol use, however, is still unclear. While Scherrer et al.[86] reported that PTSD mediates the association, Koenen et al.[82] found a direct relationship between combat and alcohol dependence after adjusting for the effects of PTSD. Similarly, while some twin studies have found a familial association between alcohol and PTSD,[87] others have not.[88,89] One VETR study tested various models to explain the relationship between combat, alcohol, and PTSD and evaluated a shared vulnerability model, in which the same genes that influence exposure to combat also influence alcohol use and PTSD symptoms.[90] The authors suggested that shared genes might reflect common underlying personality traits, such as impulsivity and sensation seeking, also associated with volunteering for and experiencing higher levels of combat,[8,91,92] vulnerability for developing alcohol use disorders,[93] and vulnerability for developing PTSD.[90]

Prevention and Treatment

Due to the elevated risk of psychopathology among war veterans, early intervention and treatment of psychiatric disorders is critical to prevent more chronic conditions. While more veterans of OIF/OEF are enrolling in VA health care (29%) compared to Vietnam veterans (10%),[12] the majority of veterans are not seeking treatment, largely because veterans are twice as likely to report concern about stigmatization and other barriers to receiving care compared to individuals in the general population.[13] Only 23–40% of veterans with symptoms of a mental disorder returning from Iraq and Afghanistan sought care,[13] and a RAND Corporation study of all branches of the military found that only about half of veterans with MDD or PTSD received treatment.[94] Veterans who seek mental health care access care very quickly, with an average of less than 3 months from leaving the military to first visit, and the average time from first visit to mental health diagnosis only 13 days.[12] The increased percentage of veterans seeking treatment and the relative speed with which they are being assessed and diagnosed opens the door to early intervention.

Although utilization of mental health care among veterans has increased since the Vietnam War, efforts have focused on improving access to evidence-based care. Several innovative strategies include integrating mental health services into primary care facilities and providing services via the Internet and telephone, which may address barriers such as stigma, transportation, and childcare.[95] To further address the perceived stigma of receiving care, the Department of Defense and VA are reframing psychiatric treatment for mental disorders into stress management training for combat stress reactions.[95]

The quality of mental health treatment has significantly improved since the Vietnam War era, with significant advances in evidenced-based treatments. Research suggests that cognitive behavioral therapy using imaginal and in vivo exposure and cognitive reprocessing therapy is most effective for combat-related PTSD. Weekly group-based exposure therapy has also been found to produce clinically significant and lasting reductions in PTSD symptoms among war veterans.[96] An initial study of the effectiveness of a virtual reality Iraq/Afghanistan exposure therapy demonstrated that 16 out of 20 patients returning from war no longer met criteria for PTSD at post-treatment.[97] A meta-analysis of pharmacotherapy for PTSD demonstrated that 59.1% of individuals showed clinical improvement compared to 38.5% who received placebo.[98] Thus, once individuals are able to access care, there is a reasonable expectation of a favorable prognosis.

Since suicide is a growing concern in the military, numerous programs have been developed to respond to suicide among military personnel. One study found that exposure to a suicide prevention program resulted in a 33% reduction in the risk for suicide.[99] This program included removing the stigma associated with seeking mental health treatment, ensuring confidentiality in treatment, strengthening social support, promoting effective coping skills, and enhancing understanding of mental health. More recent interventions include BATTLEMIND, a program that provides solders with skills to help cope with stress encountered during deployment and helps soldiers and their families readjust after returning from overseas. The Army recently developed another intervention that provides troops with education about suicidal behaviors to enable soldiers to recognize suicide risk in others to intervene.[100] In 2008, the National Institute of Mental Health and the Army began a collaborative five-year prospective study of suicide among soldiers.[59] Exploring susceptibility and resiliency factors, such as differences in soldiers' vulnerability to the stress of extended deployments, physiological responses to stress, ability to readjust to life at home, alcohol and drug use, genetic predisposition, interpersonal factors, and stressful life events, should help to inform more effective interventions.

Psychosocial Effects of War

Combat experiences early in adulthood may have lifelong ramifications in areas other than psychopathology, including socioeconomic status (educational attainment, adult income, and employment), interpersonal outcomes, and physical health. Thus, we have suggested that posttraumatic symptoms of war and combat and the political climate veterans' faced at home upon their return may have made it more difficult to resume everyday social roles and obligations and perpetuated the enduring societal costs of exposing military personnel to combat.[101] Of concern today is the possibility that veterans of OIF/OEF will face similar challenges upon their return home.

The Vietnam Era Twin Study of Aging (VETSA) project recently reported on the effects of combat exposure on lifetime educational attainment (LEA) in Vietnam veterans.[101] Twins who served in Vietnam had completed significantly fewer years of education by their 50s, and there was a negative correlation between level of combat exposure and LEA. Variables that might confound the relationship between combat and LEA were controlled for by comparing twin pairs discordant for Vietnam service; twins who served in Vietnam had significantly lower LEA than their co-twins. Greater cognitive ability and older age at the time of military induction both predicted higher LEA; after statistically controlling for these variables, the relationship between combat exposure and LEA remained significant, demonstrating that combat experience reduces lifelong educational prospects, even after cognitive ability is controlled.

Other research has documented the negative effects of military service and combat exposure on income and employment status.[10,19] Stellman and colleagues[10] assessed various social outcomes among Vietnam veterans approximately 35 years after exposure to military combat and reported significantly lower income in those exposed to high levels of combat. In a study by Prigerson et al.,[19] data from the National Comorbidity Survey revealed that combat exposure significantly contributed to current unemployment and job loss after controlling for PTSD.

In a VETR sample, higher levels of combat were associated with less eagerness to "get involved with life" after discharge and poorer adjustment to civilian life, consistent with findings from previous studies.[10] Higher combat exposure has also been linked to lower scores on activities of daily living, self-esteem, and social relationships (including personal relationships and social support).[102]

In VETSA, we found that higher levels of combat were associated with a lower number of confidants and less satisfaction with the individual's closest friendship. Intimate relationships were also affected by combat exposure. Subjects with PTSD reported greater difficulty in their sexual performance and less satisfaction with sex, but interestingly, did not differ in terms of frequency and intensity of sexual desire. Findings also suggest[103] that combat exposure in combination with PTSD was significantly associated with the quality of marriage including agreement between partners on important matters (money, friends, time spent together, etc.), amount of tension in the relationship, satisfaction with sex life, level of expressed affection, and the level of common interests and shared activities in Vietnam veterans. Another study reported that combat exposure remained related to marital satisfaction 35 years after exposure to combat.[10]

Many studies have examined the association between war trauma and physical health outcomes such as health-related quality of life, physical and social functioning, bodily pain, chronic health conditions (cardiovascular disease, gastrointestinal disease, hypertension, respiratory conditions, joint disorders, and skin conditions), activities of daily living (bathing, walking up stairs, and shopping), and sleep problems.[103–108] Selim and colleagues[104] examined the physical and mental health of approximately 887,775 participants from the 1999 Large Health Survey of Veteran Enrollees. Veterans aged 65 and older reported 4 ± 2.4 chronic conditions, with arthritis and hypertension the most prevalent (64%). The prevalence of several chronic conditions (arthritis, congestive heart failure, cancer, and stroke) increased with age. They also suggested that loss of spouse and low educational attainment could have a deleterious effect on one's emotional and physical well-being along with overall health status.[104]

A recent study examined the physical and mental health ramifications of traumatic war/combat experience in approximately 17,700 Civil War veterans via the use of archival data files.[105] The authors distinguished between "heavy combat exposure" and "intimate violence" which includes directly witnessing death, seeing the slain enemy prior to or after killing them, and witnessing comrades die. Younger veterans exposed to war trauma and veterans witnessing the death of military comrades were more likely to be diagnosed with cardiovascular, gastrointestinal, and nervous disorders. Younger enlistees had a greater risk of early mortality while prisoner of war experience predicted signs of comorbid, physical, nervous, and mortality outcomes.

Other research has documented the effects of combat exposure on hearing problems, joint disorders, skin and urinary problems, and the liability for reporting chronic health conditions such as hypertension, respiratory conditions, and sleep problems in veterans who served during the Vietnam and Gulf Wars.[10,107,108,109] One study found that among Gulf War veterans, 51% suffered from disturbed sleep, with 13% of these veterans demonstrating chronic insomnia before the war and 38% developing insomnia during the war.[109] Sleep problems persisted after returning from war, with 19% of previously noninsomniacs suffering from insomnia up to 4 weeks later. Studies have also reported a strong correlation between combat exposure and frequency of nightmares in Vietnam veterans.[110] Data from a VETR study demonstrated an association of combat exposure with overall sleep quality, waking often, and having trouble staying asleep[111] and studies have reported that combat exposure is moderately correlated with sleep onset insomnia and weakly correlated with disrupted sleep maintenance.[110] Sleep disturbances are a central feature of PTSD, with findings demonstrating that 100% of veterans with PTSD have sleep problems.[112] There is a paucity of research, however, examining the relationship between sleep problems in veterans without PTSD. A recent study found that 90% of Vietnam veterans without PTSD had clinically significant sleep disturbances, demonstrating the pervasiveness of sleep problems among veterans and suggesting that military-related factors other than PTSD might contribute to insomnia.[112]

Issues for Future Research on the Effects of Combat

In a seminal 1991 article on methodology for research on the effects of the Vietnam War, King and King[113] made seven specific recommendations for improving research on veterans. They recommend including heterogeneous samples, incorporating reliability and validity checks into data collection, explicating the trauma construct, developing the convergent and discriminant validity of PTSD, using prospective data, attending to factors that influence who served in the military and the nature of their service, and implementing a life span developmental approach. Their recommendations continue to be very relevant and a number of studies have incorporated many of the design features advocated by the Kings.

It is an important priority for future research on the effects of combat to collect predeployment data; a number of studies have undertaken such an effort. One such example is the Neurocognition Deployment Health Study,[114] in which neuropsychological data were collected from 961 male and female active-duty Army soldiers. About two-thirds of the sample was deployed to Iraq and was assessed prior to deployment and shortly after returning. About one-third did not deploy and served as a control group. Deployment to Iraq was associated with poorer performance on tasks of sustained attention, verbal learning, and visual-spatial memory as well as increased negative state affect on measures of confusion and tension. The Millennium Cohort Study is a very large and ambitious prospective health project that is investigating the long-term health effects of military service, including deployments. Motivated by questions left unanswered after the 1991 Gulf War, the Millennium Cohort Study, conducted by the Department of Defense, the Department of Veterans Affairs, and civilian researchers, was started in 2001. Almost 150,000 individuals are participating in the study.

In a number of critical ways, the wars in which the United States is currently involved share important features with the Peloponnesian War and every war since then. Combatants may be injured and exposed to life-threatening situations, and they may see comrades killed and disabled. Another risk incurred through participation in combat is that of "moral injury." Litz and colleagues[115] pointed out that combatants have confronted moral and ethical challenges throughout history. Witnessing, failing to prevent, or perpetrating acts that violate deeply held moral beliefs and expectations may be psychologically, socially, and emotionally harmful to the individual. While many of the features of war that lead to untoward outcomes have remained unchanged over millennia, there are a number of issues in contemporary conflicts that are different from other wars in the past. One important change is the larger number of women serving as combatants. According to the U.S. Census Bureau (*Statistical Abstract of the United States: 2009)*, almost 200,000 women were on active duty in the military as of September, 2007. In 1950, women comprised less that 2% of military personnel; by 2007, women represented 14% of the armed forces. There were 1.8 million female military veterans as of 2007. With a few notable exceptions, such as studies of nurses who participated in the Vietnam War (e.g., Carson and colleagues[116]), the vast majority of investigations of the effects of combat have exclusively focused on men. Undoubtedly, some of what is known about the effects of combat will be applicable to women. However, it is also very clear that there are aspects of the war environment that differentially affect women. For example, sexual assault and rape of female service personnel have been identified as extremely serious problems that have become more severe with the increasing integration of women into the armed forces. More research is urgently needed on the effects of such trauma on women and effective means of prevention.

Another factor that has varied across wars is the representativeness of the population from which combatants are drawn. During WWII there were high rates of volunteering as well as a universal draft that cast a broad net among adult men in the United States; all men between the ages of 18 and 45 were liable for military service. From 1940 to 1947, when the wartime selective service act expired, over 10 million men were inducted into the military. During the Vietnam War there was also a military draft, but an expanded number of deferral opportunities reduced the representativeness of those who were conscripted. The draft was eliminated in 1973 and all those inducted since then have been volunteers. It is likely that the circumstance under which one enters military service has some relationship to the eventual outcomes. Another dimension on which wars differ is the level of popular support. During WWII there was broad, but not unanimous, public support for the war. Veterans returning from WWII were generally warmly greeted by a grateful citizenry. Public opinion during the Vietnam War was much more sharply divided, and a high proportion of individuals (including veterans) were opposed to the war or at least ambivalent about it. Fairly widespread negative opinions about the war often translated into negative attitudes towards returning veterans of the war. It seems likely that positive public attitudes and gratitude towards veterans may help promote coping with the effects of traumatic experiences, while rejection and disapproval may serve to intensify the problems of veterans attempting to readjust to civilian life. The current wars have, thus far, attracted considerably less public opposition than the Vietnam War, perhaps reflecting in part the absence of a military draft, which allows most Americans to remain at arm's length from the suffering of the combatants. Moreover, even those who are critical of the wars do not seem to extend their disapproval to the individual service members who are involved.

Different wars are associated with differential probabilities of exposure to various types of trauma. For example, modern unconventional and guerilla wars, without clearly delineated battlefields, increase the likelihood of witnessing, failing to prevent, or perpetrating acts that conflict with an individual's ethical, moral, and spiritual principles. The probability of incurring this type of moral injury is probably elevated when combat takes place in urban or other areas in which there are large numbers of civilians present. Traumatic brain injury (TBI) has been called the signature injury of the conflicts in Iraq and Afghanistan, reflecting opposition tactics and an increased probability of surviving combat injuries due to improvements in equipment and medical care on the battlefield and beyond. The results of a survey undertaken by Schneiderman and colleagues[117] indicated that about 12% of OEF/OIF veterans reported a history consistent with mild TBI. In fact, 11% screened positive for PTSD. Accordingly, there has been considerable interest in TBI and its correlates. A recent study by Pietrzac et al.[118] found that the relationship between mild TBI and psychosocial functioning and general health ratings two years after return from deployment was mediated by PTSD. The coexistence of TBI and PTSD may present particularly difficult clinical challenges.[119] Shared symptomatic and functional features of PTSD and TBI raise important and difficult questions about mutual pathophysiology.[120]

This chapter focused primarily on mental health consequences of exposure to combat, but the effects are multifarious and are visible in many domains. For example, Elder and colleagues[121] found that overseas duty, service in the Pacific theater, and exposure to combat significantly increased the risk for relatively early mortality for WWII veterans. MacLean and Elder[66] reviewed literature on the relationship of military service and the life course from a sociological perspective. They concluded that veterans exposed to combat suffered worse outcomes than noncombat veterans and nonveterans on a wide array of psychosocial outcomes. When a society decides to send its young men and women into combat, the price to be paid may include death or physical disfigurement and disability, but may also include a lifetime of emotional suffering and a lifelong disadvantage in competing for the benefits available in our society. Society incurs a huge responsibility for caring for damaged individuals and seeking to prevent or minimize harm. Above all, it is imperative to understand the gravity and momentous consequences of the decision to send young people to war.

Acknowledgments

The Department of Veterans Affairs has provided financial support for the development and maintenance of the Vietnam Era Twin Registry (VETR). Numerous organizations have provided invaluable assistance in the conduct of this study, including: Department of Defense; National Personnel Records Center, National Archives and Records Administration; the Internal Revenue Service; National Opinion Research Center; National Research Council, National Academy of Sciences; the Institute for Survey Research, Temple University; Schulman, Ronca, and Bucuvalas, Inc. VETSA is supported by grants from NIH/NIA (R01 AG018384, R01 AG018386, R01 AG022381, and R01 AG022982). Most importantly, we gratefully acknowledge the continued cooperation and participation of the members of the VETR and their families.

References

1. Eisen, S., True, W., Goldberg, J., Henderson, W., & Robinette, C. D. (1987). The Vietnam Era Twin (VET) Registry: Method of construction. *Acta Genet Med Gemellol (Roma), 36*(1), 61–66.
2. Henderson, W. G., Eisen, S., Goldberg, J., True, W. R., Barnes, J. E., & Vitek, M. E. (1990). The Vietnam Era Twin Registry: A resource for medical research. *Public Health Rep, 105*(4), 368–373.

3. Tsuang, M., Bar, J. L., Harley, R., & Lyons, M. J. (2001). The Harvard Twin Study of Drug Abuse: What have we learned? *Harvard Review of Psychiatry*, 267–279.
4. Goldberg, J., True, W., Eisen, S., Henderson, W., & Robinette, C. D. (1987). The Vietnam Era Twin (VET) Registry: Ascertainment bias. *Acta Genet Med Gemellol (Roma), 36*(1), 67–78.
5. Kremen, W. S., Thompson-Brenner, H., Leung, Y. M., et al. (2006). Genes, environment, and time: The Vietnam Era Twin Study of Aging (VETSA). *Twin Res Hum Genet, 9*(6), 1009–1022.
6. Killgore, W. D., Cotting, D. I., Thomas, J. L., et al. (2008). Post-combat invincibility: Violent combat experiences are associated with increased risk-taking propensity following deployment. *J Psychiatr Res, 42*(13), 1112–1121.
7. Taft, C. T., Vogt, D. S., Marshall, A. D., Panuzio, J., & Niles, B. L. (2007). Aggression among combat veterans: Relationships with combat exposure and symptoms of posttraumatic stress disorder, dysphoria, and anxiety. *J Trauma Stress, 20*(2), 135–145.
8. Lyons, M. J., Goldberg, J., Eisen, S. A., et al. (1993). Do genes influence exposure to trauma? A twin study of combat. *Am J Med Genet, 48*(1), 22–27.
9. Sareen, J., Cox, B. J., Afifi, T. O., et al. (2007). Combat and peacekeeping operations in relation to prevalence of mental disorders and perceived need for mental health care: Findings from a large representative sample of military personnel. *Arch Gen Psychiatry, 64*(7), 843–852.
10. Stellman, S., Stellman, J., & Koenen, K. (2000). Enduring social and behavioral effects of exposure to military combat in Vietnam. *Ann Epidemiol, 10*(7), 480.
11. Seal, K. H., Metzler, T. J., Gima, K. S., Bertenthal, D., Maguen, S., & Marmar, C. R. (2009). Trends and risk factors for mental health diagnoses among Iraq and Afghanistan veterans using Department of Veterans Affairs health care, 2002–2008. *Am J Public Health, 99*(9), 1651–1658.
12. Seal, K. H., Bertenthal, D., Miner, C. R., Sen, S., & Marmar, C. (2007). Bringing the war back home: Mental health disorders among 103,788 U.S. veterans returning from Iraq and Afghanistan seen at Department of Veterans Affairs facilities. *Arch Intern Med, 167*(5), 476–482.
13. Hoge, C. W., Castro, C. A., Messer, S. C., McGurk, D., Cotting, D. I., & Koffman, R. L. (2004). Combat duty in Iraq and Afghanistan, mental health problems, and barriers to care. *N Engl J Med, 351*(1), 13–22.
14. Fontana, A. & Rosenheck, R. (2008). Treatment-seeking veterans of Iraq and Afghanistan: Comparison with veterans of previous wars. *J Nerv Ment Dis, 196*(7), 513–521.
15. Fontana, A. & Rosenheck, R. (1994). Traumatic war stressors and psychiatric symptoms among World War II, Korean, and Vietnam War veterans. *Psychol Aging, 9*(1), 27–33.
16. Fontana, A. & Rosenheck, R. (1994). Posttraumatic stress disorder among Vietnam Theater Veterans. A causal model of etiology in a community sample. *J Nerv Ment Dis, 182*(12), 677–684.
17. Hoge, C. W., Auchterlonie, J. L., & Milliken, C. S. (2006). Mental health problems, use of mental health services, and attrition from military service after returning from deployment to Iraq or Afghanistan. *JAMA, 295*(9), 1023–1032.
18. MacGregor, A. J., Shaffer, R. A., Dougherty, A. L., et al. (2009). Psychological correlates of battle and nonbattle injury among Operation Iraqi Freedom veterans. *Mil Med, 174*(3), 224–231.

19. Prigerson, H. G., Maciejewski, P. K., & Rosenheck, R. A. (2002). Population attributable fractions of psychiatric disorders and behavioral outcomes associated with combat exposure among US men. *Am J Public Health, 92*(1), 59–63.
20. Dohrenwend, B. P., Turner, J. B., Turse, N. A., Adams, B. G., Koenen, K. C., & Marshall, R. (2006). The psychological risks of Vietnam for U.S. veterans: A revisit with new data and methods. *Science, 313*(5789), 979–982.
21. Toomey, R., Kang, H. K., Karlinsky, J., et al. (2007). Mental health of US Gulf War veterans 10 years after the war. *Br J Psychiatry, 190,* 385–393.
22. Kessler, R. C., Chiu, W. T., Demler, O., Merikangas, K. R., & Walters, E. E. (2005). Prevalence, severity, and comorbidity of 12-month DSM-IV disorders in the National Comorbidity Survey Replication. *Arch Gen Psychiatry, 62*(6), 617–627.
23. Baker, D. G., Heppner, P., Afari, N., et al. (2009). Trauma exposure, branch of service, and physical injury in relation to mental health among U.S. veterans returning from Iraq and Afghanistan. *Mil Med, 174*(8), 773–778.
24. Shen, Y. C., Arkes, J., & Pilgrim, J. (2009). The effects of deployment intensity on post-traumatic stress disorder: 2002–2006. *Mil Med, 174*(3), 217–223.
25. Goldberg, J., True, W. R., Eisen, S. A., & Henderson, W. G. (1990). A twin study of the effects of the Vietnam War on posttraumatic stress disorder. *JAMA, 263*(9), 1227–1232.
26. Green, B. L., Grace, M. C., Lindy, J. D., Gleser, G. C., & Leonard, A. (1990). Risk factors for PTSD and other diagnoses in a general sample of Vietnam veterans. *Am J Psychiatry, 147*(6), 729–733.
27. Roy-Byrne, P., Arguelles, L., Vitek, M. E., et al. (2004). Persistence and change of PTSD symptomatology—a longitudinal co-twin control analysis of the Vietnam Era Twin Registry. *Soc Psychiatry Psychiatr Epidemiol, 39*(9), 681–685.
28. Kulka, R. A., Schlenger, W. E., Fairbanks, J. A., Hough, R. L., Jordan, B. K., Marmar, C. R., et al. (1990). Trauma and the Vietnam War generation: Report of findings from the National Vietnam Veterans Readjustment Study New York: Brunner/Mazel.
29. Kremen, W. S., Koenen, K. C., Boake, C., et al. (2007). Pretrauma cognitive ability and risk for posttraumatic stress disorder: A twin study. *Arch Gen Psychiatry, 64*(3), 361–368.
30. Thompson, W. W. & Gottesman, I. I. (2008). Challenging the conclusion that lower preinduction cognitive ability increases risk for combat-related post-traumatic stress disorder in 2,375 combat-exposed Vietnam War veterans. *Mil Med, 173*(6), 576–582.
31. Tellegen, A. (1982). Brief manual for the Multidimensional Personality Questionnaire. Unpublished manuscript. University of Minnesota.
32. Ikin, J. F., Sim, M. R., McKenzie, D. P., et al. (2007). Anxiety, post-traumatic stress disorder and depression in Korean War veterans 50 years after the war. *Br J Psychiatry, 190,* 475–483.
33. Fiedler, N., Ozakinci, G., Hallman, W., et al. (2006). Military deployment to the Gulf War as a risk factor for psychiatric illness among US troops. *Br J Psychiatry, 188,* 453–459.
34. Grayson, D. A., Marshall, R. P., Dobson, M., et al. (1996). Australian Vietnam veterans: Factors contributing to psychosocial problems. *Aust N Z J Psychiatry, 30*(5), 600–613.
35. Jordan, B. K., Schlenger, W. E., Hough, R., et al. (1991). Lifetime and current prevalence of specific psychiatric disorders among Vietnam veterans and controls. *Arch Gen Psychiatry, 48*(3), 207–215.
36. O'Toole, B. I., Marshall, R. P., Schureck, R. J., & Dobson, M. (1998). Posttraumatic stress disorder and comorbidity in Australian Vietnam veterans: Risk factors, chronicity and combat. *Aust N Z J Psychiatry, 32*(1), 32–42.

37. O'Toole, B. I., Marshall, R. P., Grayson, D. A., et al. (1996). The Australian Vietnam Veterans Health Study: III. Psychological health of Australian Vietnam veterans and its relationship to combat. *Int J Epidemiol, 25*(2), 331–340.
38. Sher, L. (2009). A model of suicidal behavior in war veterans with posttraumatic mood disorder. *Med Hypotheses, 73*(2), 215–219.
39. Glover, H. (1984). Survival guilt and the Vietnam veteran. *J Nerv Ment Dis, 172*(7), 393–397.
40. Blacher, R. S. (2000). "It isn't fair": Postoperative depression and other manifestations of survivor guilt. *Gen Hosp Psychiatry, 22*(1), 43–48.
41. Henning, K. R. & Frueh, B. C. (1997). Combat guilt and its relationship to PTSD symptoms. *J Clin Psychol, 53*(8), 801–808.
42. Okulate, G. T. & Jones, O. B. (2006). Post-traumatic stress disorder, survivor guilt and substance use—a study of hospitalised Nigerian army veterans. *S Afr Med J, 96*(2), 144–146.
43. Hendin, H. & Haas, A. P. (1991). Suicide and guilt as manifestations of PTSD in Vietnam combat veterans. *Am J Psychiatry, 148*(5), 586–591.
44. Boscarino, J. (1979). Alcohol abuse among veterans: The importance of demographic factors. *Addict Behav, 4*(4), 323–330.
45. Boscarino, J. (1980). Drinking by veterans and nonveterans: A national comparison. *J Stud Alcohol, 41*(9), 854–859.
46. Jacobson, I. G., Ryan, M. A., Hooper, T. I., et al. (2008). Alcohol use and alcohol-related problems before and after military combat deployment. *JAMA, 300*(6), 663–675.
47. Hooper, R., Rona, R. J., Jones, M., Fear, N. T., Hull, L., & Wessely, S. (2008). Cigarette and alcohol use in the UK Armed Forces, and their association with combat exposures: A prospective study. *Addict Behav, 33*(8), 1067–1071.
48. Goldberg, J., Eisen, S. A., True, W. R., & Henderson, W. G. (1990). A twin study of the effects of the Vietnam conflict on alcohol drinking patterns. *Am J Public Health, 80*(5), 570–574.
49. Smith, B., Ryan, M. A., Wingard, D. L., Patterson, T. L., Slymen, D. J., & Macera, C. A. (2008). Cigarette smoking and military deployment: A prospective evaluation. *Am J Prev Med, 35*(6), 539–546.
50. Stein, R. J., Pyle, S. A., Haddock, C. K., Poston, W. S., Bray, R., & Williams, J. (2008). Reported stress and its relationship to tobacco use among U.S. military personnel. *Mil Med, 173*(3), 271–277.
51. Biddle, D., Hawthorne, G., Forbes, D., & Coman, G. (2005). Problem gambling in Australian PTSD treatment-seeking veterans. *J Trauma Stress, 18*(6), 759–767.
52. Green, B. L., Lindy, J. D., Grace, M. C., & Gleser, G. C. (1989). Multiple diagnosis in posttraumatic stress disorder. The role of war stressors. *J Nerv Ment Dis, 177*(6), 329–335.
53. Kessler, R. C., Hwang, I., LaBrie, R., et al. (2008). DSM-IV pathological gambling in the National Comorbidity Survey Replication. *Psychol Med, 38*(9), 1351–1360.
54. Kausch, O., Rugle, L., & Rowland, D. Y. (2006). Lifetime histories of trauma among pathological gamblers. *Am J Addict, 15*(1), 35–43.
55. Scherrer, J. F., Xian, H., Kapp, J. M., et al. (2007). Association between exposure to childhood and lifetime traumatic events and lifetime pathological gambling in a twin cohort. *J Nerv Ment Dis, 195*(1), 72–78.
56. Peltzer, K., Mabilu, M. G., Mathoho, S. F., Nekhwevha, A. P., Sikhwivhilu, T., & Sinthumule, T. S. (2006). Trauma history and severity of gambling involvement among horse-race gamblers in a South African gambling setting. *Psychol Rep, 99*(2), 472–476.

57. Scherrer, J. F., Slutske, W. S., Xian, H., et al. (2007). Factors associated with pathological gambling at 10-year follow-up in a national sample of middle-aged men. *Addiction, 102*(6), 970–978.
58. Dreazen, Y. J. (2009). The military: A general's personal battle. *The Wall Street Journal*, W1 2009, March 28.
59. Kuehn, B. M. (2009). Soldier suicide rates continue to rise: Military, scientists work to stem the tide. *JAMA, 301*(11), 1111–1113.
60. Eaton, K. M., Messer, S. C., Garvey Wilson, A. L., & Hoge, C. W. (2006). Strengthening the validity of population-based suicide rate comparisons: An illustration using U.S. military and civilian data. *Suicide Life Threat Behav, 36*(2), 182–191.
61. Kang, H. K. & Bullman, T. A. (2008). Risk of suicide among US veterans after returning from the Iraq or Afghanistan war zones. *JAMA, 300*(6), 652–653.
62. Kaplan, M. S., Huguet, N., McFarland, B. H., & Newsom, J. T. (2007). Suicide among male veterans: A prospective population-based study. *J Epidemiol Community Health, 61*(7), 619–624.
63. Allen, J. P., Cross, G., & Swanner, J. (2005). Suicide in the Army: A review of current information. *Mil Med, 170*(7), 580–584.
64. Goldsmith, S. K. (2001). *Risk factors for suicide: A summary of a workshop*. National Academy Press.
65. Bullman, T. A & Kang, H. K. (1996). The risk of suicide among wounded Vietnam veterans. *Am J Public Health, 86*(5), 662–667.
66. MacLean, A. & Elder, G. H., Jr. (2007). Military service in the life course. *Annual Review of Sociology, 33*, 175–196.
67. Bell, J. B. & Nye, E. C. (2007). Specific symptoms predict suicidal ideation in Vietnam combat veterans with chronic post-traumatic stress disorder. *Mil Med, 172*(11), 1144–1147.
68. Robins, L. N., Helzer, J. E., Ratcliff, K. S., & Seyfried, W. (1982). Validity of the diagnostic interview schedule, version II: DSM-III diagnoses. *Psychol Med, 12*(4), 855–870.
69. Ginzburg, K., Ein-Dor, T., & Solomon, Z. (2009). Comorbidity of posttraumatic stress disorder, anxiety and depression: A 20-year longitudinal study of war veterans [published online ahead of print Sep 16 2009]. *J Affect Disord.*
70. Grayson, D., Dobson, M., & Marshall, R. (1998). Current combat-related disorders in the absence of PTSD among Australian Vietnam veterans. *Soc Psychiatry Psychiatr Epidemiol, 33*(4), 186–192.
71. Breslau, N., Davis, G. C., & Schultz, L. R. (2003). Posttraumatic stress disorder and the incidence of nicotine, alcohol, and other drug disorders in persons who have experienced trauma. *Arch Gen Psychiatry, 60*(3), 289–294.
72. Breslau, N. (2002). Epidemiologic studies of trauma, posttraumatic stress disorder, and other psychiatric disorders. *Canadian Journal of Psychiatry, 47*, 923–929.
73. Cottler, L. B., Compton, W. M., Mager, D., Spitznagel, E. L., & Janca, A. (1992). Posttraumatic stress disorder among substance users from the general population. *Am J Psychiatry, 149*(5), 664–670.
74. Cottler, L. B., Nishith, P., & Compton, W. M. (2001). Gender differences in risk factors for trauma exposure and post-traumatic stress disorder among inner-city drug abusers in and out of treatment. *Compr Psychiatry, 42*(2), 111–117.
75. Johnson, S. D., Striley, C., & Cottler, L. B. (2006). The association of substance use disorders with trauma exposure and PTSD among African American drug users. *Addict Behav, 31*(11), 2063–2073.

76. Resnick, H. S., Kilpatrick, D. G., Best, C. L., & Kramer, T. L. (1992). Vulnerability-stress factors in development of posttraumatic stress disorder. *J Nerv Ment Dis, 180*(7), 424–430.
77. Bremner, J. D., Southwick, S. M., Darnell, A., & Charney, D. S. (1996). Chronic PTSD in Vietnam combat veterans: Course of illness and substance abuse. *Am J Psychiatry, 153*(3), 369–375.
78. Centers for Disease Control Vietnam Experience Study. (1988). Health Status of Vietnam Veterans. I: Psychosocial characteristics. *Journal of the American Medical Society, 259*, 2701–2707.
79. Kessler, R. C., Sonnega, A., Bromet, E., Hughes, M., & Nelson, C. B. (1995). Posttraumatic stress disorder in the National Comorbidity Survey. *Arch Gen Psychiatry, 52*(12), 1048–1060.
80. Franko, D. L., Thompson, D., Barton, B. A., et al. (2005). Prevalence and comorbidity of major depressive disorder in young black and white women. *J Psychiatr Res,39*(3), 275–283.
81. Koenen, K. C., Lyons, M. J., Goldberg, J., et al. (2003). A high risk twin study of combat-related PTSD comorbidity. *Twin Res, 6*(3), 218–226.
82. Koenen, K. C., Lyons, M. J., Goldberg, J., et al. (2003). Co-twin control study of relationships among combat exposure, combat-related PTSD, and other mental disorders. *J Trauma Stress, 16*(5), 433–438.
83. Koenen, K. C., Hitsman, B., Lyons, M. J., et al. (2005). A twin registry study of the relationship between posttraumatic stress disorder and nicotine dependence in men. *Arch Gen Psychiatry, 62*(11), 1258–1265.
84. Koenen, K. C., Fu, Q. J., Ertel, K., et al. (2008). Common genetic liability to major depression and posttraumatic stress disorder in men. *J Affect Disord, 105*(1–3), 109–115.
85. Fu, Q., Koenen, K. C., Miller, M. W., et al. (2007). Differential etiology of posttraumatic stress disorder with conduct disorder and major depression in male veterans. *Biol Psychiatry, 62*(10), 1088–1094.
86. Scherrer, J. F., Xian, H., Lyons, M. J., et al. (2008). Posttraumatic stress disorder; combat exposure; and nicotine dependence, alcohol dependence, and major depression in male twins. *Compr Psychiatry, 49*(3), 297–304.
87. Xian, H., Scherrer, J. F., Grant, J. D., et al. (2008). Genetic and environmental contributions to nicotine, alcohol and cannabis dependence in male twins. *Addiction, 103*(8), 1391–1398.
88. Davidson, J., Smith, R., & Kudler, H. (1989). Familial psychiatric illness in chronic posttraumatic stress disorder. *Compr Psychiatry, 30*(4), 339–345.
89. Davidson, J. R., Tupler, L. A., Wilson, W. H., & Connor, K. M. (1998). A family study of chronic post-traumatic stress disorder following rape trauma. *J Psychiatr Res, 32*(5), 301–309.
90. McLeod, D. S., Koenen, K. C., Meyer, J. M., et al. (2001). Genetic and environmental influences on the relationship among combat exposure, posttraumatic stress disorder symptoms, and alcohol use. *J Trauma Stress, 14*(2), 259–275.
91. Wilson, J. P. (1988). Understanding Vietnam veterans. In F. M. Ochberg, (Ed.). *Post-traumatic therapy and victims of violence* (pp. 227–253). New York: Brunner/Mazel.
92. Zuckerman, M. (1991). *Psychobiology of personality*. New York: Cambridge University Press.
93. Sher, K. J. & Trull, T. J. (1994). Personality and disinhibitory psychopathology: Alcoholism and antisocial personality disorder. *J Abnorm Psychol, 103*(1), 92–102.

94. Tanielian, T. & Jaycox, L. H. (2008). *Invisible wounds of war: Psychological and cognitive injuries, their consequences, and services to assist recovery*. Santa Monica, CA: RAND Corp.
95. Marmar, C. R. (2009). Mental health impact of Afghanistan and Iraq deployment: Meeting the challenge of a new generation of veterans. *Depress Anxiety, 26*(6), 493–497.
96. Ready, D. J., Thomas, K. R., Worley, V., et al. (2008). A field test of group based exposure therapy with 102 veterans with war-related posttraumatic stress disorder. *J Trauma Stress, 21*(2), 150–157.
97. Rizzo, A. A., Difede, J., Rothbaum, B. O., et al. (2009). VR PTSD exposure therapy results with active duty OIF/OEF combatants. *Stud Health Technol Inform, 142*, 277–282.
98. Stein, D. J., Ipser, J. C., & Seedat, S. (2006). Pharmacotherapy for post traumatic stress disorder (PTSD). *Cochrane Database Syst Rev*, (1), CD002795.
99. Knox, K. L., Litts, D. A., Talcott, G. W., Feig, J. C., Caine, E. D. (2003). Risk of suicide and related adverse outcomes after exposure to a suicide prevention programme in the US Air Force: Cohort study. *BMJ, 327*(7428), 1376.
100. Army reports sharp rise in suicides in January. *The Wall Street Journal* 2009, February 5.
101. Lyons, M. J., Kremen, W. S., Franz, C., et al. (2006). Vietnam service, combat, and lifetime educational attainment: Preliminary results from the Vietnam Era Twin Study of Aging. *Research on Aging, 28*(1), 37–55.
102. Ikin, J. F., Sim, M. R., McKenzie, D. P., et al. (2009). Life satisfaction and quality in Korean War veterans five decades after the war. *J Epidemiol Community Health, 63*(5), 359–365.
103. Caselli, L. T. & Motta, R. W. (1995). The effect of PTSD and combat level on Vietnam veterans' perceptions of child behavior and marital adjustment. *J Clin Psychol, 51*(1), 4–12.
104. Selim, A. J., Berlowitz, D. R., Fincke, G., et al. (2004). The health status of elderly veteran enrollees in the Veterans Health Administration. *J Am Geriatr Soc, 52*(8), 1271–1276.
105. Pizarro, J., Silver, R. C., & Prause, J. (2006). Physical and mental health costs of traumatic war experiences among Civil War veterans. *Arch Gen Psychiatry, 63*(2), 193–200.
106. Hunt, N. & Robbins, I. (2001). The long-term consequences of war: The experience of World War II. *Aging Ment Health, 5*(2), 183–190.
107. Eisen, S. A., Neuman, R., Goldberg, J., et al. (1998). Contribution of emotionally traumatic events and inheritance to the report of current physical health problems in 4042 Vietnam era veteran twin pairs. *Psychosom Med, 60*(5), 533–539.
108. Eisen, S. A., Goldberg, J., True, W. R., & Henderson, W. G. (1991). A co-twin control study of the effects of the Vietnam War on the self-reported physical health of veterans. *Am J Epidemiol, 134*(1), 49–58.
109. Askenasy, J. J. & Lewin, I. (1996). The impact of missile warfare on self-reported sleep quality. Part 1. *Sleep, 19*(1), 47–51.
110. Neylan, T. C., Marmar, C. R., Metzler, T. J., et al. (1998). Sleep disturbances in the Vietnam generation: Findings from a nationally representative sample of male Vietnam veterans. *Am J Psychiatry, 155*(7), 929–933.
111. McCarren, M., Goldberg, J., Ramakrishnan, V., & Fabsitz, R. (1994). Insomnia in Vietnam era veteran twins: Influence of genes and combat experience. *Sleep, 17*(5), 456–461.

112. Lewis, V., Creamer, M., & Failla, S. (2009). Is poor sleep in veterans a function of post-traumatic stress disorder? *Mil Med, 174*(9), 948–951.
113. King, D. & King, L. A. (1991). Validity issued in research on Vietnam veteran adjustment. *Psychological Bulletin, 109*(1), 107–124.
114. Vasterling, J. J., Proctor, S. P., Amoroso, P., et al. (2006). The Neurocognition Deployment Health Study: A prospective cohort study of Army Soldiers. *Mil Med, 171*(3), 253–260.
115. Litz, B. T., Stein, N., Delaney, E., et al. (2009). Moral injury and moral repair in war veterans: A preliminary model and intervention strategy. *Clin Psychol Rev, 29*(8), 695–706.
116. Carson, M. A., Paulus, L. A., Lasko, N. B., et al. (2000). Psychophysiologic assessment of posttraumatic stress disorder in Vietnam nurse veterans who witnessed injury or death. *J Consult Clin Psychol, 68*(5), 890–897.
117. Schneiderman, A. I., Braver, E. R., & Kang, H. K. (2008). Understanding sequelae of injury mechanisms and mild traumatic brain injury incurred during the conflicts in Iraq and Afghanistan: Persistent postconcussive symptoms and posttraumatic stress disorder. *Am J Epidemiol, 167*(12), 1446–1452.
118. Pietrzak, R. H., Johnson, D. C., Goldstein, M. B., Malley, J. C., & Southwick, S. M. (2009). Posttraumatic stress disorder mediates the relationship between mild traumatic brain injury and health and psychosocial functioning in veterans of Operations Enduring Freedom and Iraqi Freedom. *J Nerv Ment Dis, 197*(10), 748–753.
119. Brenner, L. A., Vanderploeg, R. D, & Terrio, H. (2009). Assessment and diagnosis of mild traumatic brain injury, posttraumatic stress disorder, and other polytrauma conditions: Burden of adversity hypothesis. *Rehabil Psychol, 54*(3), 239–246.
120. Stein, M. B. & McAllister, T. W. (2009). Exploring the convergence of posttraumatic stress disorder and mild traumatic brain injury. *Am J Psychiatry, 166*(7), 768–776.
121. Elder, G., Clipp, E. C., Brown, J. S., Martin, L. R., & Friedman, H. S. (2009). The lifelong mortality risks of World War II experiences. *Research on Aging, 31*(4), 391–412.

6

Assessing the Link Between Disaster Exposure and Mental Illness

CAROL S. NORTH

Mental Health in the Aftermath of Disaster

We live in a world where horrific, unthinkable events occur with tragic regularity. The media faithfully inform us as populations of the world are bombarded by natural disasters (earthquakes, tsunamis, hurricanes, tornadoes, volcanoes), technological accidents (transportation accidents, major structural collapses), and human intentionally caused incidents including terrorist attacks (mass shootings, bombings, bioterrorism). Experts predict future increases in the incidence and magnitude of such events. Global warming is expected to intensify the frequency and severity of natural disasters in upcoming decades. Growing reliance on technological advancements for mass transportation and other needs of daily life throughout the world portends acceleration in the occurrence of mass-casualty accidents. With growing global unrest, terrorists become bolder in their attacks. The mental health sequelae of these events can be expected to take a significant toll on the populations of the world exposed to such mass casualties. Epidemiologic research has demonstrated that large numbers of survivors of major disasters can be expected to suffer serious psychiatric consequences.[1,2]

Understanding the mental health effects of trauma is, unfortunately, anything but straightforward. This is in part because exposure to trauma may not, surprisingly, be an entirely random event. It is well established that preexisting characteristics, including psychiatric disorders and personality features, increase risk for exposure to traumatic events.[3–5] These important variables may obfuscate the differentiation of mental health effects of traumatic exposure from preexisting psychological characteristics of the exposed individuals at risk for trauma. A compelling reason to study mental health effects of disasters, therefore, is that disasters in general, more than other traumatic events, may be "equal-opportunity" occurrences, striking somewhat randomly and independently of preexisting characteristics of the individuals involved.[6] This attribute of disasters minimizes the potential for confounding from preexisting characteristics responsible for selection bias for trauma exposure in studies of mental health effects of other types of trauma.[7] (An important exception to this generality was observed among Hurricane Katrina evacuees, to be discussed in more detail later.)

A growing body of disaster mental health research has clarified the types and prevalence of psychiatric disorders typically arising after exposure to various disasters. The most prevalent disorder observed in disaster-exposed populations is typically posttraumatic stress disorder (PTSD), followed by major depression.[1,6,8,9] PTSD usually presents as a comorbid disorder,[6,8,10] a consistent observation across most traumatized populations. After most disasters, the majority of survivors do not develop a psychiatric disorder, although emotional distress is an expected response for almost everyone. Postdisaster distress is therefore a normative response that should be differentiated from disaster-related psychopathology, because these distinct entities require different intervention strategies.[6,8,11]

Only certain psychiatric disorders newly arise with regularity in the postdisaster setting. Schizophrenia and bipolar disorder are not among them.[12] Although increased use of alcohol, tobacco, and illegal drugs has been reported to follow disasters,[13–18] its clinical significance is unknown and it does not regularly translate into new substance use disorders after disasters.[6,8,11,20] Neither does somatization disorder regularly commence after disasters. Somatoform symptoms (i.e., physical symptoms without medical explanation) may be difficult to distinguish from manifestations of physical injuries (i.e., somatic symptoms) after disasters. Studies carefully differentiating them have demonstrated that the onset of somatoform symptoms generally predates rather than follows disaster exposure.[20–25]

The Quandaries of Trauma Exposure in PTSD

PTSD deviates from most psychiatric diagnoses in that this disorder is defined in relation to a potentially etiologic event, a traumatic stressor (Criterion A in *DSM-IV-TR*). For other diagnoses, the symptom criteria are simply listed, and the diagnosis is established by the symptoms, without assumption, or even consideration, of etiology. PTSD thus differs from other psychiatric disorders in its reliance on more than just the symptomatic manifestations of the disorder, requiring temporal and/or contextual relation to a potentially etiologic event. This unusual requirement in the criteria establishes PTSD as a "conditional disorder," which introduces complexities for working with this disorder in both clinical practice and research studies.

Considerable controversy surrounds the traumatic stressor criterion for the diagnosis of PTSD.[26–31] Proponents for expanding the definition of the traumatic stressor criterion have lobbied for inclusion of currently nonqualifying events such as divorce,[32] financial difficulties,[33] and childbirth[34,35] among the types of traumatic stressors that would qualify an individual for consideration of the diagnosis. Suggestions to expand the stressor criterion to include such types of events have been countered with protestations over consequent diagnostic "bracket creep."[29,36] Even the requirement for posttraumatic symptoms to be referenced to a traumatic event has been challenged.[37,38] It has been suggested that the assessment of posttraumatic symptoms be conducted without specifying any association with a traumatic event[39] and also that the defining traumatic event be dropped from the definition altogether to redefine PTSD based solely on a characteristic symptom complex.[40] Disconnecting posttraumatic symptoms from the defining traumatic event in the definition of PTSD, however, is contrary to the specific temporal and contextual occurrence of symptoms related to a traumatic event that uniquely distinguishes the disorder from other syndromes and yields a homogeneous set of cases.[26,27,38,41,42]

In research and clinical practice settings alike, measurement of posttraumatic symptoms is not always conducted with regard to the contextual or temporal framework of exposure to a qualifying event. It is not clear, however, what posttraumatic symptoms represent outside the diagnostic construct of PTSD and its defining traumatic exposure criterion.[26] A common approach is to use a symptom scale of items based on the 17 symptoms listed under the diagnosis of PTSD without specifically linking them to the occurrence of a traumatic event. Including symptoms without assessing their contextual or temporal relationship to a traumatic event functionally uncouples the psychological manifestations from the defining traumatic event.[6,43] Counting otherwise common symptoms such as insomnia, difficulty concentrating, or irritability in the setting of a traumatic event may inadvertently link unrelated problems to the traumatic stressor under investigation.[6,26] This is especially likely if the symptoms were already present before the traumatic event occurred.

Precisely what constitutes a traumatic event is not the only aspect of the definition of a traumatic stressor for the diagnosis of PTSD that has garnered considerable debate. Another debatable aspect of the traumatic stressor criterion is how much personal exposure to a traumatic event is sufficient to qualify an individual for consideration of a diagnosis of PTSD. The current definition of PTSD in *DSM-IV-TR* specifies that exposure to a qualifying traumatic event entails

> ... direct personal experience of an event that involves actual or threatened death or serious injury, or threat to one's physical integrity; or witnessing an event that involves death, injury, or a threat to the physical integrity of another person; or learning about unexpected violent death, serious harm, or threat of death or injury experienced by a family member or close associate (p. 463).[44]

By this definition, therefore, people who were evacuated from the World Trade Center (WTC) after the airplanes struck the towers in the September 11, 2001 attacks might be candidates for a diagnosis of PTSD if they met the symptom criteria. People who were not directly endangered themselves but who directly observed the horrific events unfolding up close could be candidates for a PTSD diagnosis if they met the symptom criteria. Finally, people who were far away but learned of the danger to their close family members who were in the WTC when the planes struck could be candidates for a PTSD diagnosis if they met the symptom criteria.

The causal relationships between disaster exposure and ensuing psychopathology might seem obvious on the surface, but assignment of causal pathways is actually a thorny exercise. The route from a traumatic event to subsequent symptoms does not automatically proceed with direct linear causality from the event to the symptoms. Relationships between traumatic events and mental health status are not generally as simple as two-variable unidirectional models might suggest.[26] The occurrence of Midwestern floods provides an example of relationships with unanticipated causal directionalities. Midwestern flooding has been found to be associated with a 25% lifetime prevalence rate of alcohol use disorder.[20] While it might be tempting in this case to assume that alcohol abuse represents self-medication of postdisaster emotional distress, in fact the onset of virtually all of the alcohol use disorder cases was shown to have predated the disaster. The relationship between alcoholism and flooding in this study was explained by the high preexisting rates of alcohol use disorders among the population choosing to live on a flood plain where land is more affordable.

Hurricane Katrina provided another example of nonintuitive causal relationships in disaster-exposure scenarios. Those who were unable to evacuate until after the storm disproportionately represented the most disadvantaged segment of the population with the greatest preexisting poverty and chronic health and mental health and substance abuse problems predating the disaster. After the disaster this evacuee population was also distressed, traumatized, and displaced, with the same set of preexisting problems as well as potential for PTSD.[12,45] Among Hurricane Katrina evacuees presenting for psychiatric treatment at a shelter in Dallas, preexisting mental illness, including schizophrenia, mood disorders, and substance abuse, accounted for most diagnoses made by treating psychiatrists.[12]

Research on Hurricane Katrina evacuees and Midwestern flood survivors has clarified the value of restraint in assigning causal pathways to established relationships between psychopathology and disaster exposure.[12,20] Differentiating postdisaster prevalence from incidence of psychopathology after disaster—that is, determining whether the psychiatric disorder began anew after the disaster or was preexisting—readily clarifies potential causal relationships. When preexisting psychopathology accounts for the observed association of postdisaster psychopathology and disaster exposure, then the preexisting psychopathology may be a risk factor for disaster exposure, or, alternatively, it may be a selection factor for the disaster-exposed sample being examined. For example, substance use has been demonstrated to predict exposure to traumatic events leading to PTSD in drug-using populations.[46–48]

A number of carefully conducted, methodologically rigorous research studies on trauma exposure have assessed full diagnostic criteria for psychiatric disorders, documenting relatively rapid onset of PTSD among some previously healthy people directly exposed to a qualifying traumatic event.[1] Although it may be tempting to presume linear causality from disaster to psychopathology when new onset of psychiatric illness arises in the early aftermath of a disaster, even these relationships may not necessarily be clear-cut or intuitive, further supporting the application of restraint in assigning causal pathways. Other factors may play important roles in the development of postdisaster psychopathology and may even overshadow the effects of disaster exposure. Dose-response models predict greater posttraumatic responses in direct proportion to severity of trauma exposure, but these relationships are apparently not especially robust or straightforward, because they have not always been consistently and significantly demonstrated in studies examining them.[29,49–51] Furthermore, considerable inter-individual variability is apparent, with some highly exposed individuals reporting few psychological effects, yet other minimally exposed or even unexposed individuals reporting many PTSD symptoms.

Because the posttraumatic response does not manifest in perfect correspondence with exposure to trauma, it is prudent to remain circumspect in the operationalization of the definition of PTSD with regard to etiology. To assume causality in defining PTSD in the context of a traumatic event diverges from the traditional approach in diagnostic nomenclature since the introduction of *DSM-III* to follow “a descriptive approach that attempted to be neutral with respect to theories of etiology” (p. xxvi)[44] and creates problems for psychiatric nosology. Unwarranted conclusions about etiology can be avoided by specifying simply that a traumatic event is temporally associated with the psychiatric syndrome that follows, without invoking specific causality.[26] *DSM-IV-TR* has accomplished this in its definition of PTSD:

> The essential feature of posttraumatic stress disorder is the *development of* characteristic symptoms *following exposure* to an extreme traumatic stressor (emphasis added) (p. 463).[44]

Following this agnostic approach discourages premature assumption of causal relationships, encourages testing of causal hypotheses with empirical data, and circumvents reliance on unsupported conjecture and personal conviction to explain relationships among related variables. Accepting the temporal and contextual association of the traumatic exposure and subsequent posttraumatic symptoms without the burden of causal assumptions also promotes exploration of causal relationships beyond constraints of simple linear pathways dictated by etiologic definitions of diagnosis.[26,40]

Restraint in assignment of causal links applies to other psychiatric disorders as well as to PTSD in association with trauma exposure. Such restraint allowed Breslau's group to empirically examine potential causal pathways in the observed co-occurrence of substance use disorders and PTSD among people who have experienced trauma.[52] Their investigation found that although trauma exposure, PTSD, and substance use disorders occurred in association with one another, trauma exposure did not lead to substance abuse directly and was therefore not determined to represent a direct causal risk factor for substance use disorders. The association between PTSD and substance use disorders was best explained either by PTSD playing a causal role for substance abuse or by shared vulnerability factors other than trauma exposure for both disorders.

The world of disaster research was much simpler before the terrorist attacks of September 11, 2001, but even prior to the 9/11 terrorist attacks and the subsequent anthrax attacks, the relationships between trauma exposure and subsequent mental health issues were far from straightforward and incompletely characterized. The new post-9/11 era of disaster mental health brought novel complexities and challenges to this field of research requiring new ways of conceptualizing disaster mental health issues and innovations in research methods.

New Complexities for Defining Traumatic Exposure in a Post-9/11 World

In previous decades, research examining psychosocial effects of disasters largely focused on directly exposed survivors and bereaved family members. This research assembled a wealth of epidemiologic data describing types, frequencies, and predictors of mental health problems in survivor populations.[1,2] Before the Oklahoma City bombing of 1995 and especially before the terrorist attacks of September 11, 2001, disaster research proceeded with relative bliss in its examination of populations with unambiguous exposure status. In the era before the advent of these large-scale terrorist events of unprecedented magnitude on American soil, it was usually abundantly clear that people either were or were not exposed to a disaster in settings of natural disasters, technological accidents, and smaller-scale intentional incidents involving attacks with conventional weapons such as mass shootings and bombings. In those events, people not directly exposed themselves and not suffering the loss of a loved one in the event would hardly be considered victims at risk for psychopathology due to the disaster.

The September 11, 2001, attacks established a watershed in the conceptualization of exposure in disaster research.[6,53,54] Attempting to draw the lines of exposure in the September 11, 2001 attacks was an uncertain and complicated endeavor. People throughout the New York City area observed the horrific events unfolding—planes hitting the towers, the burning/smoking towers, and the towers falling—from vantage points throughout Manhattan and distances of several miles away. Additionally, the media brought images of the attacks and the ensuing catastrophic events into the lives of people all over the US and the world—almost immediately, and repeatedly in ensuing hours and days. Many of these media images were close-up and graphic, such as footage of trapped WTC workers waving distress signals from windows and victims leaping to their deaths from the towering twin infernos.

Millions of people not directly exposed to the September 11 attacks in the classic sense of the *DSM-IV-TR* trauma exposure criterion for PTSD learned of the unfolding events from media broadcasts and word of mouth. Concerns were aired that many or even most of these people would be potentially vulnerable to negative mental health sequelae. In this environment, formal efforts were made to anticipate numbers of psychiatric casualties and extent of need for mental health services.[53] Broader populations—not limited to New York City area residents, but also populations learning of the events as they unfolded throughout the US and the world—were assessed for potential mental health effects in ensuing research studies.[55–63] Mental health effects on these extended populations were reported in numbers unrivaled by research findings from any other disaster in documented world history. Authorities were quickly alerted for potential for widespread and devastating mental health consequences of this unprecedented large-scale attack on American citizens.

Research had not previously had occasion to address a disaster of this magnitude and the mental health sequelae on such large populations, creating a gap in expertise needed to address the immediate situation.[53] The extent of previous disaster research and customary methods of assessment of PTSD could not begin to address the complexities of exposure and its relation to posttraumatic sequelae confronting early efforts to estimate the extent of mental health effects of the 9/11 attacks. These issues arose from features unique to the 9/11 attacks: the unparalleled scope and magnitude of the attacks coupled with the heinous, intentional nature of the terrorist acts. In this disaster, people well outside of the traditional boundaries for direct or even indirect exposure to it may have felt vulnerable to unknown near-future and distant dangers of possible further terrorist attacks potentially aimed at them, as well as very upset over what had happened in the sites directly attacked.[64]

Disaster mental health researchers had not previously had occasion to consider the broad extent of emotional responses to such a massive disaster on populations not exposed in ways described in more "ordinary" past disasters with relatively clear-cut boundaries of exposure. After the 9/11 attacks, disaster researchers routinely began to consider populations with little or no direct personal exposure to imminent danger or direct connection to the disaster as potentially vulnerable to mental health effects, and the nation's population was surveyed for posttraumatic symptoms.[56–58,63] A fundamental difficulty of post-9/11 research was, therefore, defining disaster exposure and affected populations.

Disaster research is ordinarily difficult to conduct, but research in the early post-9/11 period faced extraordinary logistical difficulties.[53,54,65–67] An immediate barrier was that the most highly exposed population was not readily accessible for systematic sampling. Therefore, early research sampled residents of Manhattan and surrounding areas through random-digit-dial methods.[55,68,69] Although more than one-third of this Manhattan area population sample reported that they had witnessed the attacks directly ("in person"), only 13% of the sample had experienced the attacks from south of Canal street (within about 0.7 mile of the WTC complex) and only 10 of 1,570 participants (0.6% of the sample) were in the WTC complex at the time.[55,68,69] Most of those who "directly witnessed" the attacks, therefore, were among the masses throughout the New York City area with a visual line of sight of the burning towers from distances as far as many miles away. Approximately 6% of the sample had "symptoms consistent with PTSD" (i.e., reporting symptoms similar to those described in *DSM-IV* symptom criteria B, C, and D for PTSD), and those who said they "directly witnessed" the attacks were about twice as likely as others to have such symptoms.[68] In this study, PTSD symptoms, therefore, were described in a population largely without disaster exposure as conceptualized in traditional pre-9/11 disaster research.

People across the New York City area and in the Washington, DC region understandably may have considered themselves in danger during the 9/11 attacks and afterward.[64] As information spread about additional potential threats to other parts of the country, a palpable sense of vulnerability gripped the nation. Would we now be a nation of PTSD-afflicted people in the post-9/11 era? In a national study of U.S. adults conducted 3–5 days after 9/11, "substantial stress symptoms" were reported by 44% and "stress symptoms" by 90%, as rated on a questionnaire that queried the five most common PTSD symptoms among Oklahoma City bombing survivors.[56] In another study, the prevalence of "probable PTSD" (defined as exceeding a self-report posttraumatic symptom screening scale threshold) 1–2 months after 9/11 was 11% in New York City, 3% in Washington, DC, and 4% in the rest of the country including locations as far away as Houston and Los Angeles.[57] Another nationwide study reported that 17% of the U.S. population outside New York City had "symptoms of September 11-related posttraumatic stress" (on a self-report posttraumatic symptom scale with items fitted to *DSM-IV* symptom criteria B, C, and D for PTSD) at 2 months, diminishing to 6% by 6 months after the attacks.[58] In these national samples of people far away from the direct exposure zone, the posttraumatic symptoms assessed did not appear to be linked to qualifying exposures.

Interpreting the findings from these 9/11 studies requires cautious circumspection about the implications of relationships between amount of emotional upset and exposure to the disaster. The degree to which individuals are upset—or even horrified—by a traumatic event is not a valid indicator of their exposure to it. Being upset or horrified over a trauma and being exposed to trauma are two different entities. Some people without any direct or indirect exposure to a disaster occurring elsewhere may describe themselves as very upset about it and may report symptoms related to it. In this situation, the trauma experienced by direct victims represents to those unexposed not a trauma, but a stressor. Learning about trauma encountered by strangers, such as through media reports or word of mouth, is different from having direct exposure to a qualifying event for the diagnosis of PTSD. Among unrelated people, learning about other people's trauma would constitute a stressor rather than a trauma.

Posttraumatic symptoms among individuals not exposed (either directly through their own experience or indirectly through the experience of a loved one) to a disaster are inconsistent with established criteria for PTSD. Responses of individuals not personally exposed to a monumental disaster likely represent emotional distress to the event, and if most of the population after such a massive trauma experiences emotional upset, then it would be considered normative distress among individuals who are understandably upset over the events of the day.[58] Alternatively, such posttraumatic responses could represent symptoms of other disorders or problems related to preexisting difficulties or to other stressors related to the 9/11 attacks, such as financial difficulties following the 9/11 attacks in an economically stressed post-9/11 environment. The majority of people directly exposed to a traumatic event who do not meet criteria for a psychiatric disorder such as PTSD might also have symptom responses not meeting criteria for a psychiatric diagnosis that could be considered emotional distress, and if most people have such reactions, this distress might be considered normative. These distinctions are important, because the interventions needed for psychiatric disorders may differ in important ways from interventions needed for distress. Inappropriate pathologization of normative responses to traumatic events is not ultimately helpful to those who are distressed but not psychiatrically ill.

Conclusions

The understanding of mental health responses to disasters reached a new level of complexity after the 9/11 attacks. Psychiatric illness and symptoms, especially PTSD, in association with disasters requires careful consideration of the causal pathways in the observed relationships. The approach to assessment of populations after disasters requires thoughtful consideration of exposure. People without sufficient exposure to a traumatic event, even a massive event of national significance, may be distressed by it, but by definition they cannot have PTSD or posttraumatic symptoms related to an event to which they were not themselves actually exposed either directly or indirectly through loved ones. Among those who were exposed, not all symptoms necessarily represent psychopathology, and research must differentiate distress from psychopathology in these groups. When psychiatric disorders such as PTSD follow exposure to disaster, the causal relationships between trauma exposure and subsequent psychopathology are so complex that simple two-variable unidirectional models from exposure to mental health sequelae cannot adequately address them.

Three major implications of these considerations apply to disaster research methods. First, research investigations must determine ways to more definitively assess exposures and link symptoms to those exposures in sorting out the mental health effects of major disasters. Further research is needed to clarify what combination of types of events and degree of exposure will yield the most homogenous syndrome with consistent clinical characteristics, familial patterns, biological correlates, and longitudinal stability required for validation of the diagnostic criteria for PTSD.[26] Second, among those exposed, subdiagnostic distress must be differentiated from major psychiatric illness such as PTSD in determining the mental health effects of disaster exposure.[54] Third, among those with psychiatric illness following exposure to disaster, caution in assignment of causal relationships is warranted until all causal pathways and directions are examined in models incorporating all relevant variables.

Acknowledgments

This research was supported by the VA North Texas Health Care System and by National Institute of Mental Health (NIMH) Grant MH68853 to Dr. North. Points of view in this document are those of the authors and do not necessarily represent the official position of NIMH, the Department of Veterans Affairs, or the U.S. Government. The author gratefully acknowledges the efforts of Rebecca P. Smith, MD, Alina M. Surís, PhD, and Barry A. Hong, PhD, who reviewed and commented on earlier drafts of this manuscript.

References

1. Norris, F. H., Friedman, M. J., Watson, P. J., Byrne, C. M., Diaz, E., & Kaniasty, K. (2002). 60,000 disaster victims speak: Part I. An empirical review of the empirical literature, 1981–2001. *Psychiatry*, *65*(3), 207–239.

2. Norris, F. H., Friedman, M. J., & Watson, P. J. (2002). 60,000 disaster victims speak: Part II. Summary and implications of the disaster mental health research. *Psychiatry, 65*(3), 240–260.
3. Breslau, N., Davis, G. C., & Andreski, A. (1995). Risk factors for PTSD-related traumatic events: A prospective analysis. *Am J Psychiatry, 152*(4), 529–535.
4. Breslau, N., Davis, G. C., Andreski, P., & Peterson, E. (1991). Traumatic events and posttraumatic stress disorder in an urban population of young adults. *Arch Gen Psychiatry, 48*(3), 216–222.
5. Breslau, N. (1998). Epidemiology of trauma and posttraumatic stress disorder. In R. Yehuda, (Ed.). *Psychological trauma* (pp. 1–29). Washington, DC: American Psychiatric Press.
6. North, C. S. (2007). Epidemiology of disaster mental health response. In R. J. Ursano, C. S. Fullerton, L. Weisæth, et al., (Eds.). *Textbook of disaster psychiatry* (pp. 29–47). New York: Cambridge University Press.
7. Hasin, D. S., Keyes, K. M., Hatzenbuehler, M. L., Aharonovich, E. A., & Alderson, D. (2007). Alcohol consumption and posttraumatic stress after exposure to terrorism: Effects of proximity, loss, and psychiatric history. *Am J Public Health, 97*(12), 2268–2275.
8. North, C. S., Nixon, S. J., Shariat, S., Mallonee, S., McMillen, J. C., Spitznagel, E. L., et al. (1999). Psychiatric disorders among survivors of the Oklahoma City bombing. *JAMA, 282*(8), 755–762.
9. North, C. S. (2004). Psychiatric effects of disasters and terrorism: Empirical basis from study of the Oklahoma City bombing. In J. M. Gorman, (Ed.). *Fear and anxiety: The benefits of translational research* (pp. 105–117). Washington, DC: American Psychiatric Publishing.
10. North, C. S., Surís, A. M., & Adewuyi, S. (2009). PTSD and psychiatric comorbidities (in press). In D. Benedek & G. H. Wynne, (Eds.). *Clinical manual for the management of posttraumatic stress disorder*. Washington, DC: American Psychiatric Press.
11. North, C. S., Hong, B. A., & Pfefferbaum, B. (2008). P-FLASH: Development of an empirically-based post-9/11 disaster mental health training program. *Mo Med, 105*(1), 62–66.
12. North, C. S., King, R. V., Fowler, R. L., Polatin, P., Smith, R. P., LaGrone, A., et al. (2008). Psychiatric disorders among transported hurricane evacuees: Acute-phase findings in a large receiving shelter site. *Psychiat Ann, 38*(2), 104–113.
13. Joseph, S., Yule, W., Williams, R., & Hodgkinson, P. (1993). Increased substance use in survivors of the Herald of Free Enterprise disaster. *Br J Med Psychol, 66*(2), 185–191.
14. McFarlane, A. C. (1998). Epidemiological evidence about the relationship between PTSD and alcohol abuse: The nature of the association. *Addict Behav, 23*(6), 813–825.
15. Pfefferbaum, B. & Doughty, D. E. (2001). Increased alcohol use in a treatment sample of Oklahoma City bombing victims. *Psychiatry, 64*(4), 296–303.
16. Sims, A. & Sims, D. (1998). The phenomenology of post-traumatic stress disorder. A symptomatic study of 70 victims of psychological trauma. *Psychopathol, 31*(2), 96–112.
17. Smith, D. W., Christiansen, E. H., Vincent, R., & Hann, N. E. (1999). Population effects of the bombing of Oklahoma City. *Journal of the Oklahoma State Medical Association, 92*(4), 193–198.
18. Vlahov, D., Galea, S., Ahern, J., Resnick, H., & Kilpatrick, D. (2004). Sustained increased consumption of cigarettes, alcohol, and marijuana among Manhattan residents after September 11, 2001. *Am J Publ Health, 94*(2), 253–254.

19. Reference deleted in text.
20. North, C. S., Kawasaki, A., Spitznagel, E. L., & Hong, B. A. (2004). The course of PTSD, major depression, substance abuse, and somatization after a natural disaster. *J Nerv Ment Dis, 192*(12), 823–829.
21. North, C. S. (2003). Somatization in survivors of catastrophic trauma: A methodologic review. *Envir Health Pers, 110*(Suppl 4), 637–640.
22. Robins, L. N., Fishbach, R. L., Smith, E. M., Cottler, L. B., Solomon, S. D., & Goldring, E. (1986). Impact of disaster on previously assessed mental health. In J. H. Shore, (Ed.). *Disaster stress studies: New methods and findings* (pp. 22–48). Washington, DC: American Psychiatric Association.
23. Escobar, J. I., Canino, G., Rubio-Stipec, M., & Bravo, M. (1992). Somatic symptoms after a natural disaster: A prospective study. *Am J Psychiatry, 149,* 965–967.
24. Bravo, M., Rubio-Stipec, M., Canino, G. J., Woodbury, M. A., & Ribera, J. C. (1990). The psychological sequelae of disaster stress prospectively and retrospectively evaluated. *Am J Comm Psychol, 18,* 661–680.
25. Canino, G., Bravo, M., Rubio-Stipec, M., & Woodbury, M. (1990). The impact of disaster on mental health: Prospective and retrospective analyses. *Int J Ment Health, 19,* 51–69.
26. North, C. S., Surís, A. M., Davis, M., & Smith, R. P. (2009). Toward validation of the diagnosis of posttraumatic stress disorder. *Am J Psychiatry, 166*(1), 1–8.
27. Weathers, F. W. & Keane, T. M. (2007). The Criterion A problem revisited: Controversies and challenges in defining and measuring psychological trauma. *J Trauma Stress, 20*(2), 107–121.
28. Weathers, F. W. & Keane, T. M. (2007). The crucial role of Criterion A: A response to Maier's commentary. *J Trauma Stress, 20*(5), 917–919.
29. McNally, R. J. (2003). Progress and controversy in the study of posttraumatic stress disorder. *Annu Rev Psychol, 54,* 229–252.
30. Maier, T. (2007). Weathers' and Keane's, "The criterion A problem revisited: Controversies and challenges in defining and measuring psychological trauma." *J Trauma Stress, 20*(5), 915–916.
31. Spitzer, R. L., First, M. B., & Wakefield, J. C. (2007). Saving PTSD from itself in DSM-V. *J Anxiety Disord, 21*(2), 233–241.
32. Dreman, S. (1991). Coping with the trauma of divorce. *J Trauma Stress, 4*(1), 113–121.
33. Scott, M. J. & Stradling, S. G. (1994). Post-traumatic stress disorder without the trauma. *Br J Clin Psychol, 33*(Pt 1), 71–74.
34. Czarnocka, J. & Slade, P. (2000). Prevalence and predictors of post-traumatic stress symptoms following childbirth. *Br J Clin Psychol, 39*(Pt 1), 35–51.
35. Ayers, S. & Pickering, A. D. (2001). Do women get posttraumatic stress disorder as a result of childbirth? A prospective study of incidence. *Birth, 28*(2), 111–118.
36. Rosen, G. M. (2005). Traumatic events, criterion creep, and the creation of pretraumatic stress disorder. *Scientific Review of Mental Health Practice, 3,* 39–42.
37. Green, B. L. (1990). Defining trauma: Terminology and generic stressor dimensions. *J Appl Soc Psychol, 20*(2), 1632–1641.
38. Solomon, S. D. & Canino, G. J. (1990). Appropriateness of DSM-III-R criteria for post-traumatic stress disorder. *Compr Psychiatry, 31,* 227–237.
39. Resnick, H. S., Kilpatrick, D. G., Dansky, B. S., Saunders, B. E., & Best, C. L. (1993). Prevalence of civilian trauma and posttraumatic stress disorder in a representative national sample of women. *J Consult Clin Psychol, 61*(6), 984–991.
40. Maier, T. (2006). Post-traumatic stress disorder revisited: Deconstructing the A-criterion. *Med Hypotheses, 66*(1), 103–106.

41. Breslau, N., Chase, G. A., & Anthony, J. C. (2002). The uniqueness of the DSM definition of post-traumatic stress disorder: Implications for research. *Psychol Med, 32*(4), 573–576.
42. Breslau, N. (2002). Epidemiologic studies of trauma, posttraumatic stress disorder, and other psychiatric disorders. *Can J Psychiatry, 47*(10), 923–929.
43. Nemeroff, C. B., Bremner, J. D., Foa, E. B., Mayberg, H. S., North, C. S., & Stein, M. B. (2006). Posttraumatic stress disorder: A state-of-the-science review. *J Psychiatr Res, 40*(1), 1–21.
44. American Psychiatric Association. (2000). *Diagnostic and statistical manual of mental disorders.* 4th, Text Revision ed. Washington, DC: American Psychiatric Association.
45. Greenough PG, Lappi MD, Hsu EB, Fink S, Hsieh YH, Vu A, et al. (2008). Burden of disease and health status among Hurricane Katrina-displaced persons in shelters: A population-based cluster sample. *Ann Emerg Med, 51*(4), 426–432.
46. Cottler, L. B., Compton, W. M., Mager, D., Spitznagel, E. L., & Janca, A. (1992). Posttraumatic stress disorder among substance users from the general population. *Am J Psychiatry, 149*(5), 664–670.
47. Cottler, L. B., Nishith, P., & Compton, W. M., III. (2001). Gender differences in risk factors for trauma exposure and post-traumatic stress disorder among inner-city drug abusers in and out of treatment. *Compr Psychiatry, 42*(2), 111–117.
48. Johnson, S. D., Striley, C., & Cottler, L. B. (2006). The association of substance use disorders with trauma exposure and PTSD among African American drug users. *Addict Behav, 31*(11), 2063–2073.
49. Bowman, M. L. (1999). Individual differences in posttraumatic distress: Problems with the DSM-IV model. *Can J Psychiatry, 44*(1), 21–33.
50. Schnyder, U., Moergeli, H., Klaghofer, R., & Buddeberg, C. (2001). Incidence and prediction of posttraumatic stress disorder symptoms in severely injured accident victims. *Am J Psychiatry, 158*(4), 594–599.
51. Basoglu, M., Paker, M., Paker, O., Ozmen, E., Marks, I., Incesu, C., et al. (1994). Psychological effects of torture: A comparison of tortured with nontortured political activists in Turkey. *Am J Psychiatry, 151*(1), 76–81.
52. Breslau, N., Davis, G. C., & Schultz, L. R. (2003). Posttraumatic stress disorder and the incidence of nicotine, alcohol, and other drug disorders in persons who have experienced trauma. *Arch Gen Psychiatry, 60*(3), 289–294.
53. North, C. S. (2004). Approaching disaster mental health research after the 9/11 World Trade Center terrorist attacks. *Psychiatr Clin North Am, 27*(3), 589–602.
54. North, C. S. & Pfefferbaum, B. (2002). Research on the mental health effects of terrorism. *JAMA, 288*(5), 633–636.
55. Galea, S., Resnick, H., Ahern, J., Gold, J., Bucuvalas, M., Kilpatrick, D., et al. (2002). Posttraumatic stress disorder in Manhattan, New York City, after the September 11th terrorist attacks. *J Urban Health, 79*(3), 340–353.
56. Schuster, M. A., Stein, B. D., Jaycox, L., Collins, R. L., Marshall, G. N., Elliott, M. N., et al. (2001). A national survey of stress reactions after the September 11, 2001, terrorist attacks. *N Engl J Med, 345*(20), 1507–1512.
57. Schlenger, W. E., Caddell, J. M., Ebert, L., Jordan, B. K., Rourke, K. M., Wilson, D., et al. (2002). Psychological reactions to terrorist attacks:Findings from the National Study of Americans' Reactions to September 11. *JAMA, 288*, 581–588.

58. Silver, R. C., Holman, E. A., McIntosh, D. N., Poulin, M., & Gil-Rivas, V. (2002). Nationwide longitudinal study of psychological responses to September 11. *JAMA, 288*(10), 1235–1244.
59. Matt, G. E. & Vazquez, C. (2008). Anxiety, depressed mood, self-esteem, and traumatic stress symptoms among distant witnesses of the 9/11 terrorist attacks: Transitory responses and psychological resilience. *Span J Psychol, 11*(2), 503–515.
60. MacGeorge, E. L., Samter, W., Feng, B., Gillihan, S. J., & Graves, A. R. (2007). After 9/11: Goal disruption, emotional support, and psychological health in a lower exposure sample. *Health Commun, 21*(1), 11–22.
61. Otto, M. W., Henin, A., Hirshfeld-Becker, D. R., Pollack, M. H., Biederman, J., & Rosenbaum, J. F. (2007). Posttraumatic stress disorder symptoms following media exposure to tragic events: Impact of 9/11 on children at risk for anxiety disorders. *J Anxiety Disord, 21*(7), 888–902.
62. Delahanty, D. L. (2007). Are we prepared to handle the mental health consequences of terrorism? *Am J Psychiatry, 164*(2), 189–191.
63. Laugharne, J., Janca, A., & Widiger, T. (2007). Posttraumatic stress disorder and terrorism: 5 years after 9/11. *Curr Opin Psychiatry, 20*(1), 36–41.
64. DeLisi, L. E., Maurizio, A., Yost, M., Papparozzi, C. F., Fulchino, C., Katz, C. L., et al. (2003). A survey of New Yorkers after the Sept. 11, 2001, terrorist attacks. *Am J Psychiatry, 160*(4), 780–783.
65. Smith, E. M. (1996). Coping with the challenges of field research. In E. B. Carlson, (Ed.). *Trauma research methodology* (pp. 126–152). Lutherville, MD: Sidran.
66. North, C. S., Pfefferbaum, B., & Tucker, P. (2002). Ethical and methodological issues in academic mental health research in populations affected by disasters: The Oklahoma City experience relevant to September 11, 2001. *CNS Spectr, 7*(8), 580–584.
67. North, C. S. & Pfefferbaum, B. (2004). The state of research on the mental health effects of terrorism. *Epidemiol Psichiatr Soc, 13*(1), 4–9.
68. Galea, S., Ahern, J., Resnick, H., Kilpatrick, D., Bucuvalas, M., Gold, J., et al. (2002). Psychological sequelae of the September 11 terrorist attacks in New York City. *N Engl J Med, 346*(13), 982–987.
69. Galea, S., Vlahov, D., Resnick, H., Ahern, J., Susser, E., Gold, J., et al. (2003). Trends of probable post-traumatic stress disorder in New York City after the September 11 terrorist attacks. *Am J Epidemiol, 158*(6), 514–524.

7

Addiction to Drugs, Food, Gambling, Sex, and Technology

Shared Causal Mechanisms?

MARK S. GOLD, LISA J. MERLO, ADRIE W. BRUIJNZEEL, ANNA ROYTBERG, AND MICHAEL HERKOV

Introduction

Substances including alcohol, tobacco, cocaine, cannabis, and other drugs can cause changes to the brain and behavior of the user, leading to a clinical state that is popularly known as "addiction." Various factors may affect the transition from first use of a substance to dependence; however, the end result appears fairly consistent across users. Individuals of any age, race, gender, income, or education level appear remarkably similar when describing their thoughts, feelings, and behaviors related to addiction. Research has demonstrated that substances of abuse "hijack" the brain and serve as a melting pot to produce a stereotypical addictive state, with intrusive thoughts about the drugs, cravings, perseveration, pervasive and powerful drives for the drug(s), and use that often continues until loss of health, family, and/or job, or until a serious accident or death. The leading causes of death in the United States are related to alcohol and drug use, tobacco smoke exposure, and behavioral addictions. Each year, approximately 435,000 Americans die as a result of smoking and second hand smoke exposure and 85,000 die of alcohol abuse.[1]

Drugs of abuse have been extremely well studied in laboratory animals for many years. The addicted rat is a well-known model,[2] and studies have helped to explain the complex neurobiology of addiction. However, there are limitations to animal models and extrapolations. Significant individual differences exist among humans with regard to drug experimentation, drug(s) of choice, susceptibility to addiction, prognosis following intervention, and likelihood of relapse. As a result, for more than a century, clinicians have struggled to adequately evaluate and treat patients dependent on opiates, alcohol, cannabis, and other substances. However, in the past few decades there have been notable advances in basic, translational, and clinical research that have improved efforts at prevention and treatment of addiction. The most striking changes have resulted from the emergence of reliable animal models, neuroscientific investigations of drugs' effects on neurotransmitters and pathways, and neuroimaging examining the interaction between drugs and the brain.

Research has also extended to the exploration of other potentially addictive processes. Whereas most addiction studies originally focused specifically on the use of chemical substances, more studies are beginning to focus on behavioral processes (e.g., overeating, hypersexuality, pathological gambling, and excessive use of technology) that demonstrate significant parallels with chemical addiction. In one of the earliest examples, researchers demonstrated the role of classical conditioning in driving both drug-taking and eating behaviors. Faust showed that a nonhuman primate would associate an investigator's cabinet opening with the provision of morphine and Pavlov demonstrated that a dog would associate a bell with provision of food.[3–5]

Though Pavlov understood the similarities between drugs and food, many current experts have been resistant to the notion of behavioral process addictions. But, following decades of progress in addiction neurobiology and theory, there is evidence to suggest that the addiction process is remarkably similar across stimuli. The data are compelling in some cases and suggestive in others, but the debate has been colored by the fear that the "disease" status currently applied to drug addiction might be lost as behavioral processes are considered addictive.

Neurobiology

Basic Neurobiology of Addiction

In the last few decades, much research has focused on the role of the brain reward system in the development of substance abuse and dependence. Specific components (e.g., the nucleus accumbens [NAcc], the ventral tegmental area [VTA], and the neurotransmitter dopamine [DA]), have been highlighted as key contributors to the addiction process. The brain dopaminergic system has been shown to play an important role in signaling reward and establishing stimulus-reward associations.[6–10] Food intake, drug intake, gambling, and sexual behavior increase dopamine release in the striatum and dopamine receptor antagonists prevent these behaviors.[11–16] More recently, research has examined the extent to which other behaviors (e.g., eating, sexual behavior, and gambling) are also regulated through this reward circuitry.

The Role of Dopamine in Addiction

Early cocaine research focused on DA as a major incentive for continued use of substances despite associated consequences. For example, cocaine causes increases in DA, which lead to euphoria and a sense of accomplishment. Indeed, the concept of "cocaine satiety" is viewed as an oxymoron for both laboratory animals and human users. Cocaine-related research first provided basic and clinical scientists with a focus on the drive for the drug, self administration, and loss of control, by studying the role of dopamine within the NAcc. The eventual inclusion of cocaine as a potential substance of abuse forever changed addiction research, theory, nosology, and neurobiology.[17] However, morphine, cannabis, nicotine, and ethanol administration also result in increased dopamine release in the NAcc.[18,19]

While we should not trivialize addiction to a dopamine-centric model, all drugs of abuse are now understood to have consistent effects on dopamine. Indeed, the most consistent finding across neurobiological studies of addiction has been anticipation-related, self-administration-related, and abstinence-related dopamine (DA) release in the NAcc and its relationship to the addictive process. As mentioned previously, in rodent models, craving for cocaine correlates with NAcc activity.[20] Increased DA levels are associated with the initiation of drug-seeking behavior (i.e., lever pressing), while participation in drug-seeking behavior leads to further increases in dopamine level.[21] Similarly, intravenous morphine and cannabinoid administration lead to increased DA release in the NAcc,[22] and injection of nicotine into the NAcc coincides with increased extracellular levels of dopamine.[23,24] Self-administration of ethanol is associated with increased levels of extracellular DA,[25] even at low doses.[26] In addition, human studies utilizing PET scan technology have demonstrated that oral administration of alcohol results in increased extracellular DA levels.[27]

Other Neurobiological Components Associated with Addiction

Chemical addiction is a complicated process, yet the role of dopamine does not fully explain it. Drug addiction can be defined by a compulsion to seek and take drugs, a loss of control in limiting intake, and the emergence of a negative emotional state when access to the drug is prevented. This negative emotional state is hypothesized to derive from dysregulation of key neurochemical elements, related to the experiences of reward and stress, within the basal forebrain structures (e.g., ventral striatum and extended amygdala). Extensive evidence points toward an important role for the neuropeptide corticotropin releasing factor (CRF) in the negative mood state associated with drug withdrawal and stress-induced reinstatement of drug-seeking behavior. Withdrawal from drugs of abuse mediates an increased release of CRF in subregions of the extended amygdala. Withdrawal from alcohol,[28] cannabis,[29] cocaine,[30] and nicotine[31] have been shown to induce an increased release of CRF in the central nucleus of the amygdala (CeA). Discontinuation of chronic alcohol administration increases extracellular CRF levels in the bed nucleus of the stria terminalis and CRF levels return to baseline levels with alcohol intake.[32] Preclinical evidence suggests that an elevated CRF transmission during drug withdrawal contributes to heightened anxiety. Alcohol withdrawal-induced increased anxiety-like behavior in the elevated plus maze can be reversed by the administration of the nonspecific CRF1/2 receptor antagonist α-helical CRF in the lateral ventricles[33] or the CeA.[34] CRF transmission may also mediate the negative mood states associated with drug withdrawal. We reported that pretreatment with the nonspecific CRF1/2 receptor antagonist D-Phe CRF or the specific CRF1 receptor antagonist R278995/CRA0450 prevents the elevations in brain reward thresholds (e.g., dysphoric state) associated with nicotine withdrawal.[35,36]

Two recent studies investigated the role of CRF1 receptors in the negative mood state associated with morphine withdrawal. It was shown that both antagonism of CRF1 receptors in rats with the specific CRF1 receptor antagonist antalarmin and genetic deletion of the CRF1 receptor in mice prevent morphine withdrawal-induced conditioned place aversion.[37,38] Research by Heilig and colleagues reported that antagonism of CRF1 receptors with the CRF1 receptor antagonist MTIP attenuates alcohol-withdrawal-induced anxiety-like behavior, stress-induced reinstatement of alcohol-seeking behavior, and excessive alcohol consumption in alcohol-dependent animals.[39] Extensive evidence also points toward an important role for GABAergic and glutamatergic transmission in drug addiction. Drugs that increase GABAergic transmission and/or decrease glutamatergic transmission have been suggested to attenuate the rewarding effects of drugs of abuse.[40] Therefore, novel treatments that modulate CRF, dopamine, glutamate, or GABA transmission may be potential novel treatments for drug addiction.

Commonalities in Addiction Neurobiology

It is understandable why a common neurobiology for addiction to drugs has been identified. Despite varying acute effects, the long-term behavioral effects of chemical addiction are remarkably similar across substances. As mentioned previously, several components of the neurological reward system, including the nucleus accumbens, the ventral tegmental area, and the neurotransmitters (particularly dopamine) have been implicated in virtually all chemical addictions and across species.

Within animal models, chemical "addiction" results from repeated self-administration of a drug. Researchers observe the neurobiological changes that occur over time, and this has led to the understanding of basic neurobiological processes that are associated with addiction. Observing animals' self-administration patterns for drugs of abuse, variability in brain reward thresholds, development of conditioned place preference, and responses to conditioned cues has led to the norepinephrine–locus coeruleus hyperactivity theory for drug withdrawal,[41,42] and the invention of the use of clonidine as well as the dopamine depletion theory of cocaine addiction-drug withdrawal anhedonia.[43] As the basic science models have improved, so too has human research. Advances in the fields of neurobiology and neuroimaging, proteomics, nanotechnology, pharmacology, and behavioral research have all greatly impacted the addiction field. For example, with the advent of PET and fMRI studies in humans,[44] animal work was confirmed and extended. Moving forward, research to discover the characteristics of drugs and alcohol that lead to addiction should be the gold standard against which to determine which behaviors are "addictive."

Limitations of Current Knowledge

Despite the many advances in knowledge, much remains unknown regarding addiction to both chemicals and behavioral processes. It is not simply that drugs hijack the brain and cause addiction in people like lab animals. Developmental neurobiology, genetic factors, and early environment all appear critical.[45]

Every translational research model has limitations. A rat is not a human. They have similar meso-cortico-limbic systems and neurotransmitters, but a perfunctory look at their brain suggests that human abuse and addiction will be different from that seen in rats. It is difficult to model the use of cocaine or methamphetamine for sexual enhancement, or the use of tobacco for weight loss in the laboratory. A rat model for tobacco smoking has not generally been employed, and scientists have defined the addiction, withdrawal, and relapse pathways by injecting animals with nicotine. Since pharmaceutical nicotine abuse rarely occurs, and smoking tobacco involves inhalation of vapors with liberation of hundreds of active drugs and chemicals, it is hard to argue that this model adequately captures the human disease. Similarly for alcohol, most animal models have required tricking an animal with sugar or sweeteners added to the alcohol, or administering alcohol with feeding tubes. In this case, it is hard to argue that an essential element of alcohol abuse and dependence has been eliminated from the model. Without goal-directed or volitional behavior, perhaps the brain and behavior changes observed in laboratory animals are associated with the experience of repeated intoxication against the animal's will. Still, even the tobacco and alcohol models have helped us define the neurochemistry and pathways involved in reinforcement, abstinence, and reinstatement.[46,47]

Cocaine and heroin models may more closely approximate the human experience, as animals will readily self-administer these drugs. However, pharmacological factors (e.g., route of administration) are also important. Indeed, the same drug can be used by the same person with an entirely different result. For example, chewing on a coca leaf is very different from snorting cocaine powder or smoking crack cocaine. Similarly, nicotine is highly addictive when administered through cigarettes or smokeless tobacco. Yet, nicotine patches and gum are so unappealing that many state programs give them away. Finally, technologic inventions have also been applied to drugs of abuse, making them more reinforcing, compelling, and addicting.

Addiction Nosology and Behavioral Process Addictions

In the current version of the Diagnostic and Statistical Manual of Mental Disorders (DSM-IV-TR),[48] chemical addiction is separated into two distinct diagnoses: 1) substance dependence and 2) substance abuse. However, there remains disagreement within the field regarding the utility of separate diagnoses, and some have proposed combining the disorders into one dimensional category, restoring the label "addiction." The soon-to-be-released DSM-V includes several revisions to the definitions and types of substance-related disorders that were recognized in DSM-IV. Substance use disorder is "in" and substance dependence is "out."

The DSM-V Proposed Criteria for Substance Use Disorders

In DSM-V a substance-use disorder is defined as a maladaptive pattern of substance use leading to clinically significant impairment or distress, as manifested by two (or more) of the following, occurring within a 12-month period. 1) Recurrent substance use resulting in a failure to fulfill major role obligations at work, school, or home (e.g., repeated absences or poor work performance related to substance use; substance-related absences, suspensions, or expulsions from school; neglect of children or household). 2) Recurrent substance use in situations in which it is physically hazardous (e.g., driving an automobile or operating a machine when impaired by substance use). 3) Continued substance use despite having persistent or recurrent social or interpersonal problems caused or exacerbated by the effects of the substance (e.g., arguments with spouse about consequences of intoxication, physical fights). 4) Tolerance, as defined by either a need for markedly increased amounts of the substance to achieve intoxication/desired effect, or markedly diminished effect with continued use of the same amount of the substance. 5) Withdrawal, as manifested by either the characteristic withdrawal syndrome for the substance or the same (or a closely related) substance is taken to relieve or avoid withdrawal symptoms.

6) The substance is often taken in larger amounts or over a longer period than was intended. 7) There is a persistent desire or unsuccessful efforts to cut down or control substance use. 8) A great deal of time is spent in activities necessary to obtain the substance, use the substance, or recover from its effects. 9) Important social, occupational, or recreational activities are given up or reduced because of substance use. 10) The substance use is continued despite knowledge of having a persistent or recurrent physical or psychological problem that is likely to have been caused or exacerbated by the substance. 11) Craving or a strong desire or urge to use a specific substance. Severity specifiers, course specifiers, and physiological specifiers are also proposed (http://www.dsm5.org/ProposedRevisions/Pages/Substance-RelatedDisorders.aspx).

Similarities Between Chemical Addictions and Behavioral Process Addictions

Given that behavioral criteria are utilized to diagnose the substance use disorders, it makes intuitive sense to translate the criteria to other problematic behaviors. For example, it is easy to see parallels between the escalation of heroin use that characterizes a dependent individual and increased participation in gambling that characterizes a pathological gambler. Similarly, binge drinking and binge eating share much in common, and may even co-occur. Further, the relationship disruption that results from drug use corresponds to the relationship disruption that results from out of control sexual behavior,[49] and attempts to cut down and/or control the behavior can be seen among substance users and those who overuse technology. Indeed, each of the diagnostic criteria for substance use disorders can be adapted to fit these behaviors. This has opened the door for researchers to study overeating, hypersexuality, pathological gambling, and overuse of technology as addictive processes. The type and magnitude of evidence for these conceptualizations varies somewhat among the behaviors, but each has demonstrated some support. The common thread inherent in these disorders is that the symptoms are conditional on exposure. In other words, one cannot become a problem gambler if never exposed to gambling; a person cannot be addicted to eating if s/he never eats, and s/he cannot be dependent on technology if they never use it.

Overeating as an Addictive Behavior

Eating is a natural behavior that fills both physical and emotional needs. For most individuals, eating is pleasurable, relaxing, and restorative. Like alcohol, food can be a social lubricant, which facilitates personal and professional interactions, and is often the centerpiece of significant celebrations. People also eat (and overeat) for a variety of reasons (e.g., to alleviate hunger, to relax and enjoy themselves, to relieve anxiety[50] or grief,[51] to connect with companions, or as the result of conditioned responding to environmental cues). Indeed, obesity has become a worldwide epidemic, though this has occurred in too short a time for genetic mutation to fully account for the changes.[52] As a result, researchers and clinicians have hypothesized that changes in food processing and availability have led to the development of "hyperpalatable foods," which may actually serve as substances of abuse for some individuals.[16] Such individuals are believed to respond to these foods in much the same way that an individual suffering from chemical addiction responds to drugs of abuse.[53] Interestingly, drug abusers as well as patients who describe themselves as "food addicts" describe experiencing cravings. The object of desire is different, but the event is experienced similarly.

Given the obvious parallels, chemical addiction research has been adapted to explore the potential for "food addiction" among animal and human subjects. Indeed, addictions to food and chemical substances have been linked through personal stories, direct observation, and empirical studies.[54,55] For example, researchers have developed an animal model of food (sugar) addiction in rats that closely resembles that seen with drug addiction.[56] Hoebel and colleagues[57] reported that sugar has addictive properties similar to psychostimulants and opioids. They recently confirmed that there is evidence of sugar addiction,[58] and that sugared high-fat foods contribute most to weight gain. Excessive sugar intake may have a similar effect on the brain as the abuse of opioids. Colantuoni and colleagues demonstrated that the opioid receptor antagonist naloxone induces more somatic withdrawal signs in rats that had intermittent access to standard lab chow and glucose compared to control animals that received ad libitum lab chow.[59] Furthermore, naloxone decreased dopamine levels and increased acetylcholine levels in the NAcc shell of rats that received lab chow and glucose intermittently.[59] It is interesting to note that similar neurochemical changes have been detected in rats withdrawing from nicotine and morphine.[60,61]

These observations suggest that similar neurochemical mechanisms may play a role in craving for food and drugs of abuse. Imaging studies in humans also point to shared neurobiological mechanisms among the addictive behaviors. In addition, there are numerous behavioral similarities between overeating, obesity, and chemical addictions.[16,62]

Symptoms attributed to food addiction include continuing to overeat even though it may harm your health, family, or social life; eating in secret; feeling compelled to finish all the food in your line of sight; and even eating to the point of discomfort. As a result, it is easy to compare the subjective effects experienced by individuals with food addiction to those exhibited by individuals with chemical addiction. Further, perhaps due to a combination of genetic and environmental influences, children tend to have eating behaviors or attitudes that are similar to their parents. Merlo and colleagues observed this phenomenon in a study of overweight and obese adolescents and their parents/guardians. Self-reported symptoms of food addiction were associated with BMI ratings, emotional eating, overeating, and uncontrolled eating. Their cohort frequently self-reported symptoms of food addiction and eating attitudes and behaviors similar to their parents.[63]

Research has also demonstrated a complex interaction between consumption of food and drugs. Weight loss with drug use (including nicotine), and weight gain during abstinence from drug use are common observations and are often, at least anecdotally, linked to relapse. Indeed, treatment of addiction is associated with a rebound hyperphagia and weight gain.[64,65] Although the mechanism is poorly understood, it is widely accepted. Particularly in self-help programs it is recommended that hunger should be avoided when possible as it has been associated with relapse.[66]

Overeating and/or obesity may even serve as protective factors against substance use and abuse. Indeed, when food intake is restricted the neurobiological reward system demonstrates increased sensitivity to subsequently administered drugs. This appears to occur even when the potency of drugs administered remains constant, and the effect has been demonstrated with amphetamine, phencyclidine, and dizoclipine.[67] The interaction is believed to parallel the withdrawal-induced sensitization observed among experienced drug users. It appears that drugs of abuse and food compete in the brain for similar reinforcement pathways[68] and research has suggested that this might be particularly true in the case of highly palatable foods (e.g., sugars and fats).

It is not surprising, then, that the logos, cartoons, and trademarks associated with hyperpalatable foods become potent stimuli, automatically eliciting mental and physical approach responses.[53,69] Indeed, highly recognizable food trademarks can trigger brain changes similar to those triggered by drugs or drug paraphernalia when shown to a patient with a substance use disorder.[70] For example, Wang and colleagues,[68] using PET imaging and other techniques, showed that the brain responds to food and food-related stimuli similarly to the way in which it responds to drugs. An increase in extracellular dopamine due to food cues is accompanied by a relative lack of dopamine 2 receptors. This down-regulation, similar to that seen in cocaine or alcohol addictions, could lead to increased food seeking and an inability to control consumption. Such a relationship is also evident in those who gain weight when taking certain antipsychotics.[71,72]

From a neurochemical perspective, eating (like drug use) is associated with increases in DA within the NAcc. Rodent models have demonstrated that sucrose licking significantly increases DA levels in the NAcc, whereas water licking does not.[73] Similarly, recent research has demonstrated a parallel role of the D3 dopamine receptor for both food and drug reward-related behaviors.

Animals self administer glucose and also fructose but gain weight bingeing on fructose. Evidence for sugar and fructose "addiction" has come from the work of Hoebel and Avena, observing overeating addicts in early recovery and bariatric surgery patients who binge on chocolate, milk shakes, and alcohol. In summary, animal support includes:

- *Bingeing* on sugar during the first hour of access, with *escalation* of daily intake.[74]
- *Brain changes:* increased mu and D_1 receptor binding, increased D_3 receptor mRNA in the NAc and decreased D2 binding in the striatum.[74,75]
- *Withdrawal*: both behavioral and neurochemical signs such as anxiety, depression and ACh release with low DA,[59] *Cross-sensitization* with amphetamine,[76] and augmented ethanol intake.[77]
- *"Craving"* during abstinence that could lead to relapse: the "deprivation effect"[78] and "incubation effect."[79]

Hypersexuality as an Addictive Behavior

Interest in the concept of "sexual addiction" has increased recently, especially with high profile cases such as Tiger Woods. However, there remains significant disagreement among sexual behavior specialists regarding the conceptualization and definition of the disorder,[80] which has been referred to in the literature as sexual dependence, hypersexuality, compulsive sexual disorder, paraphilia-related disorder, sexual impulsivity, nymphomania, and out-of-control sexual behavior.[81]

The prevalence of sexual addiction is not well documented. Several factors make identification of the disorder difficult, resulting in a "hidden population" of individuals who suffer from this disorder. These factors include a pervasive societal stigma, shame or embarrassment among those affected that prevents them from seeking treatment, and a lack of a standardized diagnosis or method of assessment. Based upon the number of cases that present for treatment, it has been estimated that sexual addiction may affect between 3 and 6% of the U.S. population.[82]

In general, sexual addiction is defined as "recurrent, intense, sexually arousing fantasies, sexual urges, or behaviors that persist over a period of at least 6 months and do not fall under the definition of paraphilia."[83] It is also suggested that the symptoms must cause significant distress and impairment to the afflicted individual, in order to merit diagnosis. In general, individuals who are identified as sex addicts do not merely engage in more sexual behavior within a consensual monogamous relationship. Rather, the behaviors typically include compulsive masturbation, excessive viewing of pornography, multiple sexual experiences involving prostitutes or other sex addicts, engaging in multiple extra-marital affairs, and participating in "virtual sex" experiences via the Internet, webcam, or phone. Despite the significant personal and social consequences related to sexual addiction, much confusion remains within the field about its etiology and nosology. Additionally, there are no diagnostic criteria for sexual addiction included in the *Diagnostic and Statistical Manual of Mental Disorders, Fourth Edition.*[48]

The constellation of behaviors currently referred to as "sexual addiction" was first identified by Orford.[84,85] Later Carnes,[86–88] Goodman,[89] and Earle,[90] among others, continued and extended the work. For example, Carnes described these behaviors as addictive in nature, due to the individual's inability to adequately control his/her behavior, despite the risk of adverse consequences.[86] Robertson further supported this conceptualization by arguing that sexual behavior causes chemical changes in the brain similar to those changes caused by ingesting chemical substances.[91] Goodman[89,92] noted several similarities among individuals suffering from sexual addiction and substance abusers, and others pointed out that sex addicts often have comorbid chemical addictions.[82,93] However, still others conceptualize these behaviors as compulsive in nature, and perhaps symptomatic of an underlying obsessive-compulsive disorder, noting the recurrent distressing thoughts that accompany the repetitive behaviors.[94,95] Researchers have also reported higher rates of obsessive-compulsive disorder (OCD) among individuals who report compulsive sexual behavior.[96,97] Finally, the conceptualization of these behaviors as an impulse-control disturbance has also been considered,[98] and most individuals undergoing treatment are diagnosed, according to DSM-IV criteria, with an impulse control disorder, not otherwise specified.

Fortunately, more research is being conducted to explore this issue, and the body of literature that documents and describes sexual addiction is growing steadily. Indeed, the journal *Sexual Addiction and Compulsivity: The Journal of Treatment and Prevention*, has achieved 20 years of publication, and the *Comprehensive Textbook of Psychiatry* now includes a chapter on sex addiction and its treatment.[99] In an attempt to further classify and clarify the disorder, researchers have introduced various diagnostic criteria, most of which parallel the criteria for substance use disorders or pathological gambling.[86–88,100] Others have recommended independent diagnostic criteria to be applied to these behaviors.[83]

Etiology and Associated Factors

Research examining the etiology of sexual addiction has pointed to some associated factors. Presence of a trauma history, various family patterns and experiences, and exposure to unique stimulations such as "cybersex" has all been identified as potential contributors to sexual addiction. In addition, the comorbidity between sexual addiction and other addictive behaviors (particularly substance use disorders) has been highlighted.[101] Neuroscience research examining sexual addiction dates to the 1980s[102] and developments in this area have led to the identification of biological mechanisms underlying sexual addiction.[103] Indeed, it has been demonstrated that when a patient with sexual addiction thinks about sex, priming doses of dopamine are released in the nucleus accumbens.[52] The neurobehavioral outcome mimics the changes seen in the brain after an individual with chemical addiction ingests drugs or alcohol.

In addition, this appears to be a growing problem. Just as increasing the supply of available drugs of abuse would likely result in increased cases of chemical addiction, increasing the supply of available sexually explicit material may be responsible for increased cases of sexual addiction. With the introduction of "high-speed Internet," access to potential sexual partners has increased exponentially. Individuals who suffer from sexual addiction can now log on to view an ever-increasing number of pornography sites, access "virtual partners" via webcam, and meet potential partners through online chat rooms or dating sites. As a result, it appears that these behaviors have become more widespread.

Confusion and Controversy

As mentioned previously, some researchers and clinicians advocate against referring to this constellation of behaviors as an addictive disorder. They note obvious differences between sexual behavior and substance use (e.g., lack of chemical ingestion), but also point to the lack of a well-defined animal model for sexual addiction. Researchers have modeled substance use, binge episodes, development of tolerance, and the experience of withdrawal in animals. However, there is no parallel literature with regard to excessive sexual behavior in animals. For example, it has been suggested that showing pornography to laboratory animals has no effect on them. Without animal models, questions regarding the nosology of this disorder remain complicated and unanswered.

Gambling as an Addictive Behavior

Gambling can be defined as wagering money on a game of chance or some other event (e.g., sports contest) for money or other goods or services. For most people this represents a harmless social activity such as playing an office pool on the outcome of a football game, buying a lottery ticket, or visiting a local bingo parlor. Gambling is a common behavior with a large percentage of the U.S. population reporting engaging in some type of gambling within the past year.[104] However, for some individuals gambling represents an addictive behavior that leads to a host of negative consequences for the individual, their families, and society. While it is difficult to calculate the total societal costs of gambling, Grinols estimates that as much as $54 billion is associated with gambling through such things as increased crime, lost work time, bankruptcies, and financial hardships faced by the families of gambling addicts.[105] In fact, the negative societal consequences from online gambling were so severe and widespread that the U.S. Congress passed the Unlawful Internet Gambling Enforcement Act of 2006 which prohibits Americans from using electronic funds transfers, credit cards, and checks in placing bets with gambling sites worldwide.

The DSM-IV-TR defines pathological gambling as an impulse control disorder, not elsewhere classified. It is defined as:[48]

> *A. Persistent and recurrent maladaptive gambling behavior as indicated by five (or more) of the following:*
>
> *(1) is preoccupied with gambling (e.g., preoccupied with reliving past gambling experiences, handicapping or planning the next venture, or thinking of ways to get money with which to gamble)*
>
> *(2) needs to gamble with increasing amounts of money in order to achieve the desired excitement*
>
> *(3) has repeated unsuccessful efforts to control, cut back, or stop gambling*
>
> *(4) is restless or irritable when attempting to cut down or stop gambling*
>
> *(5) gambles as a way of escaping from problems or of relieving a dysphoric mood (e.g., feelings of helplessness, guilt, anxiety, depression)*
>
> *(6) after losing money gambling, often returns another day to get even ("chasing" one's losses)*
>
> *(7) lies to family members, therapist, or others to conceal the extent of involvement with gambling*
>
> *(8) has committed illegal acts such as forgery, fraud, theft, or embezzlement to finance gambling*
>
> *(9) has jeopardized or lost a significant relationship, job, or educational or career opportunity because of gambling*
>
> *(10) relies on others to provide money to relieve a desperate financial situation caused by gambling*
>
> *B. The gambling behavior is not better accounted for by a Manic Episode.*

Because of its many shared characteristics with substance use disorders (e.g., loss of control, unsuccessful attempts to quit, continued use despite negative consequences, relapse, etc.), pathological gambling is more accurately classified as an addiction.[106] Pathological gamblers, like other addicts, try to keep their problems from others. They thrive in secrecy. Problem gamblers rarely seek treatment for their symptoms or identify it as the chief complaint when visiting mental health professionals.[107,108] Other instruments and definitions of pathological gambling are frequently used. These include self-report measures such as the South Oaks Gambling Screen[109] and the National Opinion Research DSM Screen,[110] which provide cut-off scores for both problem and pathological gambling. These instruments are brief and have shown good reliability and sensitivity to identifying gambling problems. Diagnostic interviews exist, too, such as the Diagnostic Interview Schedule (DIS), which makes DSM-IV diagnoses.

Prevalence rates of pathological gambling vary considerably, depending on the specific population. Epidemiological studies of the general population estimate pathological gambling to affect approximately 1.6% of adults.[111] However, rates among adolescents are almost twice that of adults (3.9%) and rates among individuals seeking community services are as high as 17.2%.[111,112] Other populations such as the elderly, poor, and minorities are also at increased risk.[108,113]

Etiological Factors in Pathological Gambling

Like other addictions, the etiology of pathological gambling is multifactorial. Research has shown a genetic linkage in pathological gambling that may involve the D4 dopamine receptor and MAO-A and MAO-B genes.[114–116] Pathological gambling, also like substance use, appears to be perpetuated through its effects on brain reward. Experts have long known of the role that neurotransmitters such as dopamine play in use of alcohol and drugs. Specifically, drugs of abuse lead to increased dopamine in the mesolimbic reward system of the brain, including the nucleus accumbens, ventral tegmental area, and medial forebrain bundle.[117] In the last decade, a similar link has been found in the brains of pathological gamblers involving these same areas during the anticipation and action phases of gambling.[118,119] The role of dopamine in pathological gambling finds additional support in that increased gambling behavior is found among Parkinson's patients placed on dopamine agonist drugs.[120]

A number of demographic and psychosocial factors also appear to be more common among pathological gamblers. Generally, males, youth, persons with low SES, and persons who have substance and other behavior problems are at the highest risk. There also appears to be a relationship between the type of gambling and risk for developing a gambling problem with casino gambling, lottery, pull tabs, cards (outside a casino), bingo, and sports betting significantly predicting gambling pathology.[121] Research also indicates that individuals with pathological gambling are at increased risk for other psychiatric disorders. Results from the NESARC study found that persons with pathological gambling had high rates of comorbid psychiatric disorders such as alcohol use disorder (73%), drug use disorder (38%), mood disorder (49%), anxiety disorder (41%), and personality disorders (60%).[122] While many comorbid psychiatric disorders may be a consequence of pathological gambling, the high prevalence of personality disorders suggests that certain character traits may place an individual at increased risk for developing problem gambling behavior. These include high levels of sensation seeking, high levels of competitiveness, and low ability to delay gratification.[123]

Clinical Considerations

Pathological gamblers manifest cognitive distortions that may prolong their dysfunctional gambling patterns. These distortions relate to the person's belief that they are able to predict, influence, or control gambling outcomes through various techniques such as active or passive illusory control, interpretive control, and probability and predictive control.[124] As a result, treatment programs provide structured manuals and workbooks that address these issues, specifically by identifying antecedents, analyzing behavior, and assessing of consequences, relapse prevention, and self-limiting behavior.[125] Patients also receive ancillary services such as general problem solving and financial counseling in an active monitoring paradigm. Because addictions like gambling cannot be monitored through urine drug screening, professionals must utilize multiple methods such as collateral informants like family and friends, bank statements, as well as self-report.[107]

Internet Usage as an Addictive Behavior

Unlike pathological gambling, there are currently no consistent, agreed-upon criteria for what comprises Internet addiction. However, this constellation of symptoms does require exposure to a behavior. Various criteria have emerged from research studies, which reflect general definitions of impulse control disorders and addiction.[126–128] In general, the proposed criteria all include excessive use of or preoccupation with the Internet (i.e., spending more time using or thinking about using the Internet than is reasonable), significant social and/or occupational problems related to Internet use, and continued excessive use of the Internet, despite negative consequences.

Block,[129] in proposing inclusion of Internet addiction disorder (IAD) in the DSM-V, describes the disorder on a compulsive-impulsive spectrum involving excessive gaming, sexual preoccupations, and e-mail/text messaging.[129,130] In addition to the excessive use noted by other researchers, he notes that Internet addicts experience feelings of anger, tension, and/or depression when the computer is inaccessible (i.e., withdrawal symptoms), the need for more and better equipment (i.e., tolerance symptoms), and social consequences including withdrawal to the point of isolation and dishonesty/conflict with significant others.

The lack of a consistent, accepted diagnosis makes interpretation of research results difficult, as various investigators use different criteria. There are some measures for measuring IAD, including the Internet Addiction Test and Generalized Problematic Internet Use Scale (GPIUS). These are brief questionnaires that are easy to administer, with reported estimates of reliability and validity.[131,132]

While there are few national comprehensive studies on IAD in the US, researchers have suggested general prevalence rates of between 0.3 and 0.7%.[133] However, like other addictions, it is not clear if these rates are conditional upon exposure. Clearly, prevalence rates may vary considerably by age. One study of undergraduate Internet users revealed that 64.7% reported limited symptoms suggesting problematic Internet use and 8.7% met criteria for problematic use. Problem users were more likely to be males and to use online games as well as technologically sophisticated sites.[134] Prevalence rates outside the US, especially in Southeast Asia, appear to be higher. For example, South Korea views IAD as one of the nation's most serious public health issues with approximately 210,000 children (2.1% of all Korean children aged 6–19) identified as afflicted and in need of treatment. About 80% of those needing treatment may need psychotropic medications, and perhaps 20% to 24% require hospitalization.[135–137]

Etiological Factors

Research examining etiological factors in IAD compared to other addictions is rare. Generally, Internet use is thought to stimulate brain reward in a manner similar to that seen in substance abuse and pathological gambling. Psychological models include components of classical conditioning (e.g., pairing external cues like computers with internal states), and operant conditioning (e.g., reinforcing factors such as gaining and accessing information quickly and escaping conflict).[138,139]

Internet addiction disorder appears to have a high comorbidity with other psychiatric disorders. Unipolar and bipolar mood disorders, social anxiety, disruptive behavior disorders, impulse control disorders, and substance use disorders are highly represented among groups of excessive Internet users.[140,141] Ko and colleagues recently published results of a 2-year prospective study of adolescents in Taiwan.[127] While depression, ADHD, social phobia, and hostility were all found to predict the later occurrence of Internet addiction, the most significant predictors were ADHD and hostility.

Clinical Considerations

Because of the importance of computers, information technology and the Internet in social and occupational sectors of our society, abstinence models for treatment of substance disorders are not realistic for IAD. Rather, treatment paradigms must be similar to that seen in eating disorders, where the patient must learn healthy ways of interacting with the addictive stimulus. In the vast majority of cases, IAD can be treated on an outpatient basis, although hospitalization for the disorder is sometimes seen. Most treatment models involve a cognitive behavioral model designed to challenge cognitive errors and develop more adaptive functioning. These techniques include: (a) practice the opposite time; a technique pioneered by Young, it involves mapping a person's pattern of Internet use and constructing a new schedule that disrupts their normal routine so new behaviors can be introduced into that time period, (b) use external stoppers, (c) set specific goals to limit Internet time by inserting realistic time slots into their schedule, (d) abstain from a particular application, (e) use reminder cards, (f) develop a personal inventory, (g) join a support group, and (h) participate in family therapy.[142]

Relatively little research has been conducted on pharmacological interventions with IAD. Given the relationship to other addictive disorders, medications that affect dopaminergic and serotonergic systems could hold some promise.[143] Some efficacy has been associated with a combination of mood stabilizing and antipsychotic medications, although methodological constraints of the study limit interpretation of the results.[144]

Behavioral Treatments for Addictive Behaviors

It is well known that treatment paradigms for addictive disorders are very challenging. Many individuals do not self-refer for treatment (i.e., less than 10% of pathological gamblers receive treatment).[145] In addition, as recently as the early 20th century, patients with substance use disorders were considered hopeless cases, and physicians were advised against attempting to treat them. Even today, there is no "quick fix," and successful treatment requires long-term changes in lifestyle and behavior. Across the addictive disorders described in this chapter, most successful treatments entail a comprehensive effort to promote physical, emotional, and behavioral change. The treatment process typically involves a combination of interventions and supports, with a multi-pronged approach to treatment. For example, among patients with substance use disorders, behavioral therapy is generally viewed as the first-line treatment, while pharmacotherapy can be added as an adjunct, particularly for the treatment of alcohol, opioid, and stimulant dependence.[146] Participation in group therapy or self-help groups is also considered a primary component of treatment. In addition, it is clear that personality, social support, environmental factors, and motivation for change all affect treatment outcome.

Interventions for all addictive behaviors must target the exposure, the triggers for relapse, and the negative cognitions that might follow such an event, in order to prevent a lapse from escalating into a full relapse episode. Relapse is a common occurrence in the cycle of treatment for all addictive behaviors. With regard to exposure—substance use—many individuals alternate between abstinence and active use across their lives.[147,148] Similarly, the vacillation between dieting (i.e., "abstinence") and overeating (i.e., "active use") is common among individuals struggling with obesity.[149] Individuals attempting to recover from addictions to gambling, sex, or use of technology frequently show the same general pattern. As a result, long-term comprehensive treatment is considered the gold standard of care for substance use disorders. Jeffrey[149] demonstrated that the short-term nature of most interventions for obesity contributes to their failure, whereas longer treatments are associated with improved outcomes.

12-step Programs

Participation in a 12-step fellowship (e.g., Alcoholics Anonymous or Narcotics Anonymous) remains the most common route to recovery among individuals who do not attend formal treatment, and provides the foundation for most addiction treatment center programs. The 12-step fellowships are based on a program of honesty, open-mindedness, and willingness to make changes. Spiritual principles make up an important aspect of the program, though individuals from any faith-background, including agnostics and atheists, are welcome and may benefit from participation. The programs have demonstrated effectiveness in helping individuals to achieve abstinence and maintain stable sobriety.[150] They are appropriate for individuals from any racial, ethnic, socioeconomic, or religious background; they are relevant for persons with comorbid severe mental illness as well.[151]

Given the positive outcomes associated with Alcoholics Anonymous and Narcotics Anonymous, there are now 12-step fellowships designated to overeating (i.e., Overeaters Anonymous and Food Addicts Anonymous), hypersexuality (i.e., Sex and Love Addicts Anonymous), pathological gambling (i.e., Gamblers Anonymous), and overuse of the Internet (i.e., Internet Addicts Anonymous and Webaholics Anonymous). Participants report that these programs help them in much the same way that Alcoholics Anonymous and Narcotics Anonymous help. Indeed, among problem gamblers, length and activity of participation are correlated with abstinence.[152,153]

Motivational Interviewing

Before the disease concept of addiction was introduced, most interventions took on a confrontational approach (i.e., lecturing, warning, arguing, threatening, correcting). Physicians, mental health providers, family members, and friends have used these techniques to try to change individuals with substance use disorders.

However, given that these conditions reflect more than a lack of willpower, the confrontational approach is rarely successful. Thus, Miller and Rollnick[154,155] developed a new method for helping individuals with substance use disorders, termed "motivational interviewing" (MI). MI is a patient-centered, collaborative method of guiding patients by focusing on eliciting and reinforcing the patient's own personal motivations for change. It emphasizes the patient's personal choice, responsibility in changing, and current readiness to change.

MI has been demonstrated effective in helping individuals with problematic drinking and other substance use disorders, and in encouraging substance-dependent individuals to accept participation in a formal treatment program. Given the success associated with MI interventions for individuals with substance use disorders, the approach has been adopted in numerous other fields, such as overeating, risky sexual behaviors, and gambling.

Cognitive Behavioral Therapy

Cognitive behavioral therapy (CBT) has demonstrated efficacy in the treatment of substance use disorders and is used for inpatients and outpatients. The approach utilizes a combination of psychoeducation, functional analysis and behavioral assessment, modeling and skill-building, environmental modification and contingency management, coping and refusal skills training, cognitive restructuring, and various other techniques. While participating in CBT, patients learn what triggers their substance use, how to deal with craving, ways to minimize the likelihood of relapse, and how to recognize dysfunctional thinking. Other areas include self-efficacy support, skills to improve general life functioning, and planning for the future. Group CBT provides opportunities for people to confront denial, obtain strategies and support from others, share success stories, and develop a social network.

In general, participation in CBT decreases the likelihood of relapse among individuals with substance use disorders and other behavioral addictions. Given the similarities of symptoms (e.g., cravings, loss of control, influence of the environment, dysfunctional cognitions, role of contingencies, likelihood of relapse), CBT is frequently used as a part of treatment for overeating, hypersexuality, pathological gambling, and even overuse of technology, whether in an individual or group format.[153]

Relapse Prevention

Relapse is a significant concern for individuals with both substance use and behavioral addictions. Thus, implementing strategies to decrease the likelihood of relapse is considered an important part of treatment for all of these patients.

With regard to substance use, Marlatt and Gordon[156] developed a method of intervention termed "relapse prevention" which involves assessing factors that might contribute to relapse[157] as well as normalizing the struggle to maintain sobriety. Patients are coached that one slip (i.e., "lapse") does not mean that they are doomed to failure. Once high-risk situations are identified, the patient and clinician work to develop appropriate coping skills to manage these situations. Given the similarities in symptom presentation, this strategy has been shown to be effective in helping patients recover from behavioral addictions.

Pharmacological Interventions

To date, no specific drugs have been FDA approved for the treatment of behavioral process addictions. However, several classes of medications, and many medications used to treat chemical addictions, have been evaluated. One class of drugs, opioid antagonists, has shown some success for treating pathological gambling. They modulate dopaminergic transmission in the mesolimbic reward pathway. In addition to reducing craving in alcohol- and opioid-dependent patients, these drugs, given in high doses, also reduce the intensity of urges to gamble, thoughts about gambling, and the gamblingitself.[158,159] Another opioid antagonist, nalmefene, demonstrated statistically significant improvement in gambling symptoms compared with a placebo in a 16-week double-blind trial.[160] Finally, there is some short-term research on other pharmacological agents such as olanzapine, modafinil, memantine, acamprosate, and topiramate.[108]

Similarly, topiramate (which has demonstrated efficacy in managing some patients with binge drinking) has demonstrated some efficacy in the treatment of some patients with food addiction. Generally, treatments for overeating and obesity have been drugs of abuse themselves. Amphetamines, methamphetamine, cocaine, and other psychostimulants suppress appetite while fenfluramines and ecstasy can cause an overweight person to forget to eat. Other "treatments" have included antidepressants, especially dopamine-augmenting Wellbutrin and medications normally given to patients with type II diabetes. Of these, topiramate appears to be useful to consider for binge eating, as it is associated with decreased number of binge-eating episodes per week, decreased body mass index, and shortened time to recovery.[161] Sibutramine, (a medication similar to antidepressants) and orlistat (a medication referred to as the "Antabuse for overeating") have also demonstrated potential efficacy[162–164] when adherence is long term and accompanied by exercise. Still, the overwhelming evidence is that the current medications are weak compared to the drive for food, hedonic food signals, and reinforcement. The most efficacious intervention to date (though with considerable risk, costs, and reversibility issues) has been bariatric surgery and lap-banding.

Addiction as a Unitary Disease

Although drugs of abuse are diverse and affect the brain via different acute mechanisms of action, each influences the reward circuitry of the brain's limbic system by increasing dopamine release in the nucleus accumbens. As suggested by Nestler,[165] it is possible that a common molecular pathway underlies all addictions, which can be exploited to develop more effective treatments. Applied research has shown that treatment outcomes for impaired physicians do not differ based on their choice of substance;[166] physicians with addiction to opioids or crack cocaine fare as well as those with alcohol dependence. Given the high prevalence of polysubstance abuse and the fact that the same treatment appears to be effective for alcohol, opioid, marijuana, benzodiazepine, and cocaine dependence, it may be more useful to consider the treatment of addiction disorders rather than attempt to tailor interventions based on a specific drug of abuse.

As reviewed in this chapter, research is also accumulating regarding the similarities among substances and other compulsive-behavior disorders.[167] In each case, alterations in the natural reward pathway have been implicated in the tendency to continue the behavior despite negative consequences. In addition, comorbidity is common. Pathological gambling, hypersexual behavior, and compulsive eating are frequently comorbid with drug addiction and share similar neurological patterns.[93,168,169] For example, sexual addiction is often associated with abuse of cocaine[170] or other substances, and chronic masturbation while viewing pornography has been associated with abuse of erectile dysfunction medication.[171] Thus, although similar behavioral and pharmacological treatments have shown efficacy with these groups, more research is needed to clarify the process of addiction and to determine how and why addiction manifests with various behaviors and substances of abuse. In the meantime, clinicians should be vigilant for signs of "addiction transfer" in patients who are attempting sobriety, because preliminary evidence suggests that these patients may be more vulnerable to symptoms of behavioral addiction and vice versa.[64]

Conclusion

Compulsive sexual behavior, pathological gambling, hedonic overeating, and excessive use of technology are important problems, but are they addictions? In the absence of a blood, urine, or imaging test, or a well-defined animal model, controversy will reign.

Some patients clearly have a relationship with hyperpalatable foods that appears to meet DSM-IV diagnostic criteria for substance dependence. Others demonstrate a lack of control over their sexual behavior that prevents them from functioning adequately. Pathological gamblers talk of chasing the "high" from a big win, and suffer many of the same devastating consequences as individuals who structure their lives around the use of drugs. And some individuals report feeling "addicted" to various forms of technology. In each case, these individuals have an exposure to a drug, to a machine or gambling environment, or phone or computer, or food or a sexual encounter. Those exposures are necessary, but not sufficient, for an addiction. They lose control over their behavior, continue the behavior despite serious negative consequences, spend a great deal of time engaging in the behavior or recovering from it, and make countless attempts to reduce the behavior without success. We see patients who are early in the recovery from alcohol, cocaine, or other drugs begin overeating or developing sexual compulsivity. Drugs of abuse interfere in some way with food reinforcement and vice versa. Often, smokers drink and drinkers smoke. Drugs, food, sex, and gambling appear to require access to the same brain reinforcement system and neurochemicals. Process addictions are considered so inter-related that the success of the cigarette tax has stimulated tax proposals from public health and addiction experts suggesting taxing everything from fast food to sugar to cannabis to the Internet. Still, no matter the terminology that is finally agreed upon to describe these conditions and their inter-relationships, it is clear that more work is needed to understand them and to improve efforts at prevention and treatment.

References

1. Mokdad, A. H., Marks, J. S., Stroup, D. F., & Gerberding, J. L. (2004). Actual causes of death in the United States. *JAMA. 291*(10), 1238–1245.
2. Robinson, T. E. (2004). Addicted rats. *Science. 305*, 951–953.
3. Lynch, J. J., Stein, E. A., & Fertziger, A. P. (1976). An analysis of 70 years of morphine classical conditioning: Implications for clinical treatment of narcotic addiction. *J Nerv Ment Dis. 163*(1), 47–58.
4. Faust, E. S. (1900). Ueber die Ursachen der Gewohnung an Morphin. *Arch Exp Path Pharmak. 44*, 217.
5. Pavlov, I. P. (1927). *Conditioned reflexes: An investigation of the physiological activity of the cerebral cortex.*
6. Fouriezos, G., Hansson, P., & Wise, R. A. (1978). Neuroleptic-induced attenuation of brain stimulation reward in rats. *J Comp Physiol Psychol, 92*(4), 661–671.
7. Robbins, T. W. & Everitt, B. J. (1982). Functional studies of the central catecholamines. *Int Rev Neurobiol, 23*, 303–365.
8. Spyraki, C., Fibiger, H. C., & Phillips, A. G. (1982). Attenuation by haloperidol of place preference conditioning using food reinforcement. *Psychopharmacology (Berl), 77*(4), 379–382.
9. Spyraki, C., Fibiger, H. C., & Phillips, A. G. (1983). Attenuation of heroin reward in rats by disruption of the mesolimbic dopamine system. *Psychopharmacology (Berl), 79*(2–3), 278–283.
10. Wise, R. A., Spindler, J., deWit, H., & Gerberg, G. J. (1978). Neuroleptic-induced "anhedonia" in rats: Pimozide blocks reward quality of food. *Science, 201*(4352), 262–264.

11. Church, W. H., Justice, J. B., Jr., & Byrd, L. D. (1987). Extracellular dopamine in rat striatum following uptake inhibition by cocaine, nomifensine and benztropine. *Eur J Pharmacol, 139*(3), 345–348.
12. Hernandez, L. & Hoebel, B. G. (1988). Food reward and cocaine increase extracellular dopamine in the nucleus accumbens as measured by microdialysis. *Life Sci, 42*(18), 1705–1712.
13. Pfaus, J. G., Damsma, G., Nomikos, G. G., et al. (1990). Sexual behavior enhances central dopamine transmission in the male rat. *Brain Res, 530*(2), 345–348.
14. Wise, R. A. (2004). Dopamine, learning and motivation. *Nat Rev Neurosci, 5*(6), 483–494.
15. Steeves, T. D., Miyasaki, J., Zurowski, M., et al. (2009). Increased striatal dopamine release in Parkinsonian patients with pathological gambling: A [11C] raclopride PET study. *Brain, 132*(Pt 5), 1376–1385.
16. Gold, M. S. (2004). Eating disorders, overeating, and pathological attachment to food: Independent or addictive disorders? *J Addict Dis, 23*(3), 1–3.
17. Paczynski, R. P. & Gold, M. S. (2010). Cocaine and crack. In P. Ruiz & E. Strain, (Eds.). *Lowinson & Ruiz's substance abuse*: A *comprehensive textbook, 5th Edition.* Baltimore: MD: Lippincott Williams & Wilkins.
18. Gold, M. S., Kobeissy, F. H., Wang, K. K., et al. (2009). Methamphetamine- and trauma-induced brain injuries: Comparative cellular and molecular neurobiological substrates. *Biol Psychiatry, 66*(2), 118–127.
19. Liu, J., Liang, J., Qin, W., et al. (2009). Dysfunctional connectivity patterns in chronic heroin users: An fMRI study. *Neurosci Lett, 460*(1), 72–77.
20. Risinger, R. C., Salmeron, B. J., Ross, T. J., et al. (2005). Neural correlates of high and craving during cocaine self-administration using BOLD fMRI. *Neuroimage, 26*(4), 1097–1108.
21. Phillips, P. E., Stuber, G. D., Heien, M. L., Wightman, R. M., & Carelli, R. M. (2003). Subsecond dopamine release promotes cocaine seeking. *Nature, 422*(6932), 614–618.
22. Melis, M., Gessa, G. L., & Diana, M. (2000). Different mechanisms for dopaminergic excitation induced by opiates and cannabinoids in the rat midbrain. *Prog Neuropsychopharmacol Biol Psychiatry, 24*(6), 993–1006.
23. Rahman, S., Zhang, J., Engleman, E. A., & Corrigall, W. A. (2004). Neuroadaptive changes in the mesoaccumbens dopamine system after chronic nicotine self-administration: A microdialysis study. *Neuroscience, 129*(2), 415–424.
24. Balfour, D. J. (2002). Neuroplasticity within the mesoaccumbens dopamine system and its role in tobacco dependence. *Curr Drug Targets CNS Neurol Disord, 1*(4), 413–421.
25. Gonzales, R. A., Job, M. O., & Doyon, W. M. (2004). The role of mesolimbic dopamine in the development and mainentance of ethanol reinforcement. *Pharmacol Ther, 103*(2), 121–146.
26. Di Chiara, G. (1997). Alcohol and dopamine. *Alcohol Health Res World, 21*(2), 108–114.
27. Boileau, I., Assaad, J. M., Pihl, R. O., et al. (2003). Alcohol promotes dopamine release in the human nucleus accumbens. *Synapse, 49*(4), 226–231.
28. Merlo Pich, E., Lorang, M., Yeganeh, M., et al. (1995). Increase of extracellular corticotropin-releasing factor-like immunoreactivity levels in the amygdala of awake rats during restraint stress and ethanol withdrawal as measured by microdialysis. *J Neurosci, 15*(8), 5439–5447.

29. Rodriguez de Fonseca, F., Carrera, M. R., Navarro, M., Koob, G. F., & Weiss, F. (1997). Activation of corticotropin-releasing factor in the limbic system during cannabinoid withdrawal. *Science, 276*(5321), 2050–2054.
30. Richter, R. M. & Weiss, F. (1999). In vivo CRF release in rat amygdala is increased during cocaine withdrawal in self-administering rats. *Synapse, 32*(4), 254–261.
31. George, O., Ghozland, S., Azar, M. R., et al. (2007). CRF-CRF1 system activation mediates withdrawal-induced increases in nicotine self-administration in nicotine-dependent rats. *Proc Natl Acad Sci U S A, 104*(43), 17198–17203.
32. Olive, M. F., Koenig, H. N., Nannini, M. A., & Hodge, C. W. (2002). Elevated extracellular CRF levels in the bed nucleus of the stria terminalis during ethanol withdrawal and reduction by subsequent ethanol intake. *Pharmacol Biochem Behav, 72*(1–2), 213–220.
33. Baldwin, H. A., Rassnick, S., Rivier, J., Koob, G. F., & Britton, K. T. (1991). CRF antagonist reverses the "anxiogenic" response to ethanol withdrawal in the rat. *Psychopharmacology (Berl), 103*(2), 227–232.
34. Rassnick, S., Heinrichs, S. C., Britton, K. T., & Koob, G. F. (1993). Microinjection of a corticotropin-releasing factor antagonist into the central nucleus of the amygdala reverses anxiogenic-like effects of ethanol withdrawal. *Brain Res, 605*(1), 25–32.
35. Bruijnzeel, A. W., Zislis, G., Wilson, C., & Gold, M. S. (2007). Antagonism of CRF receptors prevents the deficit in brain reward function associated with precipitated nicotine withdrawal in rats. *Neuropsychopharmacology, 32*(4), 955–963.
36. Bruijnzeel, A. W., Prado, M., & Isaac, S. (2009). Corticotropin-releasing factor-1 receptor activation mediates nicotine withdrawal-induced deficit in brain reward function and stress-induced relapse. *Biol Psychiatry, 66*(2), 110–117.
37. Contarino, A. & Papaleo, F. (2005). The corticotropin-releasing factor receptor-1 pathway mediates the negative affective states of opiate withdrawal. *Proc Natl Acad Sci U S A, 102*(51), 18649–18654.
38. Stinus, L., Cador, M., Zorrilla, E. P., & Koob, G. F. (2005). Buprenorphine and a CRF1 antagonist block the acquisition of opiate withdrawal-induced conditioned place aversion in rats. *Neuropsychopharmacology, 30*(1), 90–98.
39. Gehlert, D. R., Cippitelli, A., Thorsell, A., et al. (2007). 3-(4-Chloro-2-morpholin-4-yl-thiazol-5-yl)-8-(1-ethylpropyl)-2,6-dimethyl- imidazo[1,2-b]pyridazine: A novel brain-penetrant, orally available corticotropin-releasing factor receptor 1 antagonist with efficacy in animal models of alcoholism. *J Neurosci, 27*(10), 2718–2726.
40. Markou, A. (2008). Review. Neurobiology of nicotine dependence. *Philos Trans R Soc Lond B Biol Sci, 363*(1507), 3159–3168.
41. Gold, M. S., Redmond, D. E., Jr., & Kleber, H. D. (1978). Clonidine blocks acute opiate-withdrawal symptoms. *Lancet, 2*(8090), 599–602.
42. Gold, M. S., Byck, R., Sweeney, D. R., & Kleber, H. D. (1979). Endorphin-locus coeruleus connection mediates opiate action and withdrawal. *Biomedicine, 30*(1), 1–4.
43. Dackis, C. A. & Gold, M. S. (1985). New concepts in cocaine addiction: The dopamine depletion hypothesis. *Neurosci Bio Rev, 9*, 469–477.
44. Volkow, N. D., Fowler, J. S., Wang, G. J., & Swanson, J. M. (2004). Dopamine in drug abuse and addiction: Results from imaging studies and treatment implications. *Mol Psychiatry, 9*(6), 557–569.
45. Kim, H., Neubert, J. K., San Miguel, A., et al. (2004). Genetic influence on variability in human acute experimental pain sensitivity associated with gender, ethnicity and psychological temperament. *Pain, 109*, 488–496.

46. Dani, J. A. & Heinemann, S. (1996). Molecular and cellular aspects of nicotine abuse. *Neuron, 16,* 905–908.
47. Naqvi, N. H., Rudrauf, D., Damasio, H., & Bechara, A. (2007). Damage to the insula disrupts addiction to cigarette smoking. *Science, 315,* 531–534.
48. American Psychiatric Association. (2000). *Diagnostic and statistical manual of mental disorders—4th edition text revision (DSM-IV-TR).* Washington, D. C.: American Psychiatric Association.
49. Joranby, L., Frost-Pineda, K., & Gold, M. S. (2005). Addiction to food and brain reward systems. *Sex Addict Compuls, 12*(2), 201–217.
50. Tomiyama, A. J., Mann, T., & Comer, L. (2009). Triggers of eating in everyday life. *Appetite, 52*(1), 72–82.
51. Jansen, A., Vanreyten, A., van Balveren, T., Roefs, A., Nederkoorn, C., & Havermans, R. (2008). Negative affect and cue-induced overeating in non-eating disordered obesity. *Appetite, 51*(3), 556–562.
52. Volkow, N. D. & Wise, R. A. (2005). How can drug addiction help us understand obesity? *Nat Neurosci, 8*(5), 555–560. doi:510.1038/nn1452.
53. Gold, M. S., Graham, N. A., Cocores, J. A., & Nixon, S. J. (2009). Food addiction? *J Addict Med, 3*(1), 42–45.
54. Kleiner, K. D., Gold, M. S., Frost-Pineda, K., Lenz-Brunsman, B., Perri, M. G., & Jacobs, W. S. (2004). Body mass index and alcohol use. *J Addict Dis, 23*(3), 105–118.
55. Warren, M., Frost-Pineda, K., & Gold, M. (2005). Body mass index and marijuana use. *J Addict Dis, 24*(3), 95–100.
56. Avena, N. M., Rada, P., Moise, N., & Hoebel, B. G. (2006). Sucrose sham feeding on a binge schedule releases accumbens dopamine repeatedly and eliminates the acetylcholine satiety response *Neuroscience, 139,* 813–820.
57. Hoebel, B. G., Avena, N. M., Bocarsly, M. E., & Rada, P. (2009). Natural addiction: A behavioral and circuit model based on sugar addiction in rats. *J Addict Med, 3*(1), 33–41.
58. Avena, N. M., Rada, P., & Hoebel, B. G. (2008). Evidence for sugar addiction: Behavioral and neurochemical effects of intermittent, excessive sugar intake. *Neurosci Biobehav Rev, 32*(1), 20–39.
59. Colantuoni, C., Rada, P., McCarthy, J., et al. (2002). Evidence that intermittent, excessive sugar intake causes endogenous opioid dependence. *Obes Res, 10*(6), 478–488.
60. Rada, P., Pothos, E., Mark, G. P., & Hoebel, B. G. (1991). Microdialysis evidence that acetylcholine in the nucleus accumbens is involved in morphine withdrawal and its treatment with clonidine. *Brain Res, 561*(2), 354–356.
61. Rada, P., Jensen, K., & Hoebel, B. G. (2001). Effects of nicotine and mecamylamine-induced withdrawal on extracellular dopamine and acetylcholine in the rat nucleus accumbens. *Psychopharmacology (Berl), 157*(1), 105–110.
62. Gold, M. S., Frost-Pineda, K., & Jacobs, W. S. (2003). Overeating, binge eating, and eating disorders as addictions. *Psychiatric Annals, 33*(2), 117–122.
63. Merlo, L. J., Klingman, C., Malasanos, T. H., & Silverstein, J. H. (2009). Exploration of food addiction in pediatric patients: A preliminary investigation. *J Addict Med, 3*(1), 26–32.
64. Hodgkins, C. C., Jacobs, W. S., & Gold, M. S. (2003). Weight gain after adolescent drug addiction treatment and supervised abstinence. *Psych Annals, 33*(2), 112–117.
65. Hodgkins, C. C., Cahill, K. S., Seraphine, A. E., Frost-Pineda, K., & Gold, M. S. (2004). Adolescent drug addiction treatment and weight gain. *J Addict Dis, 23*(3), 55–65.

66. Hodgkins, C., Frost-Pineda, K., & Gold, M. S. (2007). Weight gain during substance abuse treatment: The dual problem of addiction and overeating in an adolescent population. *J Addict Dis, 26* Suppl 1, 41–50.
67. Cabeza de Vaca, S. & Carr, K. D. (1998). Food restriction enhances the central rewarding effect of abused drugs. *J Neurosci, 18*(18), 7502–7510.
68. Wang, G. J., Volkow, N. D., Thanos, P. K., & Fowler, J. S. (2009). Imaging of brain dopamine pathways: Implications for understanding obesity. *J Addict Med, 3*(1), 8–18.
69. Liu, Y. & Gold, M. S. (2003). Human functional magnetic resonance imaging of eating and satiety in eating disorders and obesity. *Psychiatric Annals, 33*(2), 127–132.
70. James, G. A., Gold, M. S., & Liu, Y. (2004). Interaction of satiety and reward response to food stimulation. *J Addict Dis, 23*(3), 23–37.
71. Goudie, A. J., Cooper, G. D., & Halford, J. C. (2005). Antipsychotic-induced weight gain. *Diabetes Obes Metab, 7*(5), 478–487.
72. Yumru, M., Savas, H. A., Kurt, E., et al. (2007). Atypical antipsychotics related metabolic syndrome in bipolar patients. *J Affect Disord, 98*(3), 247–252.
73. Hajnal, A., Smith, G. P., & Norgren, R. (2004). Oral sucrose stimulation increases accumbens dopamine in the rat. *American Journal of Physiology. Regulatory, Integrative, and Comparative Physiology, 286*(1), 31–37.
74. Colantuoni, C., Schwenker, J., McCarthy, J., et al. (2001). Excessive sugar intake alters binding to dopamine and mu-opioid receptors in the brain. *Neuroreport, 12*(16), 3549–3552.
75. Spangler, R., Wittkowski, K. M., Goddard, N. L., Avena, N. M., B.G. H, & Leibowitz, S. F. (2004). Opiate-like effects of sugar on gene expression in reward areas of the rat brain. *Brain Res Mol Brain Res, 124*(2), 134–142.
76. Avena, N. M. & Hoebel, B. G. (2003). A diet promoting sugar dependency causes behavioral cross-sensitization to a low dose of amphetamine. *Neuroscience, 122*(1), 17–20.
77. Avena, N. M., Carrillo, C. A., Needham, L., Leibowitz, S. F., & Hoebel, B. G. (2004). Sugar-dependent rats show enhanced intake of unsweetened ethanol. *Alcohol, 34*(2–3), 203–209.
78. Avena, N. M., Long, K. A., & Hoebel, B. G. (2005). Sugar-dependent rats show enhanced responding for sugar after abstinence: Evidence of a sugar deprivation effect. *Physiol Behav, 84*(3), 359–362.
79. Grimm, J. W., Fyall, A. M., & Osincup, D. P. (2005). Incubation of sucrose craving: Effects of reduced training and sucrose pre-loading. *Physiol Behav, 84*(1), 73–79.
80. Gold, S. N. & Heffner, C. L. (1998). Sexual addiction: many conceptions, minimal data. *Clin Psychol Rev, 18*(3), 367–381.
81. Merlo, L. J., Carnes, S., Carnes, P. J., & Gold, M. S. (2008). Hypersexuality disorders: Addiction, compulsion, or impulsive behavior? Paper presented at: Society of Biological Psychiatry (SOBP), 63rd Annual Scientific Convention & Meeting, May 1–3, 2008; Washington, DC.
82. Carnes, P. (1991). *Don't call it love: Recovery from sexual addiction.* New York: Bantam Books.
83. Stein, D. J., Black, D. W., & Pienaar, W. (2000). Sexual disorders not otherwise specified: compulsive, addictive, or impulsive? *CNS Spectr, 5*(1), 60–64.
84. Orford, J. (1978). Hypersexuality: Implications for a theory of dependence. *Br J Addict Alcohol Other Drugs, 73*(3), 299–210.

85. Orford, J. (1985). *Excessive appetites: A psychological view of the addictions*. Chichester, UK: Wiley.
86. Carnes, P. (1983). *Out of the shadows: Understanding sexual addiction*. Minneapolis, MN: CompCare Publishers.
87. Carnes, P. J. (1988). Bars and bordellos: Sexual addiction and chemical dependency. *Professional Counselor*.
88. Carnes, P. J. (1991). Sexual addiction. *The Counselor*.
89. Goodman, A. (1992). Sexual addiction: Designation and treatment. *J Sex Marital Ther, 18*(4), 303–314.
90. Earle, R. & Earle, M. (1995). *Sex addiction: Case studies and management*. New York: Brunner Mazel.
91. Robertson, J. (1990). Sex addiction as a disease: A neurobehavioral model. *American Journal of Preventive Psychiatry & Neurology, 2*(3), 15–18.
92. Goodman, A. (1993). Diagnosis and treatment of sexual addiction. *J Sex Marital Ther, 19*(3), 225–251.
93. Black, D. W. (2000). The epidemiology and phenomenology of compulsive sexual behavior. *CNS Spectr, 5*(1), 26–72.
94. Fischer, B. (1995). Sexual addiction revisited. *The Addictions Newsletter, 2*(5), 27.
95. Coleman, E. (1990). The obsessive-compulsive model for describing compulsive sexual behavior. *American Journal of Preventive Psychiatry & Neurology, 2*(3), 9–14.
96. Black, D. W., Kehrberg, L. L., Flumerfelt, D. L., & Schlosser, S. S. (1997). Characteristics of 36 subjects reporting compulsive sexual behavior. *Am J Psychiatry, 154*(2), 243–249.
97. Raymond, N. C., Coleman, E., & Miner, M. H. (2003). Psychiatric comorbidity and compulsive/impulsive traits in compulsive sexual behavior. *Compr Psychiatry, 44*(5), 370–380.
98. Barth, R. J. & Kinder, B. N. (1987). The mislabeling of sexual impulsivity. *J Sex Marital Ther, 13*(1), 15–23.
99. Carnes, P. J. (2005). Chapter 18: Sexual addiction. In S. Sadock, (Ed.). *Comprehensive textbook of psychiatry*. Philadelphia, PA: Lippincott, Williams & Wilkins.
100. Schneider, J. P. (1991). How to recognize the signs of sexual addiction. Asking the right questions may uncover serious problems. *Postgrad Med, 90*(6), 171–174, 177–182.
101. Carnes, P. J., Murray, R. E., & Charpentier, L. (2005). Bargains with chaos: Sex addicts and addiction interaction disorder. *Sexual Addictions & Compulsivity, 12*, 79–120.
102. Milkman, H. & Sunderwirth, S. (1987). *Craving for ecstasy: The consciousness and chemistry of escape*. New York: Lexington Books.
103. Cozolino, L. (2006). *The neuroscience of human relationships: Attachment and the developing social brain*. New York: Norton.
104. Welte, J. W., Barnes, G. M., Wieczorek, W. F., Tidwell, M. C., & Parker, J. (2002). Gambling participation in the U.S.—results from a national survey. *J Gambl Stud, 18*(4), 313–337.
105. Grinols, E. L. (2004). *Gambling in America: Costs and benefits*. Cambridge, UK: Cambridge University Press.
106. Potenza, M. N. (2006). Should addictive disorders include non-substance-related conditions? *Addiction, 101*Suppl 1, 142–151.
107. Slutske, W. S. (2006). Natural recovery and treatment-seeking in pathological gambling: Results of two U.S. national surveys. *Am J Psychiatry, 163*(2), 297–302.

108. Fong, T. W. (2009). Pathological gambling: update on assessment and treatment. *Psychiatric Times, 26*(9), 20–25.
109. Stinchfield, R. (2002). Reliability, validity, and classification accuracy of the South Oaks Gambling Screen (SOGS). *Addict Behav, 27*(1), 1–19.
110. Hodgins, D. C. (2004). Using the NORC DSM Screen for Gambling Problems as an outcome measure for pathological gambling: Psychometric evaluation. *Addict Behav, 29*(8), 1685–1690.
111. Shaffer, H. J., Hall, M. N., & Vander Bilt, J. (1999). Estimating the prevalence of disordered gambling behavior in the United States and Canada: A research synthesis. *Am J Public Health, 89*(9), 1369–1376.
112. Lepage, C., Ladouceur, R., & Jacques, C. (2000). Prevalence of problem gambling among community service users. *Community Ment Health J, 36*(6), 597–601.
113. Levens, S., Dyer, A. M., Zubritsky, C., Knott, K., & Oslin, D. W. (2005). Gambling among older, primary-care patients: an important public health concern. *Am J Geriatr Psychiatry, 13*(1), 69–76.
114. Slutske, W. S., Eisen, S., True, W. R., Lyons, M. J., Goldberg, J., & Tsuang, M. (2000). Common genetic vulnerability for pathological gambling and alcohol dependence in men. *Arch Gen Psychiatry, 57*(7), 666–673.
115. Perez de Castro, I., Ibanez, A., Torres, P., Saiz-Ruiz, J., & Fernandez-Piqueras, J. (1997). Genetic association study between pathological gambling and a functional DNA polymorphism at the D4 receptor gene. *Pharmacogenetics, 7*(5), 345–348.
116. Slutske, W. S., Meier, M. H., Zhu, G., Statham, D. J., Blaszczynski, A., & Martin, N. G. (2009). The Australian Twin Study of Gambling (OZ-GAM): Rationale, sample description, predictors of participation, and a first look at sources of individual differences in gambling involvement. *Twin Res Hum Genet, 12*(1), 63–78.
117. Gold, M. S., Gold, S. T., & Herkov, M. J. (2007). Drugs and violence. In L. Kurtz, (Ed.). *Encyclopedia of violence, peace, and conflict*. San Diego: Academic Press.
118. Reuter, J., Raedler, T., Rose, M., Hand, I., Glascher, J., & Buchel, C. (2005). Pathological gambling is linked to reduced activation of the mesolimbic reward system. *Nat Neurosci, 8*(2), 147–148.
119. Crockford, D. N., Goodyear, B., Edwards, J., Quickfall, J., & el-Guebaly, N. (2005). Cue-induced brain activity in pathological gamblers. *Biol Psychiatry, 58*(10), 787–795.
120. Driver-Dunckley, E., Samanta, J., & Stacy, M. (2003). Pathological gambling associated with dopamine agonist therapy in Parkinson's disease. *Neurology, 61*(3), 422–423.
121. Welte, J. W., Barnes, G. M., Wieczorek, W. F., Tidwell, M. C., & Parker, J. C. (2004). Risk factors for pathological gambling. *Addict Behav, 29*(2), 323–335.
122. Petry, N. M., Stinson, F. S., & Grant, B. F. (2005). Comorbidity of DSM-IV pathological gambling and other psychiatric disorders: Results from the National Epidemiologic Survey on Alcohol and Related Conditions. *J Clin Psychiatry, 66*(5), 564–574.
123. Parke, A., Griffiths, M., & Irwing, P. (2004). Personality traits in pathological gambling: Sensation seeking, deferment of gratification and competitiveness as risk factors. *Addiction Research & Theory, 12*(3), 201–212.
124. Toneatto, T., Blitz-Miller, T., Calderwood, K., Dragonetti, R., & Tsanos, A. (1997). Cognitive distortions in heavy gambling. *J Gambl Stud, 13*(3), 253–266.
125. Hodgins, D. C. & Petry, N. M. (2004). Cognitive and behavioral treatments. In J. E. Grant & M. N. Potenza, (Eds.). *Pathological Gambling: A clinical guide to treatment* (pp. 169–187). Arlington, VA: American Psychiatric Publishing.

126. Shapira, N. A., Lessig, M. C., Goldsmith, T. D., et al. (2003). Problematic internet use: Proposed classification and diagnostic criteria. *Depress Anxiety, 17*(4), 207–216.
127. Ko, C. H., Yen, J. Y., Chen, C. C., Chen, S. H., & Yen, C. F. (2005). Proposed diagnostic criteria of Internet addiction for adolescents. *J Nerv Ment Dis, 193*(11), 728–733.
128. Block, J. J. (2008). Issues for DSM-V: Internet addiction. *Am J Psychiatry, 165*(3), 306–307.
129. Block, J. J. (2007). Pathological computer use in the USA. Paper presented at: International Symposium on the Counseling and Treatment of Youth Internet Addiction, 2007; Seoul, Korea.
130. Beard, K. W. & Wolf, E. M. (2001). Modification in the proposed diagnostic criteria for Internet addiction. *Cyberpsychol Behav, 4*(3), 377–383.
131. Young, K. S. (2008). *Caught in the net.* New York: John Wiley & Sons.
132. Caplan, S. E. (2002). Problematic Internet use and psychosocial well-being: Development of a theory-based cognitive-behavioral measurement instrument. *Computers in Human Behavior, 18,* 5553–5575.
133. Shaw, M. & Black, D. W. (2008). Internet addiction: Definition, assessment, epidemiology and clinical management. *CNS Drugs. 22*(5), 353–365.
134. Morahan-Martin, J. & Schumacher, P. (2000). Incidence and correlates of pathological Internet use among college students. *Computers in Human Behavior. 16*(1), 13–29.
135. Choi, Y. H. (2007). Advancement of IT and seriousness of youth Internet addiction. Paper presented at: International Symposium on the Counseling and Treatment of Youth Internet Addiction, 2007; Seoul, Korea.
136. Koh, Y. S. (2007). Development and application of K-Scale as diagnostic scale for Korean Internet Addiction. Paper presented at: International Symposium on the Counseling and Treatment of Youth Internet Addiction, 2007; Seoul, Korea.
137. Ahn, D. H. (2007). Korean policy on treatment and rehabilitation for adolescents' Internet Addiction. Paper presented at: International Symposium on the Counseling and Treatment of Youth Internet Addiction, 2007; Seoul, Korea.
138. Beard, K. S. (2005). Internet addiction: A review of current assessment techniques and potential assessment questions. *Cyberpsychology & Behavior, 8*(1), 7–14.
139. Griffiths, M. (1997). Psychology of computer use: XLIII. Some comments on "addictive use of the Internet" by Young. *Psychol Rep, 80*(1), 81–82.
140. Shapira, N. A., Goldsmith, T. D., Keck, P. E., Jr., Khosla, U. M., & McElroy, S. L. (2000). Psychiatric features of individuals with problematic internet use. *J Affect Disord, 57*(1–3), 267–272.
141. Anderson, K. J. (2001). Internet use among college students: An exploratory study. *J Am Coll Health, 50*(1), 21–26.
142. Young, K. S. (1999). Internet addiction: Symptoms, evaluation, and treatment. In L. VandeCreek, T. L. Jackson, (Ed.). *Innovations in clinical practice.* Vol *17.* Sarasota, FL: Professional Resource Press.
143. Kuzma, J. M. & Black, D. W. (2004). Compulsive disorders. *Curr Psychiatry Rep, 6*(1), 58–65.
144. Young, K. S. (2007). Cognitive behavior therapy with Internet addicts: Treatment outcomes and implications. *Cyberpsychol Behav, 10*(5), 671–679.
145. Commission NGIS. (1999). *National Gambling Impact Study Commission Final Report.* Washington, DC.
146. Foy, A. (2007). Circuit breakers for addiction. *Intern Med J, 37*(5), 320–325.
147. Hser, Y. I., Hoffman, V., Grella, C. E., & Anglin, M. D. (2001). A 33-year follow-up of narcotics addicts. *Arch Gen Psychiatry, 58*(5), 503–508.

148. Gallop, R. J., Crits-Christoph, P., Ten Have, T. R., et al. (2007). Differential transitions between cocaine use and abstinence for men and women. *J Consult Clin Psychol, 75*(1), 95–103.
149. Jeffery, R. W., Drewnowski, A., Epstein, L. H., et al. (2000). Long-term maintenance of weight loss: Current status. *Health Psychol, 19*(1 Suppl), 5–16.
150. Chappel, J. N. & DuPont, R. L. (1999). Twelve-step and mutual-help programs for addictive disorders. *Psych Clin North Am, 22*(2), 425–446.
151. Bogenschutz, M. P., Geppert, C. M. A., & George, J. (2006). The role of twelve-step approaches in dual diagnosis treatment and recovery. *Am J Addict, 15,* 50–60. doi:10.1080/10550490500419060.
152. Stewart, R. M. & Brown, R. I. (1988). An outcome study of Gamblers Anonymous. *Br J Psychiatry, 152,* 284–288.
153. Petry, N. M. (2003). Patterns and correlates of Gamblers Anonymous attendance in pathological gamblers seeking professional treatment. *Addict Behav, 28*(6), 1049–1062.
154. Miller, W. R. & Rollnick, S. (1991). *Motivational interviewing: Preparing people to change addictive behavior.* New York: Guilford Press.
155. Miller, W. R. & Rollnick, S. (2002). *Motivational interviewing: Preparing people for change.* 2nd ed. New York: Guilford Press.
156. Marlatt, G. A. & J. R. Gordon, (Eds). (1985). *Relapse prevention: Maintenance strategies in the treatment of addictive behaviors.* New York: Guilford Press.
157. Larimer, M. E., Palmer, R. S., & Marlatt, G. A. (1999). Relapse prevention. An overview of Marlatt's cognitive-behavioral model. *Alcohol Res Health, 23*(2), 151–160.
158. Grant, J. E. & Kim, S. W. (2006). Medication management of pathological gambling. *Minn Med, 89*(9), 44–48.
159. Kim, S. W. & Grant, J. E. (2001). An open naltrexone treatment study in pathological gambling disorder. *Int Clin Psychopharmacol, 16*(5), 285–289.
160. Grant, J. E., Potenza, M. N., Hollander, E., et al. (2006). Multicenter investigation of the opioid antagonist nalmefene in the treatment of pathological gambling. *Am J Psychiatry, 163*(2), 303–312.
161. Guerdjikova, A., McElroy, S. L., Kotwal, R., & Keck, P. E. (2007). Comparison of obese men and women with binge eating disorder seeking weight management *Eat Weight Disord, 12*(1), e19–23.
162. Wilfley, D. E., Crow, S. J., Hudson, J. I., et al. (2008). Efficacy of sibutramine for the treatment of binge eating disorder: A randomized multicenter placebo-controlled double-blind study. *Am J Psychiatry, 165*(1), 51–58.
163. Appolinario, J. C., Bacaltchuk, J., Sichieri, R., et al. (2003). A randomized, double-blind, placebo-controlled study of sibutramine in the treatment of binge-eating disorder. *Arch Gen Psychiatry, 60*(11), 1109–1116.
164. Golay, A., Laurent-Jaccard, A., Habicht, F., et al. (2005). Effect of orlistat in obese patients with binge eating disorder. *Obes Res, 13*(10), 1701–1708.
165. Nestler, E. J. (2005). Is there a common molecular pathway for addiction? *Nat Neurosci, 8*(11), 1445–1449. doi:1410.1038/nn1578.
166. DuPont, R. L., McLellan, A. T., White, W. L., Merlo, L. J., & Gold, M. S. (2009). Setting the standard for recovery: Physicians health programs. *Journal of Substance Abuse and Treatment, 36,* 159–171.
167. Kelley, A. E. & Berridge, K. C. (2002). The neuroscience of natural rewards: Relevance to addictive drugs. *J Neurosci, 22,* 3306–3311.
168. Dannon, P. N., Lowengrub, K., Shalgi, B., et al. (2006). Dual psychiatric diagnosis and substance abuse in pathological gamblers: A preliminary gender comparison study. *J Addict Dis, 25*(3), 49–54.

169. Wilfley, D. E., Friedman, M. A., Dounchis, J. Z., Stein, R. I., Welch, R. R., & Ball, S. A. (2000). Comorbid psychopathology in binge eating disorder: Relation to eating disorder severity at baseline and following treatment. *J Consult Clin Psychol, 68*(4), 641–649.
170. Cocores, J. A., Miller, N. S., Gold, M. S., & Pottash, A. C. (1988). Sexual dysfunction in abusers of cocaine and alcohol. *Am J Drug Alcohol Abuse, 14*(2), 169–173.
171. Graham, N. A., Polles, A., & Gold, M. S. (2007). Performance enhancing, non-prescription use of erectile dysfunction medications. *J Addict Dis, 25*(suppl 1), 61–68.

PART III

The Public's Mental Health from Youth to Older Age

Changing Landscapes or Stable Patterns?

8

Personality Pathology, Health, and Social Adjustment in Later Life

THOMAS F. OLTMANNS AND MARCI E.J. GLEASON

Personality differences play a central role in the link between mental health and public health. Several considerations are important in this regard. Neuroticism and other personality traits represent significant risk factors for many mental disorders.[1] They are especially influential in the etiology of mood and substance use disorders, both leading sources of disease burden. In their more extreme forms, certain constellations of personality problems are considered pathological in their own right, as they have a direct, negative impact on the person's social adjustment. Considerable evidence also suggests that personality and its disorders influence subjective perceptions of health, the utilization of health care resources, and the success of treatment outcomes for mental and medical conditions. Thus, it is important to understand the impact of personality traits and pathology on health and social adjustment throughout the lifespan.[2]

Longitudinal data regarding the course and outcome of personality disorders provide one important basis for understanding these important clinical problems. Many young adults who exhibit severe personality dysfunction experience significant improvement as they get older.[3,4] Serious questions remain unanswered, however, particularly with regard to the trajectory of personality disorders in later life.[5] We do not know whether personality problems re-emerge later (with either similar or modified presentations). Relationships between personality traits, personality disorders, and symptoms of other mental disorders (e.g., major depression) have not been studied prospectively in older adults.

The study described here was designed to evaluate and compare various approaches to the measurement of personality pathology in the context of a longitudinal design. Using both self-report questionnaires and informant reports, we are collecting information regarding personality traits and pathology in an epidemiologically based, representative sample of adults between the ages of 55 and 64 living in the St. Louis metropolitan area. Repeated assessments of personality, personality disorders, mood disorders, and substance use disorders will be completed at regular 2.5-year intervals.

Epidemiological data suggest that approximately 10% to 14% of the adult population in the community would meet diagnostic criteria for at least one form of personality disorder.[6,7] This percentage would increase if we include people who exhibit several features of personality disorder, even if they don't exceed the diagnostic threshold for any particular disorder.[8] Some studies of community-based samples indicate that the prevalence of personality disorders drops from approximately 20% in younger adults to less than 10% in those who are older.[9,10]

Personality disorders represent an important mental health problem for older adults, and there is a serious need for more information in this area. This population presents a number of interesting opportunities and advantages in comparison to the study of personality pathology among adolescents and young adults. One is that personality traits (and their pathological variations) are relatively more stable in older individuals. Several reviews of normal personality development have concluded that there is substantial evidence for a gradual *increase* in stability from late adolescence through the adult years, with "strong stability" being achieved after the age of 50.[11,12] Another important consideration for older adults is that they are also entering a period in their lives when the frequency of transitions and health problems will increase. The best time to study personality and personality disorders may be during periods of significant transition because the enduring behavioral and affective expressions that define the individual and distinguish individuals from one another will be exaggerated at such times.[13]

Personality traits and personality pathology are clearly related to health and general medical outcomes among younger and older adults. Patients with personality disorders consume more mental and physical health care resources than people without personality disorders.[14,15] Increased numbers of "medically unexplained symptoms" are strongly associated with personality variables such as neuroticism.[16] One study that assessed personality disorders among patients in primary practice settings found that patients with high scores on personality disorder questionnaires reported increased numbers of outpatient, emergency, and inpatient visits in the previous 6 months.[17] These data are consistent with previous suggestions that personality variables play an important role in relation to various long-term aspects of physical health.[18,19]

In addition to their impact on health, personality disorders are associated with impaired social and occupational functioning. In clinical samples, personality disorders are typically associated with impaired social functioning and increased interpersonal conflict.[20–23] Some studies also report higher levels of social impairment and interpersonal conflict among people with personality disorders in community samples.[24–28]

While there is general agreement that personality traits and personality disorders have a negative effect on health and social adjustment, there is relatively little consensus on how best to define and measure these concepts. Dissatisfaction with the traditional categorical model represented in DSM-IV stems from a number of problems, including high rates of comorbidity among the specific types of personality disorders, confusion about the relations between personality disorders and other types of mental disorders listed on Axis I of the diagnostic manual, and ambiguity regarding the boundaries between personality traits and personality disorders.[29,30]

For the past 30 years (at least), relative merits of the DSM-IV definitions of personality disorders and various alternative dimensional models of personality and personality pathology have been debated.[31,32] Consensus has not been reached, but most models share a common hierarchical structure that cuts across the DSM-IV categories consisting of three to five basic dimensions.[33,34]

Perhaps the most popular and frequently studied dimensional model of personality pathology is based on the Five Factor Model (FFM) of personality:[35,36] neuroticism, extraversion, agreeableness, conscientiousness, and openness. Each can be further sub-divided into six specific facets. Variations on these facets can be used to create descriptions of the primary features of the personality disorder categories represented in DSM-IV. For example, the symptoms of borderline personality disorder can be described in terms of extremely high levels of the neuroticism domain (especially high angry hostility, impulsiveness, vulnerability, anxiousness, and depressiveness) and a low level on conscientiousness (especially deliberation).

We chose to focus on the FFM rather than the other dimensional models because the FFM has been used extensively in longitudinal studies on personality and aging[37,38] and because extensive data are available regarding comparisons of self- and informant-report versions of the NEO PI-R.[39] To date, comparisons of the FFM and the DSM approach to personality disorders have been limited to descriptive comparisons. The two approaches are clearly correlated with each other. Specific forms of personality disorder in the DSM-IV can be described using the FFM. For example, paranoid personality disorder translates to low agreeableness (especially trust and compliance) and high neuroticism (angry hostility). The next step in comparing the systems involves examination of the *validity* of both models. Several methods study the validity of diagnostic constructs in psychiatry,[2,40–42] including genetic, treatment outcome, and laboratory studies which demonstrate an association with a more psychological, biochemical, or molecular abnormality. Another important method involves the use of longitudinal studies demonstrating a particular course or outcome.

Like other forms of mental disorder, personality pathology is defined, in part, by its impact on the person's life. If the characteristic features of personality disorder interfere with the person's ability to get along with other people and perform social roles, they become more than eccentric traits or peculiar habits, but are viewed as a form of harmful dysfunction.[43,44] Kendell[45] argued that, like other forms of disease, mental disorders should be defined in terms of their impact on increased mortality and reduced fertility. Following this logic, two crucial considerations are health and marital adjustment. Personality disorders should be expected to lead to an increase in other kinds of health problems and a decrease in the ability to manage relationships with intimate partners.

Since personality disorders are associated with problems in social adjustment and interpersonal conflict, one way to empirically compare the two major alternatives to their classification would be to determine whether one system or the other is more useful in predicting deterioration in social functioning. Older adults offer a unique opportunity to compare different models for classifying personality disorders. They have presumably achieved a relatively stable personality, and they are also on the brink of major changes in their lives. They are approaching several forms of life transition (retirement) as well as the onset of chronic health problems. Longitudinal data regarding individual differences in response to transitions provide one important window in the study of psychopathology and methods of classifying mental disorders.[3,46,47] We plan to compare the DSM and FFM models (as well as self-report and informant measures of each model) in terms of their ability to predict health and adjustment problems in a large, representative sample of mature adults.

The pathways through which personality and personality disorders influence health and social functioning may vary as a function of the specific type of personality disorder. Personality disorders do have some impact on these aspects of people's lives and the success with which they are able to adapt to major transitions, such as retirement, changes in residence, and the loss of friends and family members. Nevertheless, the ways in which personality disorders might lead to problems in adaptation remain largely unexplored. The longitudinal design of our study will allow us to address these issues. For example, people who exhibit symptoms of obsessive-compulsive personality disorder might be expected to deal successfully with the onset of a serious health problem because they are extremely high on conscientiousness (dutiful and self-disciplined). On the other hand, they might deal poorly with the transition to retirement by virtue of the same collection of personality traits (achievement striving). People who exhibit symptoms of histrionic personality disorder might adjust well following the transition to retirement because they are high on extraversion (activity and positive emotions) and openness to experience (fantasy and actions), but they would be expected to have trouble adapting to the management of a chronic health problem because they are low on conscientiousness (especially self-discipline and deliberation). For other disorders, the effects of personality on adjustment following transitions may vary as a function of moderator variables such as the quality of the person's marital relationship. We plan to explore these and other alternatives.

Design of the SPAN Study

The first phase of our prospective cohort study has been the identification of the sample and completion of baseline assessments. That process and some preliminary results are described in this chapter. The second phase of the project, not described in this chapter, involves following those people over time. Participants and their informants complete a shorter battery of questionnaires once every 6 months, focused on mood, stressful life events, transitions (retirement, change in residence), marital adjustment, sleep patterns, and social functioning.

Recruitment of Participants

The final sample size will bc 1,600 adults between the ages of 55 and 64 living in the St. Louis, MO area. The process is currently unfolding, and 1,100 participants have completed the baseline assessment as this chapter is being written. In the following pages, we describe procedures that are being followed to identify this sample and the success that we have had thus far. Within certain methodological constraints, we have done everything possible to recruit a representative sample of people living in St. Louis.

St. Louis is the 18th largest metropolitan area in the United States, with a population of approximately 2.8 million people. It is just smaller than San Francisco and Seattle and slightly larger than Pittsburgh, Baltimore, and Denver. Some observers have described it is "the most average city in the U.S."[48] It has always been known for its ethnic diversity. With the city and adjacent county combined, 30% of the population is African American, 60% is Caucasian. Only 2% is Hispanic. Approximately 7% of people living in the St. Louis area are between the ages of 55 and 64.

Participants are recruited from the city itself and surrounding suburban areas. Households are located in neighborhoods with many different socioeconomic qualities. Participants are paid $60 for their time to complete the baseline assessment instruments, and $10 for each 30-minute follow-up assessment (once every 6 months). Collateral informants are paid $30 for their first assessment and $10 for each follow-up assessment. After participants have been in the study for two and a half years and completed four of the brief follow-up exams, they will be reevaluated using the full set of personality assessment instruments (diagnostic interview, personality questionnaires, and so on).

Baseline exclusion criteria include: current history of psychosis or life-threatening illness (e.g., advanced stages of cancer), inability to read the written informed consent statement aloud, and anyone who has immediate plans to relocate outside of the St. Louis metropolitan area. To date, three people who were psychotic at the time of the baseline assessment and six people who were unable to read the consent statement have been excluded.

Potential participants are identified using telephone records purchased from Genesys Sampling Systems. We use listed (rather than unlisted) phone numbers because they can be checked against census records to ensure that someone living in the household is within our targeted age range and because they are associated with a name and address which allows us to personalize the letter explaining the study and arrangements for appointments. Use of informative advance letters is known to increase response rates in survey research.[49]

Carefully trained staff members and undergraduate students (often working during evening hours and on weekends) make these initial phone calls. Up to 12 calls (at different times of day and on the weekend) are made. After this time a second letter is sent to the household, once again asking them to call us or return a preaddressed postcard to indicate their interest in the study. Approximately 10% of those letters generate a positive response.

When a resident does answer the phone, we mention the letter, describe the study again briefly, and ask how many people in the household are within our age range. If more than one person is eligible to participate (e.g., both husband and wife), the Kish Method[50] is used to select the eligible participant. We sample without replacement. Phone contact allows us to answer questions and emphasize the importance of participation, and if the person initially refuses to participate, another request is made several weeks later where we politely ask them to reconsider. The use of "refusal converter" calls is a standard procedure in survey research because many people decline participation if they were contacted at a busy or difficult time.[49] A small percentage of these calls yields a positive response.

Transportation is provided so that participants can meet us at the university (e.g., special taxi service for people in wheelchairs). In rare instances, an interviewer is sent to the person's home to complete the assessment. Assessment sessions can be scheduled day and evening, and any day of the week to accommodate the needs of the participants. Interviews are completed face-to-face, and questionnaires can be completed on a web-based data collection site that was created for our project or by mailing paper-and-pencil forms through the mail. The process is intended to be as flexible as possible in order to maximize participation.

To date, out of those who are eligible and have been contacted, 43% have agreed to participate. This compares favorably to participation rates obtained in other recent epidemiological studies.[51] Reluctance to participate may be caused by several factors, including dramatic increases in telemarketing in the United States as well as the increased numbers of research requests that people receive. One interesting analysis of data from the Behavioral Risk Factor Surveillance Survey (BRFSS)—a health survey conducted by the U.S. Center for Disease Control—suggests that participation rates in the range of 30 to 70% have virtually no effect on bias of results.[52] Our study makes every conceivable effort to increase participation, including initial contact with an introductory letter, meaningful financial compensation, persistent efforts to contact potential participants, flexible hours for laboratory appointments, and face-to-face data collection. We are persistent and diligent while also trying to avoid unnecessary coercion or harassment of potential participants. Given the time-consuming nature of our baseline assessments (3 hours) and the fact that we are asking for their on-going participation in a longitudinal study involving both themselves and one informant, we consider our participation rate to be a significant accomplishment.

Evaluation of Possible Sampling Bias (Nonresponse)

The goal of this study is to examine the impact of personality pathology within a sample of middle-aged people as they begin to negotiate the many challenges of later life. We hope that, within certain methodological constraints, our sample will be as representative as possible, which is why we have spent considerable effort in identifying our participants using standard epidemiological methods. Our participants are in the latter stages of middle-age, and there is some reason to believe that participation rates are lower for older people. They also live in an urban area and include a relatively high proportion of men and ethnic minorities (sometimes found to be less likely to volunteer for research studies). For all of these reasons, we have continued to be concerned about various characteristics of our sample.[53]

We have worried that the people who agreed to participate might be differentially more disturbed or less disturbed than those who do not participate. Perhaps people who are lower on agreeableness or higher on neuroticism would be less inclined to participate. In order to address the influence of nonresponse on personality scores, we designed a procedure to collect personality data from people who refused to participate in the larger study, within IRB guidelines.

A short (60-item) version of our normal personality measure (the FFI) was mailed along with a cover letter to 500 people who told us on the phone that they did not want to participate. The letter said that we respected their decision not to participate in the longer version of the study, and we offered to pay them $10 to complete the shorter questionnaire and mail it back to us (with no

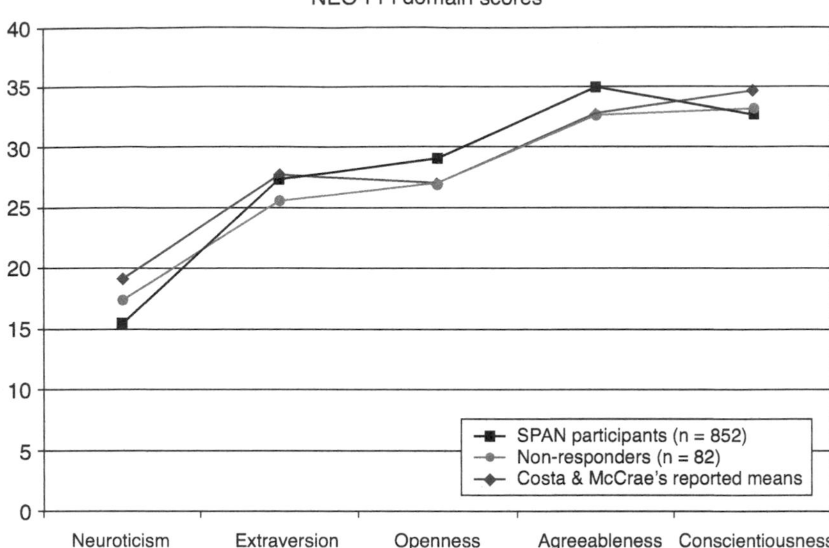

Figure 8.1 Comparison of participants and nonresponders with regard to personality scores on the Five Factor Model (NEO-PI-R).

further obligation to complete the rest of our assessment or participate in the follow-ups). We received completed questionnaires from 85 of the original nonresponders. Their scores on the five personality domains of the FFM are illustrated in Figure 8.1, along with mean scores from people who did agree to participate in the study as well as people who were used to standardize the test. Several patterns seem evident. One is that the mean scores for all three groups are quite similar, if not exactly identical, with participants producing slightly higher scores on Openness to Experience (e.g. willingness to try new activities) and Agreeableness in comparison with both the nonresponders and the original standardization sample. Second, the nonresponders score slightly lower on Extraversion than either the participants in our study or the original standardization sample. None of these differences seems to suggest important personality biases associated with nonresponse.

Oversampling of African American Men

During the first two years of the project, we collected data from approximately 700 participants. Of these, approximately 30% were African American. That proportion is very close to numbers expected on the basis of recent census data for St. Louis. Among our Caucasian participants, approximately 45% were male, also close to the expected rate in the general population. But among the African American participants, only 31% were male. Therefore, we decided to over-sample African American men.

Although racial data were not available for specific households, we did have information regarding the racial composition of sampling blocks from which our phone numbers were selected, resulting in our purchasing 300 phone numbers from three areas with high proportions (90%) of African American residents. In this sample, we included only homes for which the phone was listed in a man's name. A new letter was crafted, describing the study and emphasizing our sincere interest in including African American participants in our study. Aside from the use of this special letter and the elimination of the Kish Method to allow us to recruit only male participants, study recruitment procedures were identical. This over-sampling procedure was quite successful, yielding a participation rate in these specific sampling blocks (38%) that is quite similar to what we had found in the overall study. We decided to continue this procedure, and within five months, the proportion of African American males rose to 43%.

Recruiting Informants

Participants in the study are asked to identify someone who knows them well and who would be able to provide us with an accurate description of their personality traits, and who preferably lives with them. If that is not possible, we ask for "the person who knows you best." In order to serve as an informant, we specify that the target person and the potential informant talk at least once a month and see each other face-to-face at least once each year. Approximately half of our informants are spouses or partners, allowing us to examine marital and intimate relationships. Approximately 25% of the informants are other family members (e.g., an adult child of the target person); the rest are close friends. On average, informants have known the target person for at least 30 years. Some informants are people who do not live in St. Louis. In those cases, we collect informant data using the telephone, the Internet, or mailed questionnaires. Participants who are unwilling or unable to provide an informant are still included in the study. Only 10% of our participants have not provided informant data thus far.

Description of the Participants

Of the 1,100 target adults in the sample to date, 55% are female; all were between the ages of 55 and 64 when they entered the study (mean = 59.6, SD = 2.7 years).

With regard to race and ethnic background, 68% are Caucasian, 30% are African American, and 2% are Hispanic. Slightly more than half (56%) were born in St. Louis, 40% were born elsewhere in the US, and 4% were born outside of the US. Nearly all of the participants (92%) have lived in St. Louis for at least 20 years. Nearly two-thirds (66%) of the men and the women are employed either part time or full time. Eight percent of the men and 10% of the women are unemployed due to disability. Four percent of men and women were seeking employment at the time of their baseline assessment. Thirty-three percent of men and women have retired from at least one profession (and some of those are now working at another job). Tables 8.1 and 8.2 present additional information regarding levels of education and personal income, which are both slightly higher than expected for the population of St. Louis. Nevertheless, the sample is clearly quite diverse, and it is generally representative of middle-aged people living in this community.

When asked to describe their current marital status, 48% said that they are married, 28% are divorced, 2% are separated, 7% are widowed, and 15% have never been married. Among the 48% who had ever been divorced, 35% have been divorced only once, 10% have been divorced twice, and 3% have been divorced three to five times. Most of the participants (74%) have children (mean number is 2.4, range is 1 to 11), 42% have at least one grandchild (mean number is 3.2, range is 1 to 44), and 6% have at least one great-grandchild.

We asked a number of questions about previous life experiences, such as employment history and trouble with the police, so that we could examine connections between personality variables and these important life outcomes. Among the 33% who indicated they had been fired from a job, 67% had been fired once, 20% had been fired twice, and 5% had been fired three times. One person said he had been fired ten times. While 18% had spent at least one night in jail, 8% had been convicted of a crime. Most of those (74%) had been convicted

Table 8.1 Highest Level of Education for Participants in the SPAN Study

	Men (n = 360)	*Women (n = 444)*	*Total (n = 804)*
Less than High School	1.4%	1.4%	1.4%
High School or GED	10.0%	11.5%	10.6%
Some College	15.8%	18.9%	17.2%
Vocational School	3.9%	5.6%	4.8%
Associate's Degree	5.3%	8.1%	6.7%
Bachelor's Degree	25.0%	26.6%	26.1%
Master's Degree	21.9%	22.3%	22.0%
Doctoral Degree	7.8%	2.3%	4.8%
Professional Degree	8.1%	2.5%	5.0%
Bachelor's or More	62.8%	53.7%	57.9%

Table 8.2 Current Annual Personal Income for Participants in the SPAN Study

	Men (n = 360)	*Women (n = 444)*	*Total (n = 804)*
Under $20,000	12.7%	19.8%	16.4%
$20,000–39,999	20.1%	31.8%	26.6%
$40,000–59,999	22.9%	23.8%	23.4%
$60,000–79,999	15.2%	10.0%	12.4%
$80,000–99,999	8.3%	5.6%	6.7%
$100,000–119,999	3.3%	1.3%	2.2%
$120,000–139,999	3.3%	1.6%	2.3%
$140,000 +	11.9%	4.0%	7.7%

of a single crime. Clearly our participants experienced social and occupational impairment during their lives.

A substantial proportion of our sample (44%) indicated that they had received professional treatment for a mental disorder at some point in their life, ranging from short-term counseling for relationship problems, grief, family concerns (e.g., children's problems), and occupational issues, to long-term psychotherapy and medication for the treatment of serious mental disorders.

Assessment of Personality and Personality Disorder

Life Narrative

Our assessment process begins with a brief life narrative interview in which participants are asked to describe important features of their lives (adapted from McAdams[54]). This introductory portion of the interview is employed for several reasons: to facilitate the development of rapport with the participant, to collect information about the person's life prior to the present time, and to provide an additional perspective on the person's personality characteristics.

Semi-structured Diagnostic Interview

Every participant also completed the Structured Interview for DSM-IV Personality (SIDP-IV[55]), our primary measure of DSM-IV personality pathology. Questions in this interview are arranged by themes rather than by disorders (e.g., work style, interpersonal relationships, emotions, interests, and activities) to minimize the focus on personality pathology, which may reduce interviewer bias. Interviews were conducted by carefully trained, full-time staff members and by graduate students in clinical psychology. They typically last between 45 and 90 minutes, depending on the number of problems described by the person. Because the SIDP-IV does not have a formal training or reference manual, we relied extensively on the manual for the Personality Disorder Interview-IV[56] because it provides detailed and thoughtful descriptions of personality disorders.

Age of onset is a difficult issue that must be considered in the assessment of personality disorders (PDs) with older people. The general diagnostic criteria for a personality disorder in DSM-IV require that "the pattern is stable and of long duration and its onset can be traced back at least to adolescence or early adulthood." One major drawback of the DSM is exclusion of adult-onset personality pathology, which clearly exists.[57]

The interviewer who performs the SIDP-IV asks participants to answer questions based on what they are like when they are their usual selves. As a general rule of thumb, we suggest to participants that they focus on the past five years (following standard SIDP-IV instructions). We are using that approach for several reasons. It would be cumbersome, confusing, and time-consuming to ask the participant to describe their recent personality characteristics and then, for each item, also ask them to try to recall what they were like many years ago. For the purpose of our study, our initial personality assessments are being used to establish a baseline against which subsequent changes can be examined. We believe this is the most prudent course to follow, even though it would clearly be ideal if we did have valid information about what the person was like many years earlier as a young adult.

Multisource Assessment of Personality Pathology (MAPP)

This questionnaire includes both self-report and informant-report versions and is used as a supplementary measure of personality pathology based on the perspective outlined in DSM-IV. The self-report version of this instrument was developed from the peer nomination procedures that we used in our previous study with military recruits.[58] The revised MAPP includes items based on each of the features of ten personality disorders listed in DSM-IV. Items were constructed by translating the DSM-IV criterion sets for PDs into lay language. All of the specific PD features were rewritten into words that avoided the use of technical psychopathological terms and psychiatric jargon. A prior study found this to be reliable.[59]

We have conducted one study to compare the MAPP self-report form to two other questionnaires often used to screen for personality disorders: the PDQ-4[60] and the SCID-II questionnaire. We compared our MAPP self-report items with the PDQ-IV in a sample of 206 undergraduate students.[59] Correlations between scales ranged from 0.69 (dependent PD) to 0.87 (paranoid, borderline, and antisocial PD). The MAPP self-report scales were more conservative than the

PDQ-IV, identifying 14% of this student sample as meeting criteria for at least one form of PD, while the PDQ-IV identified 24% as having at least one PD.

NEO-Personality Inventory-Revised (NEO PI-R)

The NEO PI-R is the standard measure of the Five Factor Model (FFM) of personality (neuroticism, extraversion, openness, agreeableness, and conscientiousness),[61] providing a systematic assessment of emotional, interpersonal, experiential, attitudinal, and motivational styles. It also assesses the six traits or facets that define each domain. Taken together, the five domain scales and 30 facet scales of the NEO PI-R provide a comprehensive and detailed assessment of adult personality. It is available in two parallel versions: Form S is designed for self-reports and Form R is designed for informant reports, written in the third person for peer, spouse, or expert ratings.

Assessment of Depression, Substance Use Disorders, and Health Status

Diagnostic Interview Schedule (C-DIS)

We used the Computerized Diagnostic Interview Schedule (C-DIS-IV) screener to identify lifetime and 12-month prevalence of major depression, dysthymia, mania and hypomania, and psychosis. The C-DIS-IV[62] is an assessment that was developed for non-clinicians to collect information that could be used to generate psychiatric diagnoses according to the DSM-IV. The validity and reliability of those data indicate good agreement between diagnoses obtained by lay interviewers and clinicians.[63]

Substance Use Disorders

The MINI-International Neuropsychiatric Interview[64] is a brief, easy to administer, reliable structured interview to diagnose DSM-IV Axis I disorders. In our study, it was used to measure alcohol dependence and abuse as well as dependence and abuse associated with other drugs. In keeping with the aims of the study, the criteria for current alcohol dependence and abuse were expanded to include problems experienced across the lifetime.

Health Status

The RAND-36 Health Status Inventory (HSI) is a 36-item questionnaire that covers a wide spectrum of past four week physical and mental health.[65,66] The

HSI is widely used as an index of health status in studies that are concerned with a variety of medical conditions and outcomes. It provides scores on eight health constructs, including: physical functioning (10 items), role limitations due to physical health problems (4 items), pain (2 items), general health perceptions (5 items), emotional well-being (5 items), role limitations due to emotional problems (3 items), social functioning (2 items), and energy/fatigue (4 items).

Quality of Marital Relationship (for those participants who are currently involved in a relationship with a partner)

We use an abbreviated version of the Dyadic Adjustment Scale (DAS-4), which was developed and carefully validated to measure quality of relationships in epidemiological studies.[66] It includes four items: "How often do you discuss or have you considered divorce, separation, or terminating your relationship?" "In general, how often do you think that things between you and your partner are going well?" "Do you confide in your mate?" and "Please circle the dot which best describes the degree of happiness, all things considered, of your relationship."

Prevalence of Psychopathology and Medical Disorders

According to the C-DIS, 26% of our participants met the DSM-IV criteria for at least one episode of major depression at some point during their lives. Seventy five percent of these people had received at least some brief professional mental health treatment, though we do not know if it was specifically for depression. The rate of major depression in our sample is somewhat higher than reported in other recent epidemiological studies.[68] The lifetime prevalence rates of alcohol dependence (12%), alcohol abuse (17%), and drug dependence (9%) are also high and similar to rates that would be expected in this age group.[69] Although we screened out those individuals who were psychotic at the time of baseline assessment, 1% of our participants qualified for a lifetime diagnosis of schizophrenia or other psychotic disorder, and 2% qualified for a lifetime diagnosis of bipolar disorder.

Table 8.3 presents a list of relatively common medical disorders and the percent of our participants who indicated on the C-DIS-IV that they had been treated by a physician for one of these conditions at some point during their lives. Only 31% of the participants said that they had not experienced any of the physical illnesses listed in Table 8.3; 35% reported only one illness, 22% reported two, and 12% reported three or more. Remember that we had excluded people who said that they were very seriously ill. Although most of the people in the

Table 8.3 Percent of Participants Reporting Previous Treatment for Medical Conditions (according to the C DIS-IV)

Arthritis	25%
Asthma	11%
Bleeding Ulcer	3%
Cancer	14%
Diabetes	14%
Epilepsy	1%
Heart disease	9%
Hepatitis	5%
Stroke	3%
Tuberculosis	2%
Other serious long lasting illness	33%

sample are fairly healthy, it also includes many people who have been treated for a variety of serious illnesses at some point during their lives.

Self-Other Agreement for MAPP and NEO PI

Features of the DSM-IV personality disorders were measured using three different sources. The SIDP-IV provides an impression based on ratings made by the interviewer. The MAPP provides information on specific DSM-IV PD features separately from the point of view of the participant and also from the point of view of his or her informant. The NEO-PI can also be scored to produce PD prototype counts, using responses obtained from both the self and informant.[70] Previous work on the assessment of personality disorders suggests that while various sources of information are likely to disagree, there is also a modest amount of convergence between self-report and informant measures.[71]

Table 8.4 reports correlations among all personality disorder measures used in the SPAN Study, including the diagnostic interview (SIDP) as well as the self and informant versions of both questionnaires (the MAPP and the NEO-PI prototypes). The correlations range from low to moderate. The correlations are almost all statistically significant, but they are also consistently low. In fact, they are a bit lower than correlations typically reported in studies of self-other agreement on normal personality traits using the Five Factor Model.

Several broad patterns can be discerned among the correlations reported in Table 8.4. First, the correlations between self and informant ratings on the MAPP range between 0.17 and 0.30. These figures are quite similar to the self-other levels of agreement that were reported from our previous study comparing self-report with peer nominations for DSM-IV personality disorders in a large sample of military recruits.[58] These correlations raise important questions

Table 8.4 Correlations Between Various Sources (self and informant) and Various Instruments (MAPP and NEO-PI) for Each Type of Personality Disorder

	S-MAPP	*S-NEO*	*SIDP*	*SIDP*	*SIDP*	*SIDP*	*S-MAPP*	*S-MAPP*	*I-MAPP*	*I-MAPP*
	I-MAPP	*I-NEO*	*S-MAPP*	*I-MAPP*	*S-NEO*	*I-NEO*	*S-NEO*	*I-NEO*	*S-NEO*	*I-NEO*
PAR	0.28	0.40	0.40	0.19	0.31	0.18	0.50	0.27	0.20	0.61
SCZ	0.29	0.56	0.32	0.16	0.40	0.26	0.42	0.28	0.25	0.47
STY	0.22	0.53	0.34	0.16	0.22	0.13	0.36	0.20	0.17	0.43
ASP	0.17	0.46	0.36	0.24	0.29	0.25	0.41	0.25	0.19	0.59
BOR	0.24	0.45	0.40	0.36	0.47	0.41	0.49	0.25	0.28	0.67
HIS	0.22	0.54	0.37	0.17	0.33	0.20	0.23	0.13	0.13	0.28
NAR	0.27	0.43	0.36	0.09	0.34	0.26	0.33	0.18	0.23	0.55
AVD	0.30	0.58	0.58	0.30	0.50	0.41	0.51	0.38	0.27	0.52
DEP	0.22	0.49	0.41	0.20	0.35	0.21	0.34	0.20	0.15	0.33
OC	0.22	0.53	0.38	0.20	0.01	0.00	0.09	0.10	0.12	0.10

Note: S = self version and I = informant version of respective questionnaires. MAPP = Multisource Assessment of Personality Pathology; NEO = PD prototype count scores derived from the NEO-PI-R; SIDP = Structured Interview for DSM-IV Personality, with ratings made by the interviewer.

about whether research based exclusively on self-report provides a complete perspective on the nature of personality disorders and pathological personality traits. They suggest that a person's own description of his or her personality problems may provide a rather limited—indeed perhaps a distorted—view of this type of mental health problem.

The second obvious pattern is that self-informant correlations are consistently higher for the NEO-PI PD prototype scores than they are for the MAPP. At least two considerations may be responsible for this result. One is that the NEO-PI PD prototypes are based on a much larger number of questions than the MAPP PD scores, and may be more reliable from a psychometric point of view. Questions in the NEO-PI are also worded in a less pejorative manner, and self-other agreement on personality dimensions is typically higher for positive characteristics than for negative characteristics.

Even though self-other agreement is higher for the NEO PD prototype counts, they do not appear to have an advantage relative to the self-report MAPP if the SIDP interview is used as the criterion for evaluation (compare columns 3 and 5 in Table 8.4). Correlations between the SIDP interview and the self-report MAPP are more or less equivalent in magnitude to correlations between the SIDP interview and self-report NEO PD prototype counts. In fact, they are often just a bit higher. This is strikingly true with regard to obsessive-compulsive (OC) PD where the correlation is 0.38 for the self-MAPP with the SIDP and 0.01 for the self-report NEO and SIDP. Previous investigations have suggested that the NEO PD prototype does not accurately capture the DSM-IV definition of OCPD, and our results agree.

Fourth, scores based on the SIDP diagnostic interview are more closely related to self-report scores on the MAPP than to informant report scores on the MAPP. This result is also expected because the interviewer's ratings are based largely (though not exclusively) on answers that the participant provides to questions about the presence of personality pathology. Again, this finding is consistent with results that we have reported from the Peer Nomination Study conducted with military recruits.

Finally, the results reported in Table 8.4 indicate that for borderline personality disorder, the informant NEO PD prototype and informant MAPP work almost as well as the self-report versions of the measures for predicting interviewer ratings on the SIDP. For most of the other PDs, self-report scores are more closely related to the interviewer's rating. This result is intriguing and suggests the possibility that informant measures may be particularly useful for collecting information about the symptoms of borderline PD. Further research is necessary to determine whether the informant scores on the MAPP and NEO BPD prototype are more closely related to important outcomes in the participants' lives.

Prevalence of Personality Disorders

Table 8.5 presents detailed information regarding the presence of features of personality disorder in our sample, as reported by three different sources (self MAPP, informant MAPP, and interviewer with the SIDP-IV). The most conservative measure is the SIDP-IV interview. Semi-structured diagnostic interviews are, of course, generally considered the gold standard in epidemiological studies. Using this instrument and setting diagnostic thresholds according to DSM-IV, 9.5% of our participants met criteria for at least one form of the ten DSM-IV personality disorders. Among those people who meet criteria for at least one form of PD, 80% met criteria for only one type, 17% meet criteria for two PDs, and 3% meet criteria for three PDs. None of our participants meet criteria for more than three types of personality disorder. The most frequent diagnosis is OCPD (4.9%), followed by avoidant PD (2.9%). All of the other PDs occur in less than 1% of our participants (with the lowest being dependent and histrionic PDs, both at 0.3%).

Several previous studies have reported that personality disorder not otherwise specified (PDNOS) is an especially frequent diagnosis in clinical practice.[8] Using an empirically based standard of ten or more criteria,[72] an additional 1.2% of the participants in this community sample would meet criteria for PDNOS. The DSM-IV appendix also includes a definition of passive-aggressive PD under the heading of "criterion sets for further study." Based on the SIDP-IV results, 0.7% of our participants exceeded the diagnostic threshold for this disorder. Adding together the people who qualified for at least one of the ten primary PDs and those who qualified for PDNOS or passive-aggressive PD, we found a current prevalence of 11.9% for personality disorders among our participants.

These prevalence rates are generally consistent with several previous reports. The median prevalence rate for at least one PD of any type is 10.6% averaged across six modern studies.[73] The NESARC study reported a prevalence rate of 5.9% for borderline PD (BPD) among men and women over the age of 18,[74] substantially higher than other investigators have reported. The British National Survey of adults between the ages of 16 and 74 found that the prevalence of paranoid, schizotypal, antisocial, borderline, histrionic, narcissistic, and avoidant PDs all decreased over the lifespan. In contrast, the prevalence of schizoid and obsessive-compulsive PD increased with age.[10] This obviously reflects whether investigators report current or lifetime diagnoses.

Beyond the consideration of participants who meet DSM-IV criteria for a specific PD, Table 8.5 also indicates that our sample includes many people with subthreshold problems. Only four people were rated on the SIDP-IV interview as showing five or more features of BPD, yielding a prevalence rate of slightly less than 0.5%. Several people exhibited four or three symptoms of BPD,

Table 8.5 Number of People Who Meet a Certain Number of Criteria for Each Disorder Across Three Different Sources: MAPP Self-Report (N ≈ 920); MAPP informant report (N ≈ 798); and SIDP Interview (N ≈ 898)

	Paranoid			*Schizoid*			*Schizotypal*		
Criteria	*self*	*inform*	*SIDP*	*self*	*inform*	*SIDP*	*self*	*inform*	*SIDP*
0	343	258	757	97	129	716	426	308	780
1	264	203	102	224	210	135	225	203	89
2	159	134	20	247	190	28	153	130	19
3	63	105	11	186	123	12	61	69	8
4	42	41	6	87	68	3	23	44	1
5	31	28	2	54	54	2	16	28	1
6	9	17		22	19	2	10	10	
7	7	9		3	6		5	4	
8	2	3						3	
9							1		

	Antisocial			*Borderline*			*Histrionic*			*Narcissistic*		
Criteria	*self*	*inform*	*SIDP*	*self*	*inform*	*SIDP*	*self*	*inform*	*SIDP*	*self*	*inform*	*SIDP*
0	462	405	858	545	396	763	343	258	746	286	214	741
1	311	208	27	222	217	92	264	203	108	271	205	99
2	106	100	6	84	68	23	159	134	24	178	148	28
3	28	53	4	33	44	13	63	105	15	98	99	13
4	7	23	1	21	40	3	42	41	3	46	49	11
5	3	7	2	5	11	3	31	28	2	23	37	4
6	0	3	0	7	15	0	9	17	0	9	21	1
7	1	0	0	2	8	1	7	9	0	4	12	1
8	0	0	0	1	0	0	2	3	0	5	9	0
9	0	0	0	0	0	0	0	0	0	1	5	0

(Continues)

Table 8.5 (*Contd.*)

	Avoidant			*Dependent*			*Obsessive-Compulsive*		
Criteria	*self*	*inform*	*SIDP*	*self*	*inform*	*SIDP*	*self*	*inform*	*SIDP*
0	489	457	751	656	500	813	125	47	488
1	219	163	92	166	163	62	199	128	229
2	98	63	22	54	67	14	169	167	108
3	49	60	8	23	29	4	150	181	36
4	35	29	10	11	18	3	139	125	23
5	22	17	9	4	11	1	75	70	10
6	5	8	4	4	8	1	44	42	3
7	4	2	2	2	2		14	28	1
8					1		5	11	
9									

considered diagnostic orphans. The DSM-IV thresholds for establishing a diagnosis have frequently been described as arbitrary. One research group has argued that a broader definition of BPD using a threshold of three or more symptoms would provide a more useful definition of the disorder, improving prediction of symptom severity and interpersonal dysfunction.[75] If we employed this less conservative threshold, 2% of the participants in our study would be assigned a diagnosis of BPD. Similar findings apply to all of the other PD categories illustrated in Table 8.5.

It is also not necessary to assume that the SIDP interview is the most accurate of our assessment procedures for the identification of PD symptoms. Table 8.5 indicates that it is more conservative than the self and informant versions of the MAPP questionnaire, but it has not been established that the latter measures are less useful. One important goal of future analyses will be to compare the predictive validity of information provided by different sources (self, informant, and interviewer).

Personality and Marital Adjustment

Beyond simply counting how many people exhibit a certain number of features of personality disorders, the more important questions are concerned with the potential impact that personality pathology may have on the quality of a person's life. One interesting consideration in this regard is the formation and maintenance of intimate relationships with other adults. In our sample of participants, 49% reported that they were currently involved in an intimate relationship. Scores on several personality disorders showed small but significant correlations with this variable. Using data from the SIDP interview, there was an inverse relationship between number of symptoms of borderline PD ($r = -0.12$) and schizoid PD ($r = -0.16$) and whether or not the person was currently in a relationship. Histrionic PD was positively correlated ($r = 0.22$) with the number of previous marriages reported by participants. People who exhibited increased numbers of symptoms of BPD had also been married more times ($r = 0.12$) but were also less likely to be involved in a current relationship ($r = -0.12$).

For those participants who are currently involved in an intimate relationship with a partner, dyadic adjustment scores were negatively related to personality pathology in the participant as it was reflected in several different measures. Table 8.6 reports correlations between the participants' satisfaction with their marriages and the number of symptoms of specific personality disorders as measured by the SIDP-IV interview, the self and informant versions of the MAPP, and the self and informant NEO PD prototype counts. Most of these correlations are statistically significant, given the large sample size. This broad

Table 8.6 Correlations Between Participants' Dyadic Adjustment Scores and Personality Disorder Scores Based on Different Sources of Information for Participants Who Are in a Romantic Relationship with the Informant

	SIDP	*S-MAPP*	*I-MAPP*	*S-NEO*	*I-NEO*
Paranoid	−0.18	−0.22	−0.27	−0.27	−0.26
Schizoid	−0.20	−0.27	−0.20	−0.24	−0.23
Schizotypal	−0.20	−0.22	−0.30	−0.32	−0.27
Antisocial	−0.09	−0.18	−0.26	−0.12	−0.17
Borderline	−0.33	−0.21	−0.35	−0.28	−0.28
Histrionic	−0.04	−0.16	−0.18	0.18	0.08
Narcissistic	−0.13	−0.08	−0.26	−0.25	−0.15
Avoidant	−0.15	−0.18	−0.24	−0.22	−0.19
Dependent	−0.07	−0.10	−0.19	−0.09	−0.05
OC	−0.13	−0.13	−0.15	0.10	0.17

pattern suggests that many forms of personality pathology have an impact on the quality of intimate relationships. Perhaps most striking is the pattern for borderline PD. In three of the five columns (i.e., for the interview as well as both informant-based PD measures), the strongest correlation is for BPD.

This evidence is also consistent with the results of previous studies that have examined the connection between marital adjustment and personality disorders in younger samples of adults.[76,77] Our data indicate clearly that, although the prevalence of borderline PD and other forms of personality pathology may decrease with age, symptoms of these disorders continue to have a significant, adverse impact on the quality of social relationships.

Personality and Subjective Perceptions of Health

Beyond its impact on social adjustment, does personality pathology have a more direct association with variables related to public health? Preliminary analyses from our study have been focused on our participants' subjective perception of their own health, which provides one important predictor of future health outcomes.[78] Global self-rated health is closely connected to mortality,[79,80] and it is also closely linked to health behaviors as well as health care utilization.[81]

We combined two questions to create a composite measure of subjective perception of health. One item was the C DIS-IV general health status question: "In the last 12 months, would you describe your general health as excellent, good, fair, or poor?" The second item was the general health status question from the HSI and the HSI physical functioning scale, which is composed of questions related to the person's level of daily functioning in activities such as carrying groceries, cleaning the house, walking up stairs or around the block, and participating in sports or other strenuous physical activities.

We computed correlations between perceived health status and several other variables, including dimensional scores for the ten DSM-IV PDs (from the SIDP-IV interview), five NEO-PI domain scores, objective health indicators (i.e., number of chronic physical illnesses and physical functioning), and BDI score (as an index of depressed mood). Neuroticism, depressed mood, and number of chronic physical illnesses were negatively correlated with perceived health. Physical functioning had a significant positive correlation with perceived health. All five NEO-PI personality domains were significantly correlated with perceived health in women. Schizoid, Schizotypal, Antisocial, and Borderline PD were significantly negatively related to perceived health in both men and women.

Hierarchical linear regression was employed to examine the effect of personality pathology on perceived health when all other variables are controlled. Physical illness and functioning were entered first, and found to be predictive of perceived health for both men and women. Next, the addition of depressed mood accounted for additional variance in perceived health. Beyond that, the additional consideration of NEO-PI personality domains and personality disorders did not improve the prediction of perceived health for men. It did help for the women, however, with neuroticism significantly predicting negative perception of health. Furthermore, even after accounting for variance associated with depressed mood and neuroticism, some personality disorder scores from the SIDP interview were also associated with perceived health. More specifically, Schizoid and Antisocial PD remained significantly predictive of perceived health for women, while Borderline PD fell just short of the conventional significance level.

Like our data regarding marital relationships, our data on subjective perceptions of health indicate that personality pathology continues to have an important impact on the quality of people's lives as they move through middle age and approach the challenges of later life. Fewer people in this age range may exhibit a sufficient number of symptoms to exceed the DSM-IV thresholds for an official diagnosis of personality disorder, but the presence of several features of personality disorder is associated with poorer subjective perceptions of health, particularly among women. As the longitudinal portion of our study unfolds, we will be able to determine whether these impressions translate into more objective manifestations of disease and ultimately increased mortality.

Summary and Conclusions

Our study is the first prospective longitudinal study of the trajectory and impact of personality disorders in later life. It will allow us to evaluate the strengths and weaknesses of self-report and informant-based measures of personality pathology in terms of their ability to predict future levels of social functioning and marital adjustment (where appropriate) as well as changes in mental and physical health. We hope to learn whether some forms of personality pathology become exacerbated following challenging events and transitions. Perhaps most important, we will be able to identify those components of the DSM and FFM approaches to personality dysfunction that are most enduring and also most highly associated with impaired functioning.

Standard epidemiological methods are being used successfully to identify, recruit, and follow a diverse sample of middle-aged adults. They are representative of adults living in this typical, Midwestern city, with the exception that participants must be able to read and have a stable residence so that they can be located for follow-up assessments. Our participants report a broad range of educational, occupational, and marital experiences. Many have already been treated for serious medical conditions.

Up to the present time, data from our baseline assessments of personality, health, and social adjustment point to several preliminary conclusions:

1. Semi-structured interviews provide one important source of information regarding the presence of personality pathology. Diagnostic impressions recorded by interviewers show a significant but modest level of convergence with data collected using questionnaires completed by the participants and their informants. The level of agreement between self and informant measures is consistent with findings from previous studies. The validity of information from these different sources will be examined as the longitudinal portion of this study unfolds over the next few years.

2. Viewed from various perspectives, there is evidence of substantial personality pathology in this epidemiologically based, representative sample of middle-aged adults. The most conservative standard involves use of diagnostic interviews. Here, the proportion of people who exceed official diagnostic thresholds for some disorders, including borderline and antisocial PD, is somewhat reduced compared to rates that have been observed among younger adults.

3. Personality pathology is related in several important ways to the history and quality of our participants' intimate relationships. The most obvious pattern emerges for borderline personality disorder. People who exhibit more symptoms of BPD have been married more times than people with fewer symptoms of BPD. They are also less likely to be involved with a romantic partner at the present time. Among those people who are living with a partner, the number of BPD symptoms exhibited by the participant is inversely related to satisfaction with that relationship. That conclusion applies to the satisfaction of both the participant and the partner, and it

holds regardless of whether the participant's personality characteristics are reported by the participant or the partner.

4. Personality and personality pathology are also related to subjective perceptions of health. Number of physical illnesses, physical functioning, depressed mood, normal personality, and personality disorders all predicted self-perception of health separately. In female participants only, personality disorders predicted health perception above and beyond objective health, mood, and personality variables.

References

1. Kendler, K. & Prescott, C. (2006). *Genes, environment, and psychopathology: Understanding the causes of psychiatric and substance use disorders.* New York: Guilford Press.
2. Kendell, R. E. (2002). The distinction between personality disorder and mental illness. *Br J Psychiatry, 180,* 110–115.
3. Paris, J. (2003). *Personality disorders over time: Precursors, course, and outcome.* Washington, DC: American Psychiatric Publishing.
4. Skodol, A. (2008). Longitudinal course and outcome of personality disorders. *Psychiatr Clin North Am, 31*(3), 495–503.
5. Tackett, J., Balsis, S., Oltmanns, T., & Krueger, R. (2009). A unifying perspective on personality pathology across the life span: Developmental considerations for the fifth edition of the Diagnostic and Statistical Manual of Mental Disorders. *Dev Psychopathol, 21*(3), 687–713.
6. Lewin, T. J., Slade, T., Andrews, G., Carr, V. J., & Hornabrook, C. W. (2005). Assessing personality disorders in a national mental health survey. *Soc Psychiatry Psychiatr Epidemiol, 40*(2), 87–98.
7. Torgersen, S. (2005). Epidemiology. In J. M. Oldham, A. E. Skodol, & D. S. Bender, (Eds.). *Textbook of personality disorders.* Washington, DC: American Psychiatric Press.
8. Verheul, R. & Widiger, T. A. (2004). A meta-analysis of the prevalence and usage of the Personality Disorder Not Otherwise Specified (PDNOS) diagnosis. *J Pers Disord, 18*(4),309–319.
9. Engels, G. I., Duijsens, I. J., Haringsma, R., & van Putten, D. M. (2003). Personality disorders in the elderly compared to four younger age groups: A cross-sectional study of community residents and mental health patients. *J Pers Disord, 17*(5), 447–459.
10. Ullrich, S. & Coid, J. (2009). The age distribution of self-reported personality disorder traits in a household population. *J Pers Disord, 23*(2), 187–200.
11. Costa, P. T., Jr., McCrae, R. R., & Siegler, I. C. (1999). Continuity and change over the adult life cycle: Personality and personality disorders. In C. R. Cloninger, (Ed.). *Personality and psychopathology*. Washington, D.C.: American Psychiatric Press.
12. Shiner, R. L. (2005). A developmental perspective on personality disorders: Lessons from research on normal personality development in childhood and adolescence. *J Pers Disord, 19*(2), 202–210.
13. Caspi, A. & Moffitt, T. E. (1993). When do individual differences matter? A paradoxical theory of personality coherence. *Psycholog Inquiry, 4,* 247–271.

14. Jackson, H. J. & Burgess, P. M. (2002). Personality disorders in the community: Results from the Australian National Survey of Mental Health and Wellbeing Part II. Relationships between personality disorder, Axis I mental disorders and physical conditions with disability and health consultations. *Soc Psychiatry Psychiatr Epidemiol, 37*(6), 251–260.
15. Pilkonis, P. A., Blehar, M. C., & Prien, R. F. (1997). Introduction to the special feature: Research directions for the personality disorders: Part I. *J Pers Disord, 11*(3), 201–204.
16. Katon, W. J. & Walker, E. A. (1998). Medically unexplained symptoms in primary care. *J Clin Psychiatry, 59*Suppl 20, 15–21.
17. Hueston, W. J., Werth, J., & Mainous, A. G. 3rd. (1999). Personality disorder traits: Prevalence and effects on health status in primary care patients. *Int J Psychiatry Med, 29*(1), 63–74.
18. Friedman, H. S., Hawley, P. H., & Tucker, J. S. (1994). Personality, health, and longevity. *Curr Direct Psychol Sci, 3*(2), 37–41.
19. Shen, B. J., McCreary, C. P., & Myers, H. F. (2004). Independent and mediated contributions of personality, coping, social support, and depressive symptoms to physical functioning outcome among patients in cardiac rehabilitation. *J Behav Med, 27*(1), 39–62.
20. Kool, S., Dekker, J., Duijsens, I., de Jonghe, F., de Jong, P., & Shouws, S. (2000). Personality disorders and social functioning in depressed patients. *Soc Behav Personality, 28*, 163–176.
21. Nur, U., Tyrer, P., Merson, S., & Johnson, T. (2004). Social function, clinical symptoms and personality disturbance. *Ir J Psych Med, 21*, 18–22.
22. Skodol, A. E., Gunderson, J. G., McGlashan, T. H., et al. (2002). Functional impairment in patients with schizotypal, borderline, avoidant, or obsessive-compulsive personality disorder. *Am J Psychiatry, 159*(2), 276–283.
23. Zanarini, M. C., Frankenburg, F. R., Hennen,J., Reich, D. B., & Silk, K. R. (2005). Psychosocial functioning of borderline patients and Axis II comparison subjects followed prospectively for six years. *J Pers Disord, 19*(1), 19–29.
24. Bagge, C., Nickell, A., Stepp, S., Currett, C., Jackson, K., & Trull, T. J. (2004). Borderline personality disorder features predict negative outcomes 2 years later. *J Abnorm Psychol, 113*(2), 279–288.
25. Jackson, H. J. & Burgess, P. M. (2004). Personality disorders in the community: Results from the Australian National Survey of Mental Health and Well-Being Part III. Relationships between specific type of personality disorder, Axis I mental disorders and physical conditions with disability and health consultations. *Soc Psychiatry Psychiatr Epidemiol, 39*(10), 765–776.
26. Johnson, J. G., Cohen, P., Kasen, S., Skodol, A. E., Hamagami, F., & Brook, J. S. (2000). Age-related change in personality disorder trait levels between early adolescence and adulthood: A community-based longitudinal investigation. *Acta Psychiatrica Scandinavica, 102*(4), 265–275.
27. Oltmanns, T. F., Melley, A. H., & Turkheimer, E. (2002). Impaired social functioning and symptoms of personality disorders in a non-clinical population. *J Pers Disord, 16*(5), 438–453.
28. Ro, E. & Clark, L. A. (2009). Psychosocial functioning in the context of diagnosis: Assessment and theoretical issues. *Psychol Assess, 21*(3), 313–324.
29. Clark, L. (2007). Assessment and diagnosis of personality disorder: Perennial issues and an emerging reconceptualization. *Annu Rev Psychol, 58*, 227–257.

30. Widiger, T. A. & Mullins-Sweatt, S. N. (2005). Categorical and dimensional models of personality disorders. In J. M. Oldham, A. E. Skodol, and D. S. Bender, (Eds.). *Textbook of personality disorders.* Washington, DC: American Psychiatric Press.
31. Krueger, R. F. & Eaton, N. R. (2010). Personality traits and the classification of mental disorders: Toward a more complete integration in DSM-V and an empirical model of psychopathology. *Personality Disorders: Theory, Research, and Treatment, 1,* 97–118.
32. Trull, T. J. & Durrett, C. A. (2005). Categorical and dimensional models of personality disorder. *Annu Rev Clin Psychol, 1,* 355–380.
33. Markon, K. E., Krueger, R. F., & Watson, D. (2005). Delineating the structure of normal and abnormal personality: An integrative hierarchical approach. *J Pers Soc Psychol, 88*(1), 139–157.
34. Widiger, T. A. & Simonsen, E. (2005). Alternative dimensional models of personality disorder: Finding a common ground. *J Pers Disord, 19*(2), 110–130.
35. Saulsman, L. M. & Page, A. C. (2004). The five-factor model and personality disorder empirical literature: A meta-analytic review. *Clin Psychol Rev, 23*(8), 1055–1085.
36. Widiger, T. A. & Costa, P. T., Jr. (2002). Five-Factor model personality disorder research. In: P. T. Costa & T. A. Widiger, (Eds.). *Personality disorders and the five-factor model of personality.* 2nd ed. (pp. 59–87). Washington, DC: American Psychological Association.
37. Roberts, B. W., Walton, K. E., & Viechtbauer, W. (2006). Patterns of mean-level change in personality traits across the life course: A meta-analysis of longitudinal studies. *Psychol Bull, 132*(1), 1–25.
38. Terracciano, A., McCrae, R. R., Brant, L. J., & Costa, P. T. (2005). Hierarchical linear modeling analyses of the NEO-PI-R scales in the Baltimore longitudinal study of aging. *Psychol Aging, 20*(3), 493–506.
39. Miller, J. D., Pilkonis, P. A., & Clifton, A. (2005). Self- and other-reports of traits from the five-factor model: Relations to personality disorders. *J Pers Disord, 19*(4), 400–419.
40. Kendler, K. S. (1990). Toward a scientific psychiatric nosology. Strengths and limitations. *Arch Gen Psychiatry, 47*(10), 969–973.
41. Robins, E. & Guze, S. B. (1970). Establishment of diagnostic validity in psychiatric illness: Its application to schizophrenia. *Am J Psychiatry, 126*(7), 983–987.
42. Rounsaville, B. J., Alarcon, R. D., Andrews, G., Jackson, J. S., Kendell, R. E., & Kendler, K. (2002). Basic nomenclature issues for DSM-V. In D. J. Kupfer, M. B. First, & D. A. Regier, (Eds.). *A research agenda for DSM-V* (pp. 1–29). Washington, DC: American Psychiatric Press.
43. Robins, E. & Guze, S. (1989). Establishment of diagnostic validity in psychiatric illness. In L. N. Robins & J. E. Barrett, (Eds.). *The validity of psychiatric diagnosis* (pp. 177–197). New York: Raven Press.
44. Wakefield, J. (1999). Evolutionary versus prototype analyses of the concept of disorder. *J Abnorm Psychol, 108*(3), 374–399.
45. Kendell, R. (1975). *The role of diagnosis in psychiatry.* Oxford, England: Blackwell Scientific Publications.
46. Buka, S. L. & Gilman, S. E. (2002). Psychopathology and the life course. In J. E. Helzer & J. J. Hudziak, (Eds.). *Defining psychopathology in the 21st century: DSM-V and beyond.* Washington, DC: American Psychiatric Publishing.
47. Grilo, C. M. & McGlashan, T. H. (2005). Course and outcome of personality disorders. In J. M. Oldham, A. E. Skodol, & D. S. Bender, (Eds.). *Textbook of personality disorders.* Washington, DC: American Psychiatric Press.

48. Markus, H. R., Plaut, V. C., & Lachman, M. E. (2004). Well-being in America: Core features and regional patterns. In O. G. Brim, C. D. Ryff, & R. C. Kessler, (Eds.). *How healthy are we? A national study of well-being at midlife* (pp. 614–650). Chicago, IL: University of Chicago Press.
49. Fowler, F. J. (2002). *Survey research methods.* 3rd ed. Thousand Oaks, CA: Sage.
50. Kish, L. (1949). A procedure for objective respondent selection within the household. *J Am Statist Assoc, 44,* 380–387.
51. Galea, S. & Tracy, M. (2007). Participation rates in epidemiologic studies. *Ann Epidemiol, 17*(9), 643–653.
52. Keeter, S., Miller, C., Khout, A., Groves, R. M., & Presser, S. (2000). Consequences of reducing nonresponse in a national telephone survey. *Public Opin Q, 64,* 125–148.
53. Cottler, L. B., Zipp, J., Robins, L., & Spitznagel, E. (1987). Difficult-to-recruit respondents and their effect on prevalence estimates in an epidemiologic survey. *Am J Epidemiol, 125,* 329–339.
54. McAdams, D. P. (1993). *Stories we live by: personal myths and the making of the self.* New York: Morrow.
55. Pfohl, B., Blum, N., & Zimmerman, M. (1997). *Structured Interview for DSM-IV Personality (SIDP-IV).* Washington, DC: American Psychiatric Association.
56. Widiger, T. A., Mangine, S., Corbitt, E. M., Ellis, C. G., & Thomas, G. V. (1995). *Personality Disorder Interview–IV: A Semistructured Interview for the Assessment of Personality Disorders.* Odessa, FL: Psychological Assessment Resources, Inc.
57. Widiger, T. A. & Seidlitz, L. (2002). Personality, psychopathology, and aging. *J Res Personal, 36,* 335–362.
58. Oltmanns, T. F. & Turkheimer, E. (2006). Perceptions of self and others regarding pathological personality traits. In R. F. Krueger & J. L. Tackett, (Eds.). *Personality and psychopathology: Building bridges* (pp. 71–111). New York: Guilford.
59. Okada, M. & Oltmanns, T. F. (2009). Comparison of three self-report measures of personality pathology. *J Psychopathol Behav Assess, 31,* 280–290.
60. Hyler, S. E. (1994). *Personality Questionnaire, PDQ-IV+.* New York, NY: New York State Psychiatric Institute.
61. Costa, P. T., Jr. & McCrae, R. R. (1992). *Revised NEO Personality Inventory (NEO PI-R) and NEO Five Factor Inventory (NEO-FFI) professional manual.* Odessa, FL: Psychological Assessment Resources.
62. Robins, L. N., Cottler, L. B., Bucholz, K. K., Compton, W. M., North, C. S., & Rourke, K. M. (1999). Diagnostic Interview Schedule for the DSM-IV (DIS-IV). St. Louis, MO: Washington University School of Medicine, Department of Psychiatry.
63. Compton, W,. Cottler, L., Jacobs, J., Ben-Abdallah, A., & Spitznagel, E. (2003). The role of psychiatric disorders in predicting drug dependence treatment outcomes. *Am J Psychiatry. 160*(5), 890–895.
64. Sheehan, D., Lecrubier, Y., Sheehan, K., et al. (1998). The Mini-International Neuropsychiatric Interview (M.I.N.I.): The development and validation of a structured diagnostic psychiatric interview for DSM-IV and ICD-10. *J Clin Psychiatry, 59*(20), 22–33.
65. Hays, R. D. (1998). *RAND-36 Health Status Inventory.* San Antonio, TX: The Psychological Corporation (HBJ); 1998.
66. Hays, R. D. & Morales, L. S. (2001). The RAND-36 measure of health-related quality of life. *Ann Med, 33*(5), 350–357.
67. Sabourin, S., Valois, P., & Lussier, Y. (2005). Development and validation of a brief version of the dyadic adjustment scale with a nonparametric item analysis model. *Psychol Assess, 17*(1), 15–27.

68. Kessler, R. C., Berglund, P., Demler, O., Jin, R., Merikangas, K. R., & Walters, E. E. (2005). Lifetime prevalence and age-of-onset distributions of DSM-IV disorders in the National Comorbidity Survey Replication. *Arch Gen Psychiatry, 62*(6), 593–603.
69. Grant, B. F., Stinson, F. S., Dawson, D. A, et al. (2004). Prevalence and co-occurrence of substance use disorders and independent mood and anxiety disorders: Results from the National Epidemiologic Survey on Alcohol and Related Conditions. *Arch Gen Psychiatry, 61*(8), 807–816.
70. Miller, J., Bagby, R., Pilkonis, P., Reynolds, S., & Lynam, D. (2005). A simplified technique for scoring DSM-IV personality disorders with the five-factor model. *Assessment, 12*(4), 404–415.
71. Klonsky, E. D., Oltmanns, T. F., Turkheimer, E. (2002). Informant reports of personality disorder: Relation to self-reports and future research directions. *Clin Psychol: Sci Pract, 9*, 300–311.
72. Pagan, J., Oltmanns, T., Whitmore, M., & Turkheimer E. (2005). Personality disorder not otherwise specified: Searching for an empirically based diagnostic threshold. *J Person Disord, 19*(6), 674–689.
73. Lenzenweger, M. (2008). Epidemiology of personality disorders. *Psychiatr Clin North Am, 31*(3), 395–403.
74. Grant, B. F., Chou, S. P., Goldstein, R. B., et al. (2008). Prevalence, correlates, disability, and comorbidity of DSM-IV borderline personality disorder: Results from the Wave 2 National Epidemiologic Survey on Alcohol and Related Conditions. *J Clin Psychiatry, 69*(4), 533–545.
75. Clifton, A. & Pilkonis, P. (2007). Evidence for a single latent class of Diagnostic and Statistical Manual of Mental Disorders borderline personality pathology. *ComprPsychiatry, 48*(1), 70–78.
76. South, S. C., Oltmanns, T. F., & Turkheimer, E. (2008). Personality disorder symptoms and marital functioning. *J Consult Clin Psychol, 76*(5), 769–780.
77. Whisman, M. & Schonbrun, Y. (2009). Social consequences of borderline personality disorder symptoms in a population-based survey: Marital distress, marital violence, and marital disruption. *J Pers Disord, 23*(4), 410–415.
78. Powers, A. D. & Oltmanns, T. F. (in press). Personality pathology as a risk factor for negative health perception. *J Pers Disord.*
79. Blazer, D. G. (2008). How do you feel about...? Health outcomes in late life and self-perceptions of health and well-being. *Gerontologist, 48*(4), 415–422.
80. Vuorisalmi, M., Lintonen, T., & Jylhä, M. (2005). Global self-rated health data from a longitudinal study predicted mortality better than comparative self-rated health in old age. *J Clin Epidemiol, 58*(7), 680–687.
81. Schneider, G., Driesch, G., Kruse, A., Wachter, M., Nehen, H., & Heuft, G. (2004). What influences self-perception of health in the elderly? The role of objective health condition, subjective well-being and sense of coherence. *Arch Gerontol Geriatr, 39*, 227–237.

9

Mortality from Common Mental Disorders and Medical Conditions

WILLIAM W. EATON, MARTHA L. BRUCE, ALDEN L. GROSS, O. JOSEPH BIENVENU, ROSA M. CRUM, AND LINDA B. COTTLER

Introduction

The risk of mortality associated with a history of a mental disorder has been a long-standing interest in psychiatry.[1–4] The early literature focused on severe disorders and persons in treatment facilities. However, the relevance of these studies to the general population was limited, since only a small percentage of persons with the most common mental disorders—that is, anxiety, mood, and substance use disorders—end up in a treatment setting. The advent of population-based studies of mental disorders which include specific diagnoses (so-called "generation three" psychiatric epidemiologic studies[5]) addressed the problem of treatment bias. Now, a quarter-century since they began, these studies have sufficient person years of exposure to the risk of death to elucidate the relationship of the common mental disorders to mortality. This paper reviews literature on the four common mental disorders, summarizes what is known to date about the mortality risk they entail, and presents data on the vital status of household-residing respondents from the New Haven and Baltimore sites of the Epidemiologic Catchment Area Program. The literature on the common mental disorders was reviewed systematically (Table 9.1, taken from Eaton et al.[6]) using only studies that were prospective and based in the population, as opposed to the clinic. A standardized and replicable form of diagnosis was required for inclusion in the review. For most disorders a prior systematic review was available and was updated. Comparison is made to four prominent medical conditions available in the ECA data and to similar analyses from the National Health Interview Survey in 2000.

Table 9.1 All-cause Mortality Associated with Mental Disorders as Compared to General Population Samples Without the Disorder

	Median Relative Risk	*Interquartile Range*	*Number of Studies Found*	*Number of Studies Included*
Panic Disorder	1.9	0.8–3.2	77	4
Social Phobia	NA	NA	28	NA
Simple Phobia	NA	NA	28	NA
Major Depressive Disorder	1.7	1.3–2.2	282	14
Drug Abuse/ Dependence	2.0	1.6–2.1	610	2
Alcohol Abuse/ Dependence	1.8	1.5–2.0	913	7

NA—no sources available.
Panic (Eaton et al., 2007; Bruce et al., 1994a; Kouzis et al., 1995; Grasbeck et al., 1996).
Depression (Eaton et al., 2007; Kua, 1992; Pulska et al., 1998; Henderson et al., 1997; Gallo et al., 2005; Murphy et al., 2008; Joukamaa et al., 2001; Davidson et al., 1988; Bruce et al., 1994a; Pulska et al., 1997; Penninx et al., 1998; Kouzis et al., 1995; Saz et al., 1999; Mogga et al., 2006).
Drug abuse/dependence-(Kouzis et al., 1995; Eaton et al., 2007).
Alcohol abuse/dependence-(Eaton et al., 2007; Kouzis et al., 1995; Bruce et al., 1994a; Vaillant, 1996; Bourgkard et al., 2008; Rossow & Amundsen, 1997; Dawson, 2000).

Review of Mental Disorders and Mortality

Depression

With few exceptions and across nationalities and cultures, depressive illness and symptoms have been associated with increased risk of mortality.[7–19] These findings have generated numerous questions and hypotheses about the underlying reasons for this association. The evidence is ambiguous and is likely best addressed by a well-characterized population-based sample followed over a long period of time.

Depression is the psychiatric condition most strongly linked to suicide among older adults, although most depressed older adults die from causes other than suicide. Conwell and coworkers,[20] investigating psychological autopsies of all suicides within a geographical region, found that with increasing age, depression was more likely to be unaccompanied by other psychiatric conditions, such as substance abuse. Because suicide accounts for so little of the observed relationship between depression and mortality, it is necessary to look at how biological or psychosocial factors, or both, account for the observed relationship through pathways not resulting in suicide. The evidence to date suggests that both sets of factors contribute to mortality risk, but more information is needed about how these factors increase, mediate, or modify this risk before effective prevention and treatment interventions can be designed.

The bodily changes associated with depression may involve physiological characteristics which entail higher risk for a range of medical conditions with associated higher risk for death, such as hypertension,[21] diabetes,[22] heart problems,[23] osteoporosis,[24] stroke,[25] kidney disease,[26] and some but not all cancers.[27–31]

There is now empirical evidence that cerebrovascular disease confers vulnerability to a variety of syndromes, including depression, other mood syndromes, and psychosis, but also cognitive impairment and peripheral neurologic signs.[32] The clinical presentation of vascular depression has been characterized and resembles that of a medial frontal lobe syndrome with prominent psychomotor retardation, apathy, and pronounced disability. Depression in persons with vascular stigmata or cerebrovascular lesions identified through neuroimaging has poor outcomes, including persistence of depressive symptoms, unstable remission of depression, and increased risk for dementia.[33–34] The consistent evidence of the increase of cardiovascular causes of death with depression lends support to a biological explanation for the depression-mortality link, even though these same associations might also be explained, in part, by psychosocial factors.

Psychosocial factors linked to depression and relevant to mortality risk include d*ecision-making capacity, motivation, and behavioral compromise.* Depression interferes with making decisions that require considering complex or multiple sets of data, a central aspect of executive functioning.[35] Several investigators have found that older persons with depression perform particularly poorly on tests of executive functioning, specifically in terms of sustained effort and response inhibition.[36–37] Older depressed persons have slowed information-processing speed, diminished set-shifting and problem-solving abilities, and greater difficulty initiating novel responses than younger depressed persons. These deficits further diminish the ability of older depressed persons to accomplish the tasks related to health promotion and treatment over time. The motivational symptoms of depression may affect health behaviors by diminishing one's intent to do anything, especially related to asymptomatic conditions. Symptoms of hopelessness or worthlessness may distort self-perceived efficacy in preventing illness or the perceived value of preventive health behaviors. Older adults suffering from depressive disorders often have compromised behavioral competence even when depressive symptoms subside. Even when depression remits, executive functions are not normalized, although they improve to some extent.[38] Depression is a relapsing disorder, with incomplete remissions. Remaining symptoms sometimes include diminished interest in activities, low energy, somatic complaints, psychomotor retardation, and insomnia; all of which contribute to compromised function. The interaction of executive dysfunction with depression severity has been found to be a strong contributor to disability.[36] The long-standing need to depend on others for health care and fulfillment of personal needs may make it difficult for depressed elders to maintain or further develop their behavioral repertoire.

These characteristics of depression—impaired decision making, lack of motivation, and behavioral compromise—suggest several mechanisms of the psychosocial impact of depression on mortality, including poor preventive health behaviors (e.g., smoking, exercise, weight loss),[39–43] increased risk of disease (e.g., hypertension[21]), decreased access and help-seeking behaviors,[44] poorer treatment and adherence behaviors across different types of diseases and conditions,[41, 45–48] onset or exacerbation of disability,[49–50] and self-neglect or "passive suicide."[51–52]

In the systematic review of depression and mortality, 14 studies met the inclusion criteria (Table 9.1). The median value for which depressive disorder raises risk for all-cause mortality was about 70% (relative risk of 1.7), with an interquartile range of relative risks of 1.3–2.2 (Table 9.1).

Anxiety

The relationship of anxiety disorders to premature death, particularly cardiovascular death, has been the subject of a number of studies in recent decades. All of these studies have employed symptom and trait scales or retrospective diagnoses. Panic disorder has been studied most extensively in this respect, and the data are compelling for higher cardiovascular mortality in persons with panic disorder and/or agoraphobia.[53–56] Haines et al.[57] reported that elevated scores on the phobic anxiety subscale of the Crown-Crisp index[58] predicted death from subsequent ischemic heart disease in men; these results were replicated in subsequent studies[59] in men and women. Kawachi and colleagues reported an increase in subsequent sudden cardiac death in men who endorsed nonspecific anxiety symptoms from the Cornell Medical Index.[60–61] These included positive responses to the following five questions: "Do strange people or places make you afraid?"; "Are you considered a nervous person?"; "Are you constantly keyed up and jittery?"; "Do you often become suddenly scared for no good reason?"; and "Do you often break out in a cold sweat?" In addition, Kubzansky et al. reported that worry, a primary symptom of generalized anxiety disorder, predicted subsequent cardiovascular disease.[62] Shipley et al. recently reported that high anxiety proneness (neuroticism) was a predictor of subsequent death from cardiovascular disease.[63]

An interesting possibility is that the relationship of anxiety to mortality depends on age. In young people, for whom accidents and injuries are important causes of death, anxiety is protective from death due to these causes;[64] later in life anxiety is associated with raised risk for death associated with chronic illnesses like heart attack and stroke, as discussed above.

Panic, generalized anxiety, and agoraphobic disorders/symptoms, and the closely related personality trait neuroticism,[65] are associated with low autonomic flexibility[66–68] and thus heart rate variability. Since low heart rate variability is a risk factor for sudden death in patients with a variety of cardiac conditions, some have suggested this as a plausible mechanism by which anxiety disorders could increase risk for sudden cardiac death.[69–70]

We were unable to find any credible estimates for the association of mortality with social phobia or simple phobia. Three of the four studies on panic disorder and mortality were from different sites and time periods of the Epidemiologic Catchment Area Program. The median relative risk for death linked to panic disorder was 1.9, with interquartile range of 0.8–3.2 (Table 9.1). These meager results for anxiety disorders may reflect a raised risk for some individuals and lower risk for others, depending, for example, on age.[64]

Alcohol

Individuals with diagnosed alcohol dependence (or alcoholism) are more likely to die prematurely than the general population. Liskow et al. showed that overall age-adjusted standardized mortality among men with alcoholism was 2.5 times higher, and 5.5 times higher for those between the ages of 35–44 relative to men in the general population.[71] Characteristics associated with mortality among those with alcoholism include lower educational level, less psychosocial functioning, and greater severity of psychopathology.[71] Analyses in specific geographic areas have provided population-based evidence of strong links of alcohol problems with suicide and homicide.[72–73] In addition, ethnic minorities in the US in alcohol treatment appear to be at increased risk of death compared to the general population.[74] However, much of what we know about alcohol use disorders and mortality come from treatment samples.[75–81] With relatively few exceptions,[82–83] there has been a paucity of data on specific patterns of alcohol problems from longitudinal population-based samples. In addition, few if any studies have examined subgroups with comorbid psychiatric conditions.

Some population-based studies that have examined mortality by alcohol diagnostic category have demonstrated risk variations based on alcohol consumption levels. Dawson, in a cross-sectional study, showed that differences in mortality were found among individuals with and without alcohol dependence depending on consumption patterns.[84] Although increased risk of death has been found for those with alcohol use disorders, and heavy consumption, a recent meta-analysis has provided evidence that even those with relatively low consumption levels may have higher mortality, particularly among younger subgroups.[85] There is also evidence that mortality risk differs for women and other subgroups.[86]

Moderate alcohol use is associated with a reduced risk of death from cardiovascular disease,[14,86] but not other diseases,[86] and the relationship of alcohol use level with all-cause mortality has not been clarified.[85,87–88] Although there is a frequently described J-shaped relationship of moderate drinking with cardiovascular mortality, heavy drinking is associated with an increased risk of death from cardiovascular disease.[89] In a longitudinal study from Russia, binge drinkers (160 grams of alcohol per drinking occasion) as compared with nonbinge drinkers (those who drank less than 80 grams of alcohol) had an adjusted relative risk of dying from coronary heart disease of 1.27 (CI, 0.81–1.99); those who frequently drank heavily (≥3 times/week and at least 120 grams per occasion), had an adjusted relative risk of 1.61 (1.04–2.50) for total mortality, and 2.05 (1.09–3.86) for cardiovascular disease mortality.[89] Consumption as well as drinking pattern must be considered in the assessment of death by cardiovascular causes, as well as all-cause mortality.[14,90]

For alcohol use disorder, 913 titles were generated by the search terms and 148 were examined closely. All but seven studies were eliminated because they included only persons under treatment for alcohol abuse/dependence. The range of relative risks for mortality ranged from 1.4 in the US to 3.3 in Norway, with a median of 1.8 (Table 9.1). Two of the seven studies were conducted outside the US (i.e., in France and Norway), and both of these were in the high quartile.

Other Psychoactive Drugs and Drug Disorders

Within the US alone, approximately 7,000 individuals use an illegal drug or engage in non-medical use of drugs such as marijuana, cocaine, stimulants, sedatives, or heroin each day.[91] For psychoactive drugs other than tobacco and alcohol, unintentional overdose is a primary contributor to mortality.[92–94] Minority status, sex, and geographic location impact risk for fatal overdose.[95] Coffin and colleagues abstracted death records from the chief medical examiner in New York City to evaluate deaths due to accidental overdose and found that opiates, cocaine, or alcohol accounted for 97.8% of deaths.[93] Polydrug use was responsible for 57.8% of deaths.

There are many studies based upon decedents alone, as in reports based upon the U.S. Drug Abuse Warning Network (DAWN)[96] or studies in which the experience of specific groups are compared with overall mortality rates (e.g., via indirect standardization and standardized mortality rate [SMR]). For example, DAWN provided surveillance data on drug-related deaths based on reports from medical examiners and coroners in 122 U.S. jurisdictions in 2003.[96] The DAWN data, relying on reports from medical examiners and coroners at the time of the substance user's death, does not offer information on critical antecedent factors such as substance abuse history, treatment episodes, or comorbid physical and mental health conditions, assessed years before the death.

Almost all longitudinal evidence on U.S. mortality attributable to drugs such as cocaine has come from research on cases in treatment, and institutional or hospitalized samples. These data, representing the tip of iceberg, has overrepresented the more severe end of the drug dependence spectrum. As such, drug-associated mortality risk estimates from these studies overstate the public health significance of illegal and extra-medical drug use with respect to mortality. Data from these types of samples are informative but do not provide information about individuals who haven't had health problems that resulted in treatment or hospitalization. Among the available data, mortality rates vary depending on the population under study. Degenhardt and colleagues reviewed the literature related to nonAIDS mortality among injection drug users and calculated crude mortality rates.[97] The ten U.S.-based studies represented 16,575 participants. Of the ten U.S. studies, only two did not focus on a treatment population; one followed injection drug users for 1.8 years and the other followed drug and alcohol dependent participants on welfare for 8 years. Among a sample of substance abusing inpatient veterans, standardized mortality rates were 2.4% higher than their age-, sex- and race-matched general population counterparts (24% vs. 9%).[79] These veterans were "older" at the time of admission: 72% were between 55 and 64 years of age, while the rest were 65 and older. Virtually all (90%) of these substance users had at least one medical diagnosis in their prior treatment episode in addition to their substance use diagnosis. Joe and Simpson calculated crude mortality rates among a cohort of 297 male opioid addicts 12 years post enrollment in substance abuse treatment, and reported 13.8 death/1,000 person years, which was calculated to be 6.9 times the rate of an age-matched general population sample.[98] Hser and colleagues followed 581 male heroin users for 33 years post admission to a California compulsory drug treatment program to assess the natural history of heroin use.[99] At the 10 year follow-up 14% had died; at the second follow-up 20 years later 28% had died; and 49% had died by the 33 year follow-up.

Chronic conditions, such as asthma, hypertension, liver disease, and heart conditions, have been documented among substance users without primary care.[100] A comparison of substance-abusing patients with controls from the same HMO shows that substance abuse patients were more likely to have been diagnosed with pain, asthma, chronic obstructive pulmonary disease, hypertension, and cirrhosis than controls.[101]

Population-based studies focusing on mortality among individuals with drug use disorders are almost nonexistent. For drug use disorders the systematic search yielded 610 titles, but most were eliminated because they included only persons under treatment for drug abuse/dependence. Two met our criteria, and both were from the ECA program (relative risk of mortality of 1.6 and 2.3, median 2.0 in Table 9.1).

Methods

The Epidemiologic Catchment Area program[102] and its data collection procedures have been described before.[103] In New Haven 5,034 adults age 18 and older living in a 13-town region of the greater New Haven community of approximately 300,000 were interviewed, representing 77% of the respondents designated in the multistage sampling procedure. The design included a deliberate oversample of the elderly. Vital status through 1990 was determined by searching the Connecticut state mortality data, the National Death Index, and published obituaries in local newspapers for the years 1988–1990.

The Baltimore ECA follow-up sample consisted of 3,481 household-residing individuals sampled probabilistically from 175,211 household residents of Eastern Baltimore for participation in the Baltimore site of the Epidemiologic Catchment Area (ECA) Program. Persons over the age of 65 were purposely oversampled by designating all members of the household for interview, as well as whomever in the household was designated from a random selection. A total of 4,238 persons were designated for the sample and 3,481 (82%) completed the interview. Vital status for all individuals in the baseline survey was obtained through 2003 from the National Death Index Plus, and supplemented by field work for deaths in 2004. Forty-two percent of the sample interviewed in 1981 had died by the time of the interview in 2004.

The National Health Interview Survey in 2000 (NHIS 2000) was used as a comparison study. The NHIS is a nationally representative stratified multistage clustered area probability sample of households and noninstitutional group quarters. The sample consisted of 100,618 civilians living in the United States in 2000. The NHIS survey has been administered annually since 1956 through the National Center for Health Statistics (NCHS), which is part of the Centers for Disease Control and Prevention (CDC). The NHIS provides mortality data through 2003 which can be linked to NHIS public use files for respondents interviewed between 1986 and 2000. The 2000 survey year was selected for this study because of the availability of mortality data but also because of the inclusion of questions relating to mental health. Questions about physical conditions were of the form, "Have you ever been told by a doctor or other health professional that you had [condition]?" Presence of mental health problems was established using the question, "What condition or health problem causes you to have difficulty with [names of respondent-specified activities]?" which were followed up with, "How long have you had [condition]?"

The interviews in both ECA sites were built around the Diagnostic Interview Schedule.[104] Simple questions about lifetime occurrence of four health conditions were drawn from the National Health Interview Survey at the time, identically for the New Haven and Baltimore ECA sites. For example, the question about stroke was: "Have you ever had a stroke?"

Results

The ECA samples include a higher proportion of elderly than the NHIS, due to oversampling of the elderly in the former, but there were no strong differences between the ECA and NHIS samples by race, sex, or educational attainment (Table 9.2). Using weighted estimates for the age distribution that were post-stratified to the 1980 census, the age distributions were similar between the ECA and NHIS. The ECA samples had weighted prevalences of each of the four chronic medical conditions which were about three times as high as the NHIS, presumably reflecting the different age distributions as well as differences in question formats between the two surveys. The prevalence of self-reported emotional conditions in the NHIS was very low (1.4%).

Persons over the age of 65 at baseline were over 30 times more likely to die during the follow-up periods than younger persons, in unadjusted (not shown) and adjusted models (Table 9.2). The patterns are similar in both the ECA and the NHIS samples. The hazard ratios for deaths of females were about 70% of those for males in both samples. There was no significant difference in mortality by race. College-educated persons were less likely to die during the follow-up, in both samples, but there was no significant difference by occupational status (ECA only).

The effect of chronic medical conditions on risk for death is evident and statistically significant for all four chronic conditions in both samples, but it is much stronger for the NHIS sample. This difference is not due to the different age distributions because the parameters are adjusted for age. It is possibly due to more precise wording of the questions, which taps a subpopulation of persons with a more severe or impairing form of the disorder.

In the ECA sample there are moderate but statistically significant raised risks for death for persons who at baseline met criteria for major depressive disorder, phobic disorder, alcohol abuse or dependence, and drug abuse or dependence. The strongest effect is for drug abuse or dependence (Table 9.3: RR = 1.6, 95% CI, 1.1–2.4), and the weakest effect is for phobia, with only a 10% increase in risk. The estimated relative risk for panic disorder is 1.5 but the 95% confidence interval includes 1.0. For the NHIS, the estimated effect of emotional problems

Table 9.2 Characteristics of Respondents at Two ECA Sites in 1981, and the NHIS in 2000

	New Haven (n = 5,034)	*Baltimore (n = 3,481)*	*Combined ECA (n = 8,515)*	*National NHIS 2000 (n = 72,23)*
		Percentages		
Age in 1981, Unweighted (Weighted)				
18–29	16.0 (28.2)	26.6 (30.2)	20.3 (28.9)	22.0
30–44	16.8 (25.6)	22.7 (22.8)	19.2 (24.6)	31.8
45–64	16.0 (29.6)	24.2 (28.9)	19.3 (29.4)	30.0
65 and older	51.2 (16.6)	26.5 (18.1)	41.1 (17.2)	16.2
Female	59.0	62.0	60.3	52.1
White	88.8	63.0	78.2	81.3
Education				
Less than high school	23.2	28.4	25.4	7.8
High school	41.6	53.0	46.3	61.1
College/Post-graduate	35.1	18.6	28.3	31.2
Chronic Conditions				
Cancer	5.5 (3.5)	4.5 (3.5)	5.0 (3.5)	0.6
Heart	7.8 (4.2)	14.2 (12.7)	10.4 (7.2)	2.3
Stroke	3.9 (1.9)	3.5 (2.7)	3.7 (2.2)	0.8
Diabetes	7.2 (3.9)	7.8 (6.9)	7.5 (5.1)	1.6
Any Chronic Condition	19.4 (11.0)	22.9 (20.5)	20.8 (14.5)	4.3
Occupational Rank in Percentile (Mean)	49.2	38.9	45.1	NA
Mental Disorders				
Depression/Anxiety/ Emotional Problem	N/A	N/A	N/A	1.36%
Major Depression	5.4	4.4	5.0	N/A
Panic Disorder	1.2	1.4	1.3	N/A
Phobia	7.3	24.8	14.4	N/A
Alcohol or Drug Problem	N/A	N/A	N/A	0.02
DSM-III Alcohol Abuse/ Dependence	8.4	12.6	10.1	N/A
DSM-III Drug Abuse/ Dependence	3.6	4.8	4.2	N/A
"Other Mental Problem"	N/A	N/A	N/A	0.09
Any Mental Health Disorder	19.2	35.6	25.9	1.4%

For comparison, both unweighted and weighted proportions of persons in each age category and of chronic medical conditions in the ECA are shown.

Table 9.3 Adjusted Hazard Ratios for Mortality at Two ECA Sites and NHIS

	ECA		*NHIS*	
	HR	*CI*	*HR*	*CI*
Age in 1981				
18–29	1.0	—	1.0	—
30–44	1.9	1.4, 2.5	2.3	1.6, 3.4
45–64	9.9	7.7, 12.7	6.9	4.8, 9.9
65 and older	31.7	24.8, 40.6	36.2	25.9, 50.7
Female	0.7	0.6, 0.8	0.6	0.6, 0.7
White	0.9	0.8, 1.0	1.0	0.8, 1.1
Education				
Less than high school	1.0	—	1.0	—
High school	0.9	0.8, 0.9	0.7	0.6, 0.8
College/Post-graduate	0.7	0.6, 0.8	0.5	0.4, 0.6
Chronic Conditions				
Cancer	1.5	1.3, 1.7	5.2	4.2, 6.6
Heart	1.7	1.5, 1.9	2.4	2.1, 2.8
Stroke	1.8	1.6, 2.1	2.5	2.0, 3.0
Diabetes	1.7	1.5, 1.9	4.1	3.6, 4.8
Any Chronic Condition	1.8	1.6, 1.9	4.0	3.6, 4.6
Occupational Rank in Percentile (Mean)	1.0	1.0, 1.0	—	—
Mental Disorders				
Depression/Anxiety/Emotional Problem	—	—	1.9	1.4, 2.6
Major Depression	1.2	1.0, 1.6	—	—
Panic Disorder	1.5	0.9, 2.3	—	—
Phobia	1.1	1.0, 1.2	—	—
Alcohol or Drug Problem	—	—	4.9	1.1, 20.6
DSM-III Alcohol Abuse/Dependence	1.4	1.2, 1.6	—	—
DSM-III Drug Abuse/Dependence	1.6	1.1, 2.4	—	—
"Other Mental Problem"	—	—	3.3	0.9, 12.6
Any Mental Health Disorder	1.2	1.1, 1.4	2.0	1.4, 2.7

Values for covariates are from the model with "any mental health disorder."
Estimates from ECA are adjusted for age, sex, ethnicity, years of education, and occupational rank.
Estimates from NHIS 2000 are adjusted for age, sex, ethnicity, and years of education.

is larger than the ECA but the confidence intervals are very wide, due to the small sample of individuals reporting disorders.

Adjustment for age, sex, ethnicity, years of education, and occupational rank results in higher relative risk of death associated with the common mental disorders, compared to unadjusted rates, for both the ECA (Figure 9.1) and NHIS (Figure 9.2) samples. This occurs because the mental disorders are more prevalent in young persons, but death is more common in old persons. For both samples, the adjustment process has the opposite effect for the chronic medical

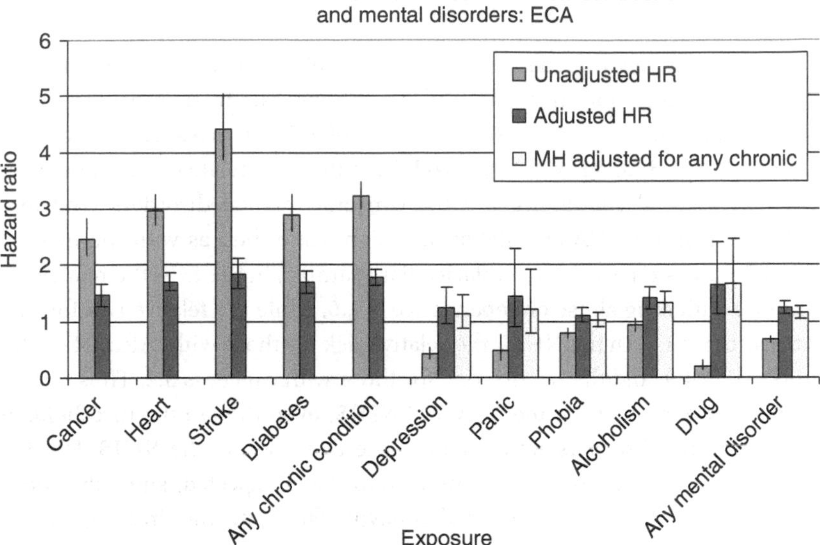

Figure 9.1 All adjusted estimates are adjusted for age, sex, years of education, ethnicity, and occupational rank. "MH adjusted for Any Chronic" estimates are further adjusted for the presence of any chronic medical condition.

conditions, because these are more likely to occur in older persons. In the ECA sample, further adjustment for the presence of any of the four chronic medical conditions (Figure 9.1) has negligible effects on relative risks for mental disorders, indicating that the effects of mental disorders and chronic medical conditions are largely independent of one another.

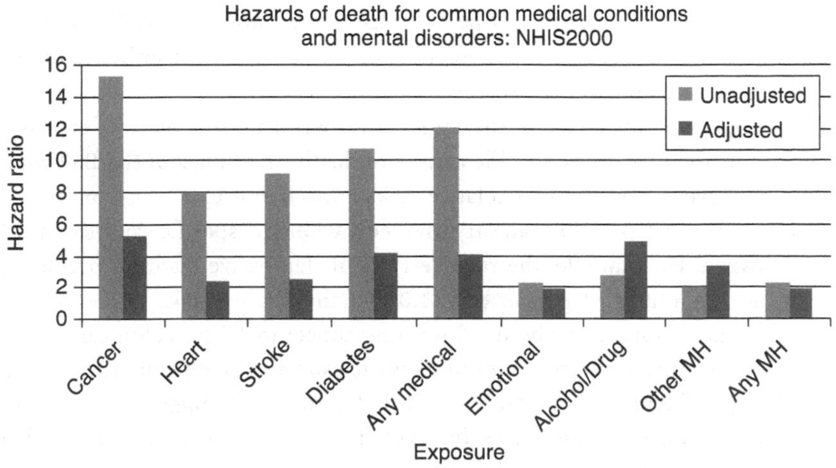

Figure 9.2 Adjusted estimates are adjusted for age, sex, years of education, and ethnicity.

Discussion

In the ECA, the relative risks for mortality for both the common medical conditions and the common mental disorders are moderate in size, statistically significant, and similar in magnitude (range of relative risks of 1.2 for major depression to 1.8 for stroke). In the NHIS samples the relative risks for both the common medical conditions and the common mental disorders tend to be higher than in the ECA and statistically significant; but, as with the ECA, the overall impression is one of similarity. For example, in the ECA the relative risk for those with drug abuse or dependence is 1.6, while the relative risk for those with cancer is 1.5. In the NHIS, the relative risk for those with "Alcohol or Drug Problem" is 4.9, and the relative risk for those with cancer is 5.2. Thus, the patterns are similar between the ECA and NHIS, even though the thresholds for presence of the disorders are broader in the ECA than in the NHIS. However, the difference is not so great as might have been expected, since the mental disorders are not typically thought of as having fatal outcomes in comparison to the medical conditions, which are typically conceived as being life threatening.

This is a preliminary analysis based on two ECA sites (New Haven, Connecticut and Baltimore, Maryland). In the future, with funding from the National Institute on Drug Abuse, two other sites will be added (Raleigh-Durham, North Carolina and St. Louis, Missouri) and all the respondents will be followed through the National Death Index through 2008. The total number of person-years of exposure in the combined four sites will be more than 350,000. The effect of adding the two sites and extending the follow-up period will be to narrow the confidence intervals. There may be differences in the parameter estimates between the estimates presented here and the estimates from the four sites due to the different population composition: The combined four sites will include a significant number of persons from rural areas, as well as persons from the south (North Carolina). The more diverse samples and enhanced precision will add credibility to the results.

An important advantage of the larger number of person years of exposure will be the ability to study specific causes of death. In studies of the Baltimore ECA, we have discovered that relative risks consequent to a common mental disorder such as depression can vary markedly when the specific causes of death are analyzed. For example, the relative risk for depressive disorder predicting any cancer is a little bit greater than 1.0; but the relative risks for the several specific cancers vary from about 1.0 for lung cancer to 4.6 for colon cancer and 3.5 for breast cancer. Relative risks for specific causes of death will provide clues to etiology of both mental and physical disorders by suggesting common etiologic pathways. Relative risks for specific causes of death will also aid in justifying and targeting prevention efforts.

References

1. Editor. (1984). Mortality in lunatic asylums. *American Journal of Insanity, 4,* 253–258.
2. Malzburg, B. (1952). Rates of discharge and rates of mortality among first admissions to the New York civil state hospitals. *Ment Hyg, 36,* 104–120.
3. Babigian, H. M. & Odoroff, C. L. (1969). The mortality experience of a population with psychiatric illness. *Am J Psychiatry, 126,* 470–480.
4. Colton, C. W. & Manderscheid, R. W. (2006). Congruencies in increased mortality rates, years of potential life lost, and causes of death among public mental health clients in eight states. *Prev Chronic Dis, 3,* A42.
5. Dohrenwend, B. P. & Dohrenwend, B. S. (1982). Perspectives on the past and future of psychiatric epidemiology: The 1981 Rema Lapouse lecture. *Am J Public Health, 72,* 1271–1279.
6. Eaton, W. W., Martins, S. S., Nestadt, G., Bienvenu, O. J., Clarke, D., & Alexandre, P. (2008). The burden of mental disorders. *Epidemiol Rev, 30,* 1–14.
7. Black, S. A. & Markides, K. S. (1999). Depression symptoms and mortality in older Mexican Americans. *Ann Epidemiol, 9,* 45–52.
8. Bruce, M. L. & Leaf, P. J. (1989). Psychiatric disorders and 15-month mortality in a community sample of older adults. *Am J Public Health, 79,* 727–730.
9. Bruce, M. L., Leaf, P. J., Rozal, G. P., Florio, L., & Hoff, R. A. (1994a). Psychiatric status and 9-year mortality data in the New Haven Epidemiologic Catchment Area Study. *Am J Psychiatry, 151,* 716–721.
10. Gallo, J. & Rabins, P. (1999). Depression without sadness: Alternative presentations of depression in late life. *Am Fam Physician, 60,* 820–826.
11. Kouzis, A., Eaton, W. W., & Leaf, P. J. (1995). Psychopathology and mortality in the general population. *Soc Psychiatry Psychiatr Epidemiol, 30,* 165–170.
12. Saz, P., Launer, L. J., Dia, J. L., De-La-Camara, C., Marcos, G., & Lobo, A. (1999). Mortality and mental disorders in a Spanish elderly population. *Int J Geriatr Psychiatry, 14,* 1031–1038.
13. Penninx, B. W., Guralnik, J. M., Mendes de Leon, C. F., Pahor, M., Visser, M., Corti, M. C., et al. (1998). Cardiovascular events and mortality in newly and chronically depressed persons > 70 years of age. *Am J Cardiol, 81,* 988–994.
14. Puddey, I. B., Rakic, V., Dimmitt, S. B., & Beilin, L. J. (1999). Influence of pattern of drinking on cardiovascular disease and cardiovascular risk factors—a review. *Addiction, 94,* 649–663.
15. Schulz, R., Beach, S. R., Ives, D. G., Martire, L. M., Ariyo, A. A., & Kop, W. J. (2000). Association between depression and mortality in older adults: The Cardiovascular Health Study. *Arch Intern Med, 160,* 1761–1768.
16. Schulz, R., Drayer, R. A., & Rollman, B. L. (2002). Depression as a risk factor for non-suicide mortality in the elderly. *Biol Psychiatry, 52,* 205–225.
17. Sharma, V. K., Copeland, J. R., Dewey, M. E., Lowe, D., & Davidson, I. (1998). Outcome of the depressed elderly living in the community in Liverpool: A 5-year follow-up. *Psychol Med, 28,* 1329–1337.
18. Whooley, M. A. & Browner, W. S. (1998). Association between depressive symptoms and mortality in older women: Study of osteoporotic fractures research group. *Arch Intern Med, 158,* 2129–2135.
19. Zheng, D., Macera, C. A., Croft, J. B., Giles, W. H., Davis, D., & Scott, W. K. (1997). Major depression and all-cause mortality among white adults in the United States. *Ann Epidemiol, 7,* 213–218.

20. Conwell, Y., Duberstein, P. R., Cox, C., Herrmann, J. H., Forbes, N. T., & Caine, E. D. (1996). Relationships of age and Axis I diagnoses in victims of completed suicide: a psychological autopsy study. *Am J Psychiatry, 153,* 1001–1008.
21. Meyer, C. M., Armenian, H. K., Eaton, W. W., & Ford, D. E. (2004). Incident hypertension associated with depression in the Baltimore Epidemiologic Catchment area follow-up study. *J Affect Disord, 83,* 127–133.
22. Mezuk, B., Eaton, W. W., Albrecht, S., & Golden, S. (2008). Depression and type 2 diabetes over the lifespan: A meta-analysis. *Diabetes Care, 31,* 2383–2390.
23. Pratt, L. A., Ford, D. E., Crum, R. M., Armenian, H. K., Gallo, J. J., & Eaton, W. W. (1996). Depression, psychotropic medication and risk of heart attack: Prospective data from the Baltimore ECA Follow-up. *Circulation, 94,* 3123–3129.
24. Mezuk, B., Eaton, W. W., Golden, S. H., Wand, G., & Lee, B. H. (2008). Depression, antidepressants and bone mineral density in a population-based cohort. *J Gerontol A Biol Sci Med Sci, 63,* 1410–1415.
25. Larson, S., Owens, P., Ford, D., & Eaton, W. (2001). Depressive disorders, dysthymia and risk of stroke: A thirteen follow-up from the Baltimore ECA. *Stroke, 32,* 1979–1983.
26. Hedayati, S. S., Jiang, W., O'Connor, C. M., et al. (2004). The association between depression and chronic kidney disease and mortaliaty among patients hospitalized with congestive heart failure. *Am J Kidney Dis, 44,* 207–215.
27. Gallo, J. J., Armenian, H. K., Ford, D. E., Eaton, W. W., & Khachaturian, A. S. (2000). Major depression and cancer: The 13-year followup of the Baltimore Epidemiologic Catchment Area sample. *Cancer Causes Control, 11,* 751–758.
28. Ford, D. E., Mead, L. A., Chang, P. P., Cooper-Patrick, L., Wang, N. Y., & Klag, M. J. (1998). Depression is a risk factor for coronary artery disease in men: The precursors study. *Arch Intern Med, 158,* 1422–1426.
29. Mykletun, A., Bjerkeset, O., Dewey, M., Prince, M., Overland, S., & Stewart, R. (2007). Anxiety, depression, and cause-specific mortality: The HUNT study. *Psychosom Med, 69,* 323–331.
30. Onitilo, A. A., Nietert, P. J., & Egede, L. E. (2006). Effect of depression on all-cause mortality in adults with cancer and differential effects by cancer site. *Gen Hosp Psychiatry, 28,* 396–402.
31. Penninx, B. W., Beekman, A. T., Honig, A., Deeg, D. J., Schoevers, R. A., van Eijk, J. T., et al. (2001). Depression and cardiac mortality: Results from a community-based longitudinal study. *Arch Gen Psychiatry, 58,* 221–227.
32. Taylor, W. D., Steffens, D. C., & Krishnan, K. R. (2006). Psychiatric disease in the twenty-first century: The case for subcortical ischemic depression. *Biol Psychiatry, 60,* 1299–1303.
33. Alexopoulos, G. S., Kiosses, D. N., Heo, M., Murphy, C. F., Shanmugham, B., & Gunning-Dixon, F. (2005). Executive dysfunction and the course of geriatric depression. *Biol Psychiatry, 58,* 204–210.
34. Krishnan, K. R., Taylor, W. D., McQuoid, D. R., et al. (2004). Clinical characteristics of magnetic resonance imaging-defined subcortical ischemic depression. *Biol Psychiatry, 55,* 390–397.
35. Kim, S. Y., Karlawish, J. H., & Caine, E. D. (2002). Current state of research on decision-making competence of cognitively impaired elderly persons. *Am J Geriatr Psychiatry, 10,* 151–165.

36. Alexopoulos, G. S., Kiosses, D. N., Klimstra, S., Kalayam, B., & Bruce, M. L. (2002). Clinical presentation of the "depression-executive dysfunction syndrome" of late life. *Am J Geriatr Psychiatry, 10,* 98–106.
37. Lockwood, K. A., Alexopoulos, G. S., & van Gorp, W. G. (2002). Executive dysfunction in geriatric depression. *Am J Psychiatry, 159,* 1119–1126.
38. Murphy, C. F. & Alexopoulos, G. S. (2004). Longitudinal association on initiation/perservation and severity of geriatric depression. *Am J Geriatr Psychiatry, 12,* 50–56.
39. Anda, R., Williamson, D., Escobedo, L., Mast, E., Giovino, G., & Remington, P. (1990). Depression and the dynamics of smoking. A national perspective. *JAMA, 264,* 1541–1545.
40. Escobedo, L. G., Anda, R. F., Smith, P. F., Remington, P. L., & Mast, E. E. (1990). Sociodemographic characteristics of cigarette smoking initiation in the United States. Implications for smoking prevention policy. *JAMA, 264,* 1550–1555.
41. Kronish, I. M., Rieckmann, N., Halm, E. A., Shimbo, D., Vorchheimer, D., Haas, D. C., et al. (2006). Persistent depression affects adherence to secondary prevention behaviors after acute coronary syndromes. *J Gen Intern Med, 21,* 1178–1183.
42. Murphy, J., Horton, N., Monson, R., Laird, N., Sobol, A., & Leighton, A. (2003). Cigarette smoking in relation to depression: Historical trends from the Stirling County Study. *Am J Psychiatry, 160,* 1663–1669.
43. van Gool, C., Kempen, G., Penninx, B., Geef, D., Beekman, A., & van Eijk, T. (2003). Relationship between changes in depressive symptoms and unhealthy lifestyles in late middle aged and older persons: Results from the Longitudinal Aging Study Amsterdam. *Age and Ageing, 32,* 81–87.
44. Desai, M. M., Bruce, M. L., & Kasl, S. V. (1999). The effects of major depression and phobia on stage at diagnosis of breast cancer. *Int J Psychiatry Med, 29,* 29–45.
45. Fusar-Poli, P., Lazzaretti, M., Ceruti, M., Hobson, R., Petrouska, K., Cortesi, M., et al. (2007). Depression after lung transplantation: Causes and treatment. *Lung, 185,* 55–65.
46. Lustman, P. J., Freedland, K. E., Griffith, L. S., & Clouse, R. E. (1998). Predicting response to cognitive behavior therapy of depression in type 2 diabetes. *Gen Hosp Psychiatry, 20,* 302–306.
47. Rieckmann, N., Kronish, I. M., Haas, D., Gerin, W., Chaplin, W. F., Burg, M. M., et al. (2006). Persistent depressive symptoms lower aspirin adherence after acute coronary syndromes. *Am Heart J, 152,* 922–927.
48. Smith, A., Krishnan, J. A., Bilderback, A., Riekert, K. A., Rand, C. S., & Bartlett, S. J. (2006). Depressive symptoms and adherence to asthma therapy after hospital discharge. *Chest, 130,* 1034–1038.
49. Bruce, M. L., Seeman, T. E., Merrill, S. S., & Blazer, D. G. (1994). The impact of depressive symptomatology on physical disability: MacArthur Studies of Successful Aging. *Am J Public Health, 84,* 1796–1799.
50. Vaccarino, V., Kasl, S. V., Abramson, J., & Krumholz, H. M. (2001). Depressive symptoms and risk of functional decline and death in patients with heart failure. *J Am Coll Cardiol, 38,* 199–205.
51. Abrams, R. C., Lachs, M., McAvay, G., Keohane, D. J., & Bruce, M. L. (2002). Predictors of self-neglect in community-dwelling elders. *Am J Psychiatry, 159,* 1724–1730.
52. Lachs, M. S., Williams, C. S., O'Brien, S., Pillemer, K. A., & Charlson, M. E. (1998). The mortality of elder mistreatment. *JAMA, 280,* 428–432.

53. Coryell, W., Noyes, R., & Clancy, J. (1982). Excess mortality in panic disorder. A comparison with primary unipolar depression. *Arch Gen Psychiatry, 39*, 701–703.
54. Coryell, W., Noyes, R., & House, J. D. (1986). Mortality among outpatients with anxiety disorders. *Am J Psychiatry, 143*, 508–510.
55. Fleet, R. P. & Beitman, B. D. (1998). Cardiovascular death from panic disorder and panic-like anxiety: A critical review of the literature. *J Psychosom Res, 44*, 71–80.
56. Smoller, J. W., Pollack, M. H., Wassertheil-Smoller, S., Jackson, R. D., Oberman, A., Wong, N. D., et al. (2007). Panic attacks and risk of incident cardiovascular events among postmenopausal women in the Women's Health Initiative Observational Study. *Arch Gen Psychiatry, 64*, 1153–1160.
57. Haines, A. P., Imeson, J. D., & Meade, T. W. (1987). Phobic anxiety and ischaemic heart disease. *Br Med J (Clin Res Ed), 295*, 297–299.
58. Crown, S. & Crisp, A. H. (1966). A short clinical diagnostic self-rating scale for psychoneurotic patients: The Middlesex Hospital Questionnaire. *Br J Psychiatry, 112*, 917–923.
59. Kawachi, I., Colditz, G. A., Ascherio, A., Rimm, E. B., Giovannucci, E., Stampfer, M. J., et al. (1994). Prospective study of phobic anxiety and risk of coronary heart disease in men. *Circulation, 89*, 1992–1997.
60. Brodman, K., Erdman, A. J., & Wolff, H. G. (1949). *Manual for the Cornell Medical Index Health Questionnaire*. New York: Cornell University Medical College.
61. Kawachi, I., Sparrow, D., Vokonas, P. S., & Weiss, S. T. (1994). Symptoms of anxiety and risk of coronary heart disease. The Normative Aging Study. *Circulation, 90*, 2225–2229.
62. Kubzansky, L. D., Kawachi, I., Spiro, A., Weiss, S. T., Vokonas, P. S., & Sparrow, D. (1997). Is worrying bad for your heart? A prospective study of worry and coronary heart disease in the Normative Aging Study. *Circulation, 95*, 818–824.
63. Shipley, B. A., Weiss, A., Der, G., Taylor, M. D., & Deary, I. J. (2007). Neuroticism, extraversion, and mortality in the UK Health and Lifestyle Survey: A 21-year prospective cohort study. *Psychosom Med, 69*, 923–931.
64. Lee, W. E., Wadsworth, M. E., & Hotopf, M. (2006). The protective role of trait anxiety: A longitudinal cohort study. *Psychol Med, 36*, 345–351.
65. Bienvenu, O. J. & Stein, M. B. (2003). Personality and anxiety disorders: a review. *J Personal Disord, 17*, 139–151.
66. Eysenck, H. J. & Eysenck, M. W. (1985). *Personality and individual differences: A natural science approach*. New York: Plenum.
67. Hoehn-Saric, R., McLeod, D. R., Funderburk, F., & Kowalski, P. (2004). Somatic symptoms and physiologic responses in generalized anxiety disorder and panic disorder: An ambulatory monitor study. *Arch Gen Psychiatry, 61*, 913–921.
68. Kawachi, I., Sparrow, D., Vokonas, P. S., & Weiss, S. T. (1995). Decreased heart rate variability in men with phobic anxiety (data from the Normative Aging Study). *Am J Cardiol, 75*, 882–885.
69. Gorman, J. M. & Sloan, R. P. (2000). Heart rate variability in depressive and anxiety disorders. *Am Heart J, 140*, 77–83.
70. Sheps, D. S. & Sheffield, D. (2001). Depression, anxiety, and the cardiovascular system: The cardiologist's perspective. *J Clin Psychiatry, 62* Suppl 8, 12–16.
71. Liskow, B. I., Powell, B. J., Penick, E. C., Nickel, E. J., Wallace, D., Landon, J. F., et al. (2000). Mortality in male alcoholics after ten to fourteen years. *J Stud Alcohol, 61*, 853–861.

72. Pridemore, W. A. & Chamlin, M. B. (2006). A time-series analysis of the impact of heavy drinking on homicide and suicide mortality in Russia, 1956–2002. *Addiction, 101,* 1719–1729.
73. Rivara, F. P., Mueller, B. A., Somes, G., Mendoza, C. T., Rushforth, N. B., & Kellermann, A. L. (1997). Alcohol and illicit drug abuse and the risk of violent death in the home. *JAMA, 278,* 569–575.
74. Costello, R. M. (2006). Long-term mortality from alcoholism: A descriptive analysis. *J Stud Alcohol, 67,* 694–699.
75. Bunn, J. Y., Booth, B. M., Cook, C. A., Blow, F. C., & Fortney, J. C. (1994). The relationship between mortality and intensity of inpatient alcoholism treatment. *Am J Public Health, 84,* 211–214.
76. Callahan, C. M. & Tierney, W. M. (1995). Health services use and mortality among older primary care patients with alcoholism. *J Am Geriatr Soc, 43,* 1378–1383.
77. Feuerlein, W., Kufner, H., & Flohrschutz, T. (1994). Mortality in alcoholic patients given inpatient treatment. *Addiction, 89,* 841–849.
78. Hurt, R. D., Offord, K. P., Croghan, I. T., Gomez-Dahl, L., Kottke, T. E., Morse, R. M., et al. (1996). 3rd mortality following inpatient addictions treatment. Role of tobacco use in a community-based cohort. *JAMA, 275,* 1097–1103.
79. Moo, R. H., Brennan, P. L., & Mertens, J. R. (1994). Mortality rates and predictors of mortality among late-middle-aged and older substance abuse patients. *Alcohol Clin Exp Res, 18,* 187–195.
80. Rossow, I. & Amundsen, A. (1997). Alcohol abuse and mortality: A 40-year prospective study of Norwegian conscripts. *Soc Sci Med, 44,* 261–267.
81. Vaillant, G. E. (1996). A long-term follow-up of male alcohol abuse. *Arch Gen Psychiatry, 53,* 243–249.
82. Ojesjo, L., Hagnell, O., & Otterbeck, L. (1998). Mortality in alcoholism among men in the Lundby Community Cohort, Sweden: A forty-year follow-up. *J Stud Alcohol, 59,* 140–145.
83. Neumark, Y. D., Van Etten, M. L., & Anthony, J. C. (2000). "Alcohol dependence" and death: Survival analysis of the Baltimore ECA sample from 1981 to 1995. *Subst Use Misuse, 35,* 533–549.
84. Dawson, D. A. (2000). Alcohol consumption, alcohol dependence, and all-cause mortality 4. *Alcohol Clin Exp Res, 24,* 72–81.
85. White, I. R., Altmann, D. R., & Nanchahal, K. (2002). Alcohol consumption and mortality: Modeling risks for men and women at different ages. *BMJ, 325,* 191.
86. Corrao, G., Rubbiati, L., Bagnardi, V., Zambon, A., & Poikolainen, K. (2000). Alcohol and coronary heart disease: A meta-analysis. *Addiction, 95,* 1505–1523.
87. Rehm, J. (2000). Alcohol consumption and mortality: What do we know and where should we go? *Addiction, 95,* 989–999.
88. Rehm, J. & Sempos, C. T. (1995). Alcohol consumption and all-cause mortality. *Addiction, 90,* 471–480.
89. Malyutina, S., Bobak, M., Kurilovitch, S. G. V., & Simonova, G. N. Y. M. M. (2002). Relation between heavy and binge drinking and all-cause and cardiovascular mortality in Novosibirsk, Russia: A prospective cohort study. *Lancet, 360,* 1488–1454.
90. Makela, P. & Paljarvi, T. P. K. (2005). Heavy and nonheavy drinking occassions, all-cause and cardiovascular mortality hospitalizations: A follow-up study in a population with a low consumption level. *J Stud Alcohol, 66,* 722–728.

91. Substance Abuse and Mental Health Services Administration. (2007). *Results from the 2006 National Survey on Drug Use and Health: National Findings (Office of Applied Studies, NSDUH Series H-32, DHHS Publication No. SMA 07–4293).*
92. Neumark, Y. D., Van Etten, M. L., & Anthony, J. C. (2000). "Drug dependence" and death: Survival analysis of the Baltimore ECA sample from 1981 to 1995. *Subst Use Misuse, 35,* 313–327.
93. Coffin, P. O., Galea, S., Ahern, J., Leon, A. C., Vlahov, D., & Tardiff, K. (2003). Opiates, cocaine and alcohol combinations in accidental drug overdose deaths in New York City, 1990–98. *Addiction, 98,* 739–747.
94. Demetriades, D., Gkiokas, G., Velmahos, G. C., Brown, C., Murray, J., & Noguchi, T. (2004). Alcohol and illicit drugs in traumatic deaths: Prevalence and association with type and severity of injuries. *J Am Coll Surgeons, 199,* 687–692.
95. Bernstein, K. T., Bucciarelli, A., Piper, T., Gross, C., Tardiff, K., & Galea, S. (2007). Cocaine- and opiate-related fatal overdose in New York City, 1990–2000. *BMC Public Health, 7,* 31.
96. Drug Abuse Warning Network. (2005). *Area profiles of drug-related mortality.* Rockville, Maryland, Department of Health and Human Services.
97. Degenhardt, L., Hall, E., & Warner-Smith, M. (2006). Using cohort studies to estimate mortality among injecting drug users that is not attributable to AIDS. *Sex Transm Infect, 82,* 56–63.
98. Joe, G. W. & Simpson, D. D. (1987). Mortality rates among opioid addicts in a longitudinal study. *Am J Public Health, 77,* 347–348.
99. Hser, Y. I., Hoffman, V., Grella, C. E., & Anglin, M. D. (2001). A 33-year follow-up of narcotics addicts. *Arch Gen Psychiatry, 58,* 503–508.
100. De Alba, I., Samet, J. H., & Saitz, R. (2004). Burden of medical illness in drug- and alcohol-dependent persons without primary care. *Am J Addictions, 13,* 33–45.
101. Mertens, J. R., Lu, Y. W., Parthasarathy, S., Moore, C., & Weisner, C. M. (2003). Medical and psychiatric conditions of alcohol and drug treatment patients in an HMO: comparison with matched controls. *Arch Int Med, 163,* 2511–2517.
102. Eaton, W. W., Regier, D. A., Locke, B. Z., & Taube, C. A. (1981). The Epidemiologic Catchment Area Program of the National Institute of Mental Health. *Public Health Reports, 96,* 319–325.
103. Eaton, W. W. & Kessler, L. G. (1985). *Epidemiologic field methods in psychiatry: The NIMH Epidemiologic Catchment Area Program.* Orlando: Academic Press, Inc.
104. Robins, L. N., Helzer, J. E., Croughan, J., & Ratcliff, K. S. (1981). National Institute of Mental Health Diagnostic Interview Schedule: Its history, characteristics, and validity. *Arch Gen Psychiatry, 38,* 381–389.

10

Child Mental Health

Status of the Promise, the Reality, and the Future of Prevention

JOHN N. CONSTANTINO

Introduction

It is common for clinicians and scientists to embark on careers in the field of child mental health on the premise that early intervention offsets lifetime risk. There exists a progressively accumulating body of knowledge that the origins of a majority of life-course-persistent mental disorders—including schizophrenia, major depression, substance dependence, and personality disorder—are traceable to childhood. But knowing that a psychiatric condition has its origins in childhood and having the ability to alter the course of subsequent development are two different matters. Single-gene neurodegenerative disorders such as Rett syndrome and Huntington's disease are striking examples of our field's limitations in the ability to halt the progression of disease even when its causal genetic determinants can be known at the time of birth. Elucidation of the downstream mechanisms of pathogenesis for such disorders is still being intensely pursued with the hope that someday preventive intervention will be possible in the way that has been successful in yet another single-gene disorder, phenylketonuria (PKU). Since the pathogenic mechanism in PKU involves interaction with a ubiquitous-but-removable dietary exposure, successful preventive intervention of the catastrophic developmental effects of this inherited condition is a reality.

The Genetic and Environmental Structure of Behavioral Abnormality in Childhood

The past two decades of behavioral genetic research have variously dampened and then raised hopes for this type of preventive intervention for child psychiatric conditions. The overwhelming conclusion from studies of twins, families, and adoptees has been that serious adverse behavioral outcomes are highly inherited, though mathematical modeling has suggested that *additive* rather than Mendelian patterns of inheritance are responsible for the causal effects. Nevertheless, this series of discoveries, that genetic influences exert substantial main effects on behavioral outcome, has propelled the pouring of resources for psychiatric research into the search for susceptibility genes, in hopes that a way will be found to interrupt the pathogenic mechanisms influenced by those genes, in the manner that has generated successful dietary intervention for PKU, and the prospect of pharmacologic intervention for fragile X syndrome.[1] Psychiatric genetics has been additionally driven by the possibility that embedded within the sizeable estimates for inherited influence in twin and family studies there exist substantial proportions of variance attributed by interactions between genetic susceptibilities and *unmeasured* environmental factors. This has engendered hope that, despite estimates for common environmental influence hovering near zero (across hundreds of studies) for most psychiatric conditions, there is a preventive role for interventions targeting parameters of environmental risk that have been inferred from sociologic and psychologic observations for centuries.

A landmark study by Caspi and colleagues[2] illustrated this possibility by showing that variation in a single gene known to regulate monoamine neurotransmission (monoamine oxidase A, MAO-A) modulated the deleterious effects of an environmental factor—child maltreatment—which is a known predictor of life-course-persistent antisocial behavior.[3] This was observed despite the *absence* of a main effect of the gene by itself on antisocial outcome. Since the discovery of that interaction in that particular sample, dozens of studies have attempted to replicate this discovery, and although the results have been mixed, they generally support the original finding, including the possible *protective* effect of lower-risk alleles in conferring resilience in the face of child maltreatment. Recent studies have also suggested that the magnitude-of-effect of inherited variation in risk or resiliency (whether incurred by allelic variations in MAO-A, other genes regulating monoamine pathways such as *catechol-O-methyl transferase* [COMT], 5-hydroxyindoleacetic acid [*5-HIAA*], or other parameters of genetic risk) varies as a function of the presence or absence of numerous modifying factors such as gender, ethnicity, and the severity of adversity of life events. Other studies have demonstrated the manner in which other parameters of inherited risk may be intensified or attenuated by variation in the environment, as is the case for the effect of poverty on IQ,[4] and the presence-in-the-home versus absence-from-the-home of antisocial fathers on their sons' behavioral outcome.[5]

Other studies involving larger, genetically informative designs in which adverse environmental influences were specifically measured and the *totality* of genetic influence was considered (e.g., twin and sibling designs) have indicated a) that some of the variance in abnormal behavioral outcome attributed to genetic factors was operating via environmental mechanisms;[6] and b) that, when specifically measured, child maltreatment exerts deleterious effects on a variety of psychiatric syndromes independent of inherited liabilities for those adverse outcomes. Recently, Jonson-Reid, Constantino, and colleagues[7] obtained official-report child maltreatment data from state administrative records on over 4,000 epidemiologically ascertained twins whose behavioral outcome was known. *Independent* main effects of maltreatment and inherited liability on antisocial development were confirmed, and were highly statistically significant, as summarized in Figure 10.1, which depicts proportion of children with clinical-level externalizing symptoms as a function of history of officially-reported child maltreatment and gradations in level of inherited liability for externalizing behavior abnormality. Externalizing behaviors in that analysis (encompassing disruptive, aggressive, and antisocial behaviors) were ascertained by the Child Behavior Checklist, a well-validated dimensional parent-report measure of general psychopathology. A subsequent clinically ascertained sample of singleton children ascertained from families affected by alcohol dependence (thereby at *combined* inherited and environmental risk for antisocial development), yielded highly similar results.[7]

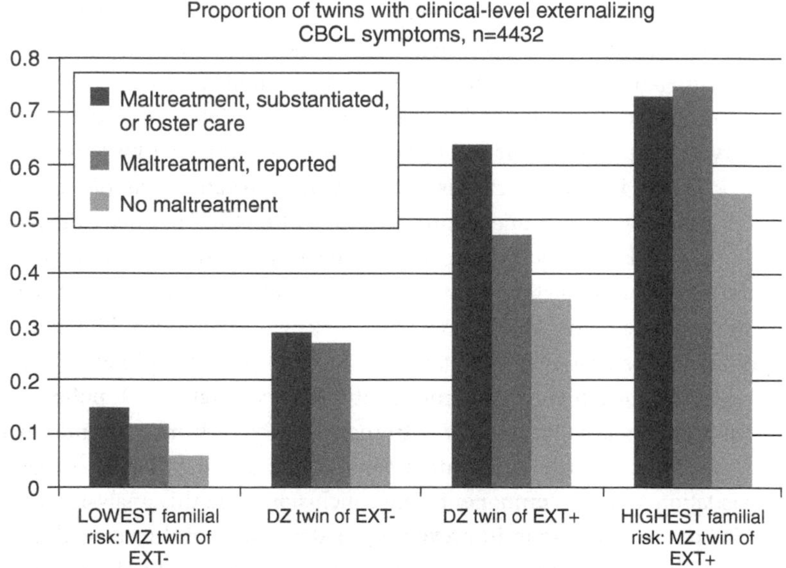

Figure 10.1 Proportion of twins with clinical-level externalizing Child Behavior Check List (CBCL) symptoms. Adapted from Jonson-Reid et al., *J Am Acad Child Adolesc Psychiatry*.

Insights on Causality from Direct Attempts to Prevent Behavioral Abnormalities in Children

In separate lines of research involving demonstrations of the effects of early intervention, longitudinal studies of children followed from the 1980s indicated that child maltreatment might be preventable by supporting young fragile families, that the behavioral outcomes of those children could be improved by preventing maltreatment, and that high quality early childhood education (including large-scale government-sponsored programs for young children at risk, such as Head Start) could confer further lasting protection from future outcomes such as school drop-out, delinquency, and adult criminality. As these longitudinal study samples have been followed to adulthood, however, it has become apparent that some of the positive effects may wane over time,[8] especially when support is not continuous, or when subjects are repeatedly exposed to adverse environmental exposures (including direct trauma, family stress, illicit drugs and alcohol, neighborhood and community disintegration) as they approach adulthood. In addition, even for the most promising preventive intervention programs, fundamental questions remain about the salient ingredients of successful programs, which children benefit most (and for which outcomes), the required dosage and duration for successful effects, and how to publicly implement expensive interventions developed in the context of research programs. It can take decades to resolve such controversies with respect to any single domain of preventive intervention, and this must be balanced with pressing current needs to address obvious aggregations of risk in the current generation of children.

A recent review of one successful component of many early childhood preventive intervention programs, *home visitation*, recently published by Howard and Brooks-Gunn,[9] is instructive in this regard. Home visitation was pioneered by Olds and colleagues[10] in studies of disadvantaged first-time mothers; those who could be engaged to participate in regular meetings with nurse home-visitors exhibited significant reductions in the rates of officially reported maltreatment of their children. The review by Howard and Brooks-Gunn, however, illustrates the complexities and shortcomings of taking successful preventive interventions to scale in larger community-based demonstration projects. Table 10.1, published in their report and reproduced below, summarizes results from 13 randomized-controlled studies of early intervention for children at risk which incorporated home visitation as a key component. The conclusion from this analysis was that the effects of home visitation in preventing maltreatment and its sequelae were highly variable, and dependent on the professional background of home visitors, profile of risk of the families, and program components accompanying home visitation.

A paraprofessional home visitation program, the Parents As Teachers program, was implemented universally as an entitlement-by-statute in the State

Table 10.1 The Effects of Home-Visiting Programs on Child Abuse, Health, Parenting, and Depression

Program	*Substantiated Child Abuse and Neglect*	*Parent Report Child Abuse and Neglect*	*Child Health and Safety*	*Home Environment*	*Parenting Responsivity and Sensitivity*	*Parenting Harshness*	*Depression and Parenting Stress*	*Child Cognition*
NFP-Elmira	Yes		Yes	No	Yes	Yes	No	Mixed
NFP-Memphis			Yes	No	Mixed		No	Mixed
NFP-Denver				Yes	Yes		No	Mixed
Hawaii Healthy Start	No	No	No	No	No		Mixed	No
HFA-San Diego		Yes	No	No	No	Yes	Mixed	Mixed
HFA-Alaska	No	Yes	No	Yes	No	Mixed	Mixed	Yes
HFA-New York	No	Yes	No			Yes	Mixed	
Early Head Start			Yes	Yes	Yes	Yes	Yes	Yes
IHDP				Yes	Yes	Yes	Yes	Yes
CCDP			No	No	No	No	No	Mixed
Early Start	No	Yes	Yes		Yes	Yes	No	
Queensland Program			No	Yes	Yes		Mixed	
Netherlands Program					Yes		No	

Note: "Mixed" indicates that findings were Isolated to specific sites or subgroups. Blank boxes indicate that the outcome was not examined for a particular program.
From Howard, K. S. and J. Brooks-Gunn, (2009). The role of home-visiting programs in preventing child abuse and neglect. *Future Child*, 19(2): p. 119–46.
NFP=Nurse Family Partnership.
HFA=Healthy Families America.
IHDP=Infant Health and Development Program.
CCDP=Comprehensive Child Development Program.

Table 10.2 Extent of Participation of Women with Legal Custody of Infants and Toddlers in Paraprofessional Home Visitation, Stratified by Level of Risk and Implementation of a Group-Based "Engagement Protocol" (EP) to Engage Them in Home Visitation

	Urban Low-Income (ULI)	*ULI + Engagement Protocol (EP)*	*ULI + Additional Social Risk + EP*	*ULI + Drug*	*ULI + Drug + EP*
Size of cohort (families)	100	50	50	100	70
Mean # home visits completed per year	1.7	10.5	9.2	0	14.6

of Missouri over two decades ago, and further illustrates ways in which potentially effective interventions struggle in the achieving of intended outcomes during the implementation phase. In the urban core of St. Louis City, for example, less than 20% of eligible families with infants participate in the program, resulting in the families and infants at highest risk for maltreatment and its consequences not being reached by the program. It has been proven possible to substantially raise the rates of participation in this entitlement program using group-based engagement strategies,[11] even among families at extremely high risk (including parents in voluntary substance recovery programs who have retained custody of their young children—see Table 10.2 above, Constantino et al., manuscript in preparation). However, it is not yet known whether targeting families whose children are at the very *highest* risk for psychopathologic outcomes can exert successful main effects on long-term outcome.

Elucidating the Nature of Inherited Liabilities that Confer Susceptibility to Complex Psychiatric Syndromes

Powerful biological risk factors are at play in the development of many psychiatric syndromes and, in subsets of vulnerable children, may not be surmountable by even very extensive preventive intervention efforts, as learned in the outcome studies of the Infant Health and Development program. Life-course longitudinal studies of the outcomes of children with inherited, maladaptive variations in critical aspects of personality, are sobering reminders of the forces of nature that are at play in the development of psychiatric syndromes. For example, there exist specific variations in affect regulation, autonomic arousal, and callous-unemotional behavior that appear to be heritable, highly stable from early childhood through adulthood, with robust biological correlates (measured via electrophysiology and neuroimaging), and predict very serious patterns of behavioral abnormality that may be substantially independent of variation in life experience.[12] Such factors may underlie the more pronounced heritability of antisocial behavior when measured as a life-course-persistent characteristic in adulthood than when measured in childhood.[13]

The knowledge of this potent effect of inherited factors on enduring psychiatric syndromes, and early findings on associations between abnormal behavior and monoamine neurotransmitter systems in humans and in nonhumans,[2,14] sustained strong interest in the search for susceptibility genes for major psychiatric disorders. The last 5 years have witnessed a rapid proliferation in the technology for extensive molecular exploration of the genome and have resulted in a set of newly completed large-scale genome-wide association studies (GWAS) for most serious life-course-persistent psychiatric disorders. The overwhelming conclusion of these studies—most of which have examined the effect of individual genetic variations in a *univariate* sense (at sample sizes in the 1,000–5,000 range)—is that common allelic variations tend to contribute small or negligible proportions of total variance to the trait of interest (some identified in genome-wide association studies may, in fact, represent "synthetic associations" generated by rare variants in linkage disequilibrium with GWAS markers[15]), that rare variants sometimes account for inherited psychiatric syndromes in families, but that in general only a small proportion of total variance in psychiatric disorder outcome is explainable on the basis of genetic variants identifiable within samples of the sizes currently available for study. This is the typical pattern for "complex diseases" (other examples of which include diabetes and hypertension).

The questions of whether rare genetic variations converge on specific genes (which would have been expected to manifest themselves in linkage analysis if variation in a given gene conferred a high enough population attributable risk), participate in epistatic interactions that increase magnitude of effect or population attributable risk or both, or operate via "final common pathway" neural mechanisms (e.g., that might be observable by neuroimaging) are still being actively pursued. The take-home message, however, is that behavior is complex and highly evolved, that there appear to be multiple genetic pathways to any given psychiatric syndrome, that disparate psychiatric syndromes partially overlap with respect to genetic variation (e.g., schizophrenia, bipolar disorder, autism[16]), that rare mutations exert significant influences for some affected individuals, and that more precise elucidation of the mechanisms of inherited risk may require sample sizes an order of magnitude larger than what are currently available for molecular genetic research. Clearly, at the time of this writing, specific molecular genetic variations are nowhere near as predictive as simple family psychiatric histories in predicting risk for psychiatric disorders in practical terms.

Implications for the Current Generation of Children

Thus, in the absence of specific molecular risk markers, and in the absence of specifically discernible pathogenic mechanisms for child psychiatric syndromes, it will be important for the field of child psychiatry to consider shifting some of its contemporary focus (and resource allocation) from the molecular to the socio-environmental, as will be described below. Child psychiatrists typically lack expertise in psychosocial prevention strategies and have not generally been trained to think of evidence-based components of preventive intervention as tools of their trade, especially for the younger siblings of their clinically identified patients. An agenda to allow the behavioral science of prevention to reach its next level is warranted.

It stands to reason, however, that if a psychiatric condition is multifactorial in its origin, it is likely that effective preventive intervention will need to be comprehensive in its approach and sensitive to the timing of various impacts at different phases of development. Since disparate causes for psychopathology become highly intercorrelated in the population,[7] this also indicates that, for children at highest risk, numerous elements of preventive intervention at multiple junctures in development will offer the greatest chance of enduring effects. *The lesson of the scientific literature on preventive intervention is that one-time inoculation with singular, time-limited interventions may not be potent enough to prevent psychiatric syndromes.* Serious attention to the comprehensiveness of intervention, its dosage, and duration are warranted, and exclusive restriction of funded research efforts to highly focused modules of care—while scientifically appealing—contrasts with the reality that there exists a multiplicity of forces impinging on the development of children at risk. The manner in which those forces accumulate and interact over time is not well understood, but it is increasingly clear that an exclusive pursuit of univariate relationships will likely distort understanding of the "real-world" phenomenology of risk and resilience.

Harnessing the Current Scientific Knowledge Base in Devising Prevention Strategies

In practical terms, what do we know about preventive intervention? It is known that many chronic mental health conditions have origins early in childhood. It is known that *some* of the most compelling environmental parameters of risk include child maltreatment, family conflict and adversity, victimization by peers in school age, early exposure to drugs and alcohol, and neighborhood/community factors such as gang culture in adolescence. There are evolving methods to minimize these risks in a univariate sense[9,17,18] but few programs definitively address *more* than one factor, and few programs address the multiplicity of factors that predispose to any one environmental hazard (e.g., the *combination* of parental stress, parental substance use, and environmental deprivation predisposing to child maltreatment). We know that mitigation of these risks appears to have direct short-term effects on child behavior, and those programs that do address multiple factors are more likely to incur long-term benefits.[8,19]

At the extreme, competent foster care and adoption have proven capable of remarkable long-term benefits to many children[20,21] and encompass the hope that environmental support—comprehensively delivered over years of time— can effect lasting change. We know that *infants* in specific adverse environments with specific profiles of inherited liability to mental illness (ascertainable using family history methods) experience officially reported maltreatment and develop psychiatric syndromes at rates that are up to an order of magnitude higher than what occurs in the general population. Recently it has also been learned that inherited profiles of early childhood behavior may profoundly distort early life experiences necessary for normal social and emotional development. An example is abnormal eye tracking[21a], which result, essentially, in gene-environment correlations that have become a specific target of early intervention strategies, in this case to ensure intervals of visual/social engagement with people that might otherwise rarely occur. Finally, we know that although universal prevention can be prohibitively expensive, the testing of targeted preventive intervention strategies are well within reach, especially given the precision with which marked elevation in risk can be ascertained.

Cost-effective *titration* of specific components of preventive intervention to families at varying risk level is in the early stages of exploration. An example is the parent education paradigm, *Triple P*, which implements community-based and large-group education efforts for families at minimal risk, but judiciously employs individually administered intensive skills training for higher-risk families or families in crisis. Both have demonstrated intervention effects in preliminary controlled trials.[22] The principles across delivery methods are the same: to promote social competence and emotional self-regulation in children via (1) ensuring a safe, engaging, and responsive caregiving environment, (2) promoting a positive learning environment, (3) using assertive discipline, (4) maintaining reasonable expectations, and (5) taking care of oneself as a parent.

These are also principles of successful *clinical* interventions for children with child psychiatric conditions, and innovative hybrids of preventive and therapeutic interventions are being developed for young children at risk for enduring psychopathology,[23] to attempt to apply the relevant therapies *before* the conditions develop. Finally, the magnitude-of-effect of initiating clinical treatment at the earliest sign of onset of a psychiatric condition remains unknown,[24] and is a critical agenda for child psychiatric research. For those conditions clearly remediable by treatment, it may be most effective to deliver care only after the condition has developed. But for those conditions known to be influenced by the environment, and whose clinical course is minimally modified by currently available treatments, there is almost no choice but to begin at the beginning and ameliorate any and every possible parameter of deleterious influence from the time of early childhood.

In conclusion, there are few, if any, smoking guns (genes), and few if any one-time inoculations for child psychopathology. Behavior is complex and multifactorial; for some children, life outcome is deleteriously affected by an array of adverse family-environmental factors that are modifiable, but only when efforts are sustained, comprehensive, and organized around the needs of individual families (not bureaucracies). This chapter has considered preventive intervention approaches that typically exist only in research programs or in fragmented patchworks in the community; they include parenting education, home visitation, early childhood education, downward extension (earliest application) of cognitive-behavioral interventions for children, parents, or dyads, foster care, the clinical care of parents, and the earliest implementation of mental health care for the earliest signs of psychiatric illness.

Although promising effects have been identified in randomized controlled trials for each of these interventions, they are often short-term, highly focused, and rarely address issues of neighborhood context or parental mental health/substance use impairment that are real-world correlates of serious combined genetic and environmental risk. The current generation of specialists in child mental health—clinicians and researchers alike—need to be trained in these methods and to be kept apprised of the advancing frontier of preventive intervention. In a next phase of development of our field, concerted efforts to elucidate which interventions, when in development, targeted toward whom, sustained at what dosage, and at what duration, will bring about cost-effective improvements in which major public mental health problems. Embedding such efforts in genetically informative and/or developmentally informative sampling designs will ensure that the agenda of separating "baby from bathwater" in preventive intervention will itself contribute to the steady advancement of behavioral neuroscience.

Acknowledgments

This work was supported, in part, by the U.S. Health Resources and Services Administration HRSA 04–062 (Healthy Tomorrows Partnership for Children) and by a gift from an anonymous donor.

References

1. Dolen, G., Osterweil, E., Rao, B. S., et al. (2007). Correction of fragile X syndrome in mice. *Neuron, 56*(6), 955–962.
2. Caspi, A., McClay, J., Moffitt, T. E., et al. (2002). Role of genotype in the cycle of violence in maltreated children. *Science, 297*(5582), 851–854.

3. Gilbert, R., Widom, C. S., Browne, K., Fergusson, D., Webb, E., & Janson, S. (2009). Burden and consequences of child maltreatment in high-income countries. *Lancet, 373*(9657), 68–81.
4. Turkheimer, E., Haley, A., Waldron, M., D'Onofrio, B., & Gottesman, II. (2003). Socioeconomic status modifies heritability of IQ in young children. *Psychol Sci, 14*(6), 623–628.
5. Blazei, R. W., Iacono, W. G., & McGue, M. (2008). Father-child transmission of antisocial behavior: The moderating role of father's presence in the home. *J Am Acad Child Adolesc Psychiatry, 47*(4), 406–415.
6. D'Onofrio, B. M., Slutske, W. S., Turkheimer, E., et al. (2007). Intergenerational transmission of childhood conduct problems: A Children of Twins Study. *Arch Gen Psychiatry, 64*(7), 820–829.
7. Jonson-Reid, M., Presnall, N., Drake, B., Fox, L., Bierut, L., Reich, W., Kane, P., Todd, R. D., Constantino, J. N. (2010). Effects of child maltreatment and inherited liability on antisocial development: an official records study. *J Am Acad Child Adolesc Psychiatry, 49*(4), 321–332.
8. Eckenrode, J., Campa, M., Luckey, D. W., et al. (2010). Long-term effects of prenatal and infancy nurse home visitation on the life course of youths: 19-year follow-up of a randomized trial. *Arch Pediatr Adolesc Med, 164*(1), 9–15.
9. Howard, K. S. & Brooks-Gunn, J. (2009). The role of home-visiting programs in preventing child abuse and neglect. *Future Child, 19*(2), 119–146.
10. Olds, D., Henderson, C. R., Jr., Cole, R., et al. (1998). Long-term effects of nurse home visitation on children's criminal and antisocial behavior: 15-year follow-up of a randomized controlled trial. *JAMA, 280*(14), 1238–1244.
11. Constantino, J. N., Hashemi, N., Solis, E., et al. (2001). Supplementation of urban home visitation with a series of group meetings for parents and infants: Results of a "real-world" randomized, controlled trial. *Child Abuse Negl, 25*(12), 1571–1581.
12. Glenn, A. L., Raine, A., Venables, P. H., & Mednick, S. A. (2007). Early temperamental and psychophysiological precursors of adult psychopathic personality. *J Abnorm Psychol, 116*(3), 508–518.
13. Lyons, M. J., True, W. R., Eisen, S. A., et al. (1995). Differential heritability of adult and juvenile antisocial traits. *Arch Gen Psychiatry, 52*(11), 906–915.
14. Suomi, S. J. (2006). Risk, resilience, and gene x environment interactions in rhesus monkeys. *Ann N Y Acad Sci*, 1094, 52–62.
15. Dickson, S. P., Wang, K., Krantz, I., Hakonarson, H., & Goldstein, D. B. (2010). Rare variants create synthetic genome-wide associations. *PLoS Biol, 8*(1), e1000294.
16. Rzhetsky, A., Wajngurt, D., Park, N., & Zheng, T. (2007). Probing genetic overlap among complex human phenotypes. *Proc Natl Acad Sci U S A*, 104(28), 11694–11699.
17. Brotman, L. M., Gouley, K. K., Huang, K. Y., et al. (2008). Preventive intervention for preschoolers at high risk for antisocial behavior: Long-term effects on child physical aggression and parenting practices. *J Clin Child Adolesc Psychol, 37*(2), 386–396.
18. Osterling, K. L. & Austin, M. J. (2008). Substance abuse interventions for parents involved in the child welfare system: Evidence and implications. *J Evid Based Soc Work, 5*(1–2), 157–189.
19. Conduct Problems Prevention Research Group. (2007). Fast track randomized controlled trial to prevent externalizing psychiatric disorders: Findings from grades 3 to 9. *J Am Acad Child Adolesc Psychiatry, 46*(10), 1250–1262.
20. Kessler, R. C., Pecora, P. J., Williams, J., et al. (2008). Effects of enhanced foster care on the long-term physical and mental health of foster care alumni. *Arch Gen Psychiatry, 65*(6), 625–633.

21. Smyke, A. T., Zeanah, C. H., Jr., Fox, N. A., & Nelson, C. A., 3rd. (2009). A new model of foster care for young children: The Bucharest early intervention project. *Child Adolesc Psychiatr Clin N Am, 18*(3), 721–734.
21a. Chawarska, K., Volkmar, F., Klin, A. (2008). Limited attentional bias for faces in toddlers with autism spectrum disorders. *Arch Gen Psychiatry, 67*(2), 178–185.
22. Prinz, R. J., Sanders, M. R., Shapiro, C. J., Whitaker, D. J., & Lutzker, J. R. (2009). Population-based prevention of child maltreatment: The U.S. Triple p system population trial. *Prev Sci, 10*(1), 1–12.
23. Luby, J. L. (2009). Early childhood depression. *Am J Psychiatry,* 166(9), 974–979.
24. Molina, B. S., Hinshaw, S. P., Swanson, J. M., et al. (2009). The MTA at 8 years: Prospective follow-up of children treated for combined-type ADHD in a multisite study. *J Am Acad Child Adolesc Psychiatry, 48*(5), 484–500.

PART IV

Issues that Shape the Debate about Public Mental Health

11

Stigma of Mental Illness

A Global View

NORMAN SARTORIUS

Introduction

Stigma is attached to mental illness wherever mental illness is recognized. It is pervasive, and will mark those who have the illness as well as their families, the institutions providing treatment, medications and other means of treatment of mental illness, as well as staff who are engaged in mental health services.[1] The stigma attached to mental disorders and to the work in the field of psychiatry makes the discipline less attractive for undergraduate and postgraduate students. Stigma is the main obstacle to the provision of mental health care and the main reason for the low priority of mental health programs in most parts of the world. The stigma of mental illness confers the notion that people who have it are dangerous and that psychiatric treatments are, at best, bringing temporary relief, not cure. What is even worse is that the population at large sees people who have a mental illness as being of low (if any) value to society and that, consequently, anything that could be done for them is too expensive.

In 1996, the World Psychiatric Association (WPA) launched a project that was to explore and diminish the stigma related to schizophrenia.[1] More than 20 countries joined this global program; many of them are continuing to implement it. The WPA venture did weaken the stigma of schizophrenia in the countries in which the program had been underway; perhaps more importantly, it created a fund of knowledge about ways in which stigma can be prevented, diminished, or removed. This chapter will describe lessons that were learned in the conduct of the WPA program—lessons that are very similar to those that were produced by other focused or general efforts to fight stigma related to mental illness.[2,3]

Selecting Targets for the Program

Targets for programs aiming to reduce stigma are usually selected on the grounds of logical reasoning. In view of the fact that many people use public transportation, posters declaring that mental illness is like any other illness are often placed on buses, subway carriages, and other vehicles. Knowing that many people listen to the radio, brief messages are added to the most popular programs. Having established that many attitudes are formed in young age, anti-stigma materials are distributed in schools. Similar interventions have for a long time been in the center of anti-stigma campaigns, occasionally resulting in a change of attitudes and sometimes in a change of behavior. Although something is achieved in these ways, it has gradually become clear that anti-stigma programs must use a different strategy, a different way of deciding about the priorities for anti-stigma programs.

The leaders of the program against stigma in Calgary[1] conducted their work guided by a committee that included people who had mental illness as well as their families. Discussions with them about the anti-stigma program made it clear that as far as they were concerned, and at that point in time, the main problem that emerged as a consequence of stigmatization was not that school children had a bad opinion about mentally ill people. Rather, they felt that the first priority should be given to a change in health services because they were discriminated against when seeking medical help. They were not against the radio and other media programs with anti-stigma messages, but they felt that it was necessary and urgent to deal with specific consequences of stigma by working with the staff of the health care institutions who were often not even aware that their behavior was discriminatory and offensive. The Calgary anti-stigma team did so, and the behavior of health service staff changed to the great satisfaction of those who sought help.[i]

The Calgary example triggered a change in the way other centers in the WPA program worked. Defining the target for anti-stigma programs in collaboration with the people who were being stigmatized—the mentally ill—became accepted as the rule. This strategy proved to be very useful not only because it often dealt with a specific disturbing problem but also because it convinced people with mental illness that the leaders of the program listen to them and focus on their problems rather than on issues that might have been found to be important elsewhere or at a different time. While activities such as mental health education

i. The complaints about the discrimination in the health services was discussed with the responsible authorities as well as with the staff of health services and could be to a large extent removed; the Calgary experience also served as the basis for action at the federal level.

in schools and the use of media were not discarded, they were used as a complementary rather than as a primary focus of action.

The Calgary experience was important for yet another reason. The fact that something could be done—without much delay—about a problem that was of concern to people with mental illness resulted in the empowerment of the group leading the anti-stigma activities in Calgary. This is not a trivial finding: the fact that programs against stigma must be of long duration, with repeated boosters, means that burn-out of the program leaders and others engaged in anti-stigma work is a real and serious risk for the continuation of activities. It also means that finding ways of maintaining enthusiasm and energy of the leading team, for example, by selecting activities that have a good chance of success in the near future, should be given particular attention.

These two lessons—selecting a target population jointly with the patients and their families, and giving priority to work that is likely to be successful—were precious in the further development of the WPA program.

Whom Should an Anti-Stigma Program Address?

Programs relying on major open access media address a large population. Thus, of necessity, messages addressed to the large population cannot focus on issues of particular relevance for a smaller group that might be of crucial importance in the effort to decrease discrimination or in other ways improve the quality of life of people with mental illness. If messages and work are concentrating on a smaller (often homogenous) group, it is possible to use language that the group considers "their" language to address specific behaviors or attitudes of members of the group. If the focus of efforts is on smaller groups, it is also possible to organize meetings in which people with a mental illness can participate, thus, using the most effective method of diminishing the stigma—personal contacts—between those whose attitudes and behavior are to be changed and the stigmatized persons.

Focusing on individuals who are in positions of influence in a setting is often a better investment for reducing stigma than a widespread campaign because influential people can take action that will be congruent with the change of attitudes that was achieved by working with them. Popular artists and others who are in the center of attention frequently turn out to have a direct experience of mental illness in their family or in themselves. Convincing them that they can and should contribute to the diminution of stigma takes a great amount of effort and time but pays off once they join the programs.

In some instances campaigns are planned in consultation with representatives of people with mental illness or with their families. Such work, it is felt, ensures that the views and needs of those most concerned will be taken into account and that the programs will be focused on their needs. This bi-directional, participatory way of proceeding is certainly better than acting without any consultation of the patients and their families. Yet, most of the organizations that claim to represent people with mental illness and their interests have a relatively small membership and do not represent the vast silent majority of the people concerned. For example, several years ago when we consulted an organization that claimed to be the world organization of "survivors of psychiatry" (i.e., people who had experienced mental illness and received treatment for it), the organization had some 100 members. While their views and ideas were valuable it is hardly possible to imagine that they represent the 600 million people in the world who are suffering from mental illnesses. Similarly, when we were preparing the World Congress of Psychiatry in Madrid in 1996 we were hoping to have sessions that would be organized by one or more organizations of people with mental illness and their relatives which would address problems of wide, international, or global significance. Groups whom we were able to find felt that they could address the problems of great local significance but not issues that would surpass their immediate local experience.

Focus of Anti-Stigma Campaigns

In a number of instances anti-stigma programs address stigma of mental illness, apparently oblivious of the fact that mental illnesses have different forms and that those who suffer from them are not homogenous. When asked, the general public describes people with mental illness as persons who have delusions and hallucinations, who are often violent and dangerous. Yet, the majority of people who have mental illnesses do not have any of these characteristics. The distinction between psychiatric disorders is important in the construction of anti-stigma programs, but also in making policies and plans for mental health and other social services. No one would think of having a single program to deal with influenza and malaria, although both are infectious diseases. The prevention of malaria may rely on mosquito nets, insecticides, sanitation of water, and other measures, vastly different from the advice that would be given to the population that is to be protected against influenza. Some of the actions against both diseases will be similar in nature—for example, reducing the fever or educating health staff about immunology. However, most of what the health services do will be specifically directed to one or the other of these two communicable diseases.

The same principle should be considered in building programs against stigma. The needs for service and help as well as the stigma attached to depression are different from the needs for service and the stigma attached to mental retardation. While certain principles and activities will be the same or very similar, the majority of measures must be specific for the two conditions if we want to help the people who suffer from them. Little is gained by lumping all mental disorders into a single group: Programs that combat stigma should be composed keeping this in mind.

Duration of Programs Against Stigma

The most often used forms of work against stigma are campaigns of a limited duration. While they might be of some value—for example in improving, temporarily, the attitudes towards people with mental illness—their longer term effect is rarely noticeable. Prejudice and discrimination have been around a long time and confirmed many times and in many situations. To think that a one-year campaign will erase centuries or decades of instruction and experience is at best naïve. Additionally, short-term campaigns often raise hopes and involve people who suffer from mental illness in an active way. The abrupt cessation of activities and support at the end of the campaign further confirms the self-stigma and the feeling that behavior of society cannot be changed. Work against stigma must be permanent and long lasting, being an essential task of health and social services. There are numerous parts of routine services that can contribute to stigmatization and subsequent discrimination of people with mental illness. Services have to examine their manner of work, the language that staff uses, the location of services, their hours of work, and a number of other facets of their functioning to ensure that they are not creating or maintaining stigma by their work and behavior. Collaboration with patients who use the services, and their families, can be invaluable in this respect and should be fostered. Apart from giving hints about ways to improve service, the consultation with end-users of services also contributes to users' self-confidence and a confirmation that they are respected by staff of mental health services.

Criteria for the Evaluation of Success of Anti-Stigma Programs

The classical way of evaluating the success of anti-stigma campaigns is the measurement of attitudes to mental illness and people who suffer from it before and after the interventions against stigma. While these measurements are of interest they often say little about the changes of quality of life and other main goals of anti-stigma programs. A much more telling way of assessing what has been achieved is to examine behavior of those surrounding the mentally ill and its changes. If a program against stigma increases the numbers of people who can find housing, find paid employment, or actively participate in community life, it can be said that the program was successful even if the attitudes of the population have not changed much. The most important source of information about the changes in the life of people with mental illness created by work against stigma are those who have or have had mental illness and their caregivers. An elementary task of a mental health service should therefore be the creation of a system of communication with patients that will be simple and effective so that changes can be monitored and that action can be directed by the effects that the program is producing.

Those two principles, that 1) the success of anti-stigma programs is measured by changes in behavior and of the world that surrounds the patients and their families, including also changes such as amendments of the legislation reducing discrimination, and 2) the users of services should be seen as partners and allies in improving the services, are gradually becoming accepted. They should remain among the central goals of all those interested in evaluating the effects of programs against stigma.

Place of Mental Health Professionals in Anti-Stigma Programs

For a very long time mental health professionals were seen as natural leaders of anti-stigma efforts. It was felt that they knew the most about mental illness and that they would be vitally interested in diminishing stigmatization—if for no other reason than because stigma's reach goes beyond the people with mental illness. It also invades the mental health service system and influences the priority that the society gives to mental health care. More recent work, and in particular reports from patients and their families, showed that mental health professionals usually do not involve themselves in anti-stigma efforts and that they often contribute to stigmatization by their behavior and statements. Examples of this are many. Mental health professionals might use the argument that mentally ill people are dangerous when they are pressing for more resources in order to improve mental health facilities. They will use expressions that are insulting for people with mental illness or confirm prejudices. They fail to use "people first" language, and speak of schizophrenics instead of saying "people with schizophrenia" and refer to or label wards as "dangerous." In the course of educating medical students and students of other health professions they will be disrespectful to patients whom they involve in teaching.

Arguments that psychiatrists use to show that mental health services can be provided in developing countries are not free of underlying prejudice. A chief argument that is often put forward is that treatment is cheap and can be provided by simply training personnel at the primary health care level. This may be perfectly true and has been shown to be so in well done research; however, this does not mean that such a fact should be the basis for the request to provide services to people with mental illness. By using the fact that little money is needed to provide care as their most important argument, psychiatrists are also confirming the widely held opinion that people with mental illness are of little value. If people with mental illness were considered equal to people without mental illness, the argument for an improvement (or provision) of services would be based on the ethical imperative to provide care to all people. The fact that treatment can be inexpensive would be secondary and follow the decision of the authorities to help an important group of people to live a life of quality. The argument that soldiers should be vaccinated against a particular disease is not based on the fact that the vaccine is cheap. Rather, it is based on the conviction that soldiers must be kept healthy in order to contribute to the defense of their country.

Ultimate Goals of Anti-Stigma Programs

The ultimate goal of anti-stigma programs is often to ensure that the general population, and in particular those who are in the immediate environment of people with mental illness, become more tolerant, and more likely to accept that people with mental illness may behave differently from others. This goal is certainly worthy but reaching it is not sufficient. Anti-stigma programs should aim at a more distant objective: to ensure that people with mental illness are fully integrated into their community, and that they remain part of it. That goal implies that the community must change in its behavior, and that people with mental illness must accept to abide by the same rules and take on responsibilities in the community to the level of their capacity. In Spain, for example, there is no separate Mental Health Act. The rules about coercion are valid for all citizens, regardless of whether they have a diagnosis of a mental disorder or not.

The Role of Family Members and People with Mental Illness in Anti-Stigma Programs

One of the most significant changes in anti-stigma program strategies is the realization that patients and family members must take an active part in the fight against stigma. Their first and most difficult task is often to get rid of self-stigmatization and to regain self-confidence.[5] Though this is not an easy task, it is necessary to give high priority to activities that will make it possible to carry it out. An example of such an activity is the education of patients in presentation skills so that they can speak with confidence about their disorder, their experience, and their needs. Patients who are educated in "speakers' bureaus" are then ready to meet groups of people in schools or at places of business, to talk about stigma, its meaning, and its consequences. Their intervention has a powerful effect on attitudes toward mentally ill people among those they meet. Additionally, speaking about the issue significantly contributes to the self-confidence and the sense of their own value that is often diminished by people who had a mental illness Members of the families of mentally ill people have a rich experience and knowledge about the management of mental illness and about living with a person who suffers from a mental illness. Yet, their experience is rarely used to educate students of health professions, such as medical or nursing students. Here again, involving family members in teaching does not only benefit the students but also contributes to the recognition of the family members' own value and contributions.

Stigma and the Treatment of Mental Illness

If treatment of mental illness were easy and fully effective it would be much easier to remove stigma and prejudice against people with mental illness. This was clearly the case with tuberculosis—once a stigmatizing disease, which presently does not suffer from the additional burden of stigma. Leprosy has also become much less frightening and people with leprosy have become more acceptable in society since effective treatment was made generally available. Unfortunately, the treatment of mental illness is not yet perfect. Thus, it is necessary to think about ways in which treatment of mental disorders can contribute to the reduction of stigmatization and its consequences.

Treatment of psychotic disorders with antipsychotic medications was a major step forward in psychiatry. While such treatment effectively contributes to the reduction of symptoms, the medications themselves have side-effects which are not only very disagreeable but also mark the person as someone who is in treatment for a mental disorder or a psychiatric disorder. More recently developed psychotropic medications have fewer side-effects of this type and are therefore more acceptable to patients and less likely to have outward signs that can lead to stigma. Their cost, however, often makes them inaccessible to patients, particularly those who are poor. The place in which treatment is provided can also contribute to stigmatization and the efforts to shift treatment from mental health institutions, for example, psychiatric hospitals, to primary health care centers or community-based organizations, are important and welcome. The notion that it is important to discuss the treatment modalities and their effects as well as side effects with patients and their families is gradually gaining ground, which is helping to manage the illness in a manner that is most useful for the patient.

The discussion about treatment and the search for ways to provide the treatment in which patients participate is new for most of the mental health specialists.

The acceptance of this strategy has to be incorporated into medical school training and developed further in postgraduate training. It must also become the norm of behavior among all others who participate in inpatient and outpatient care, in rehabilitation and in work with relatives and others.

Concluding Remarks

Advances of psychiatry and in the field of neurosciences have been most impressive and in many ways revolutionary. This progress could make the life of people with mental illness and their families much better and at the same time ensure that people with mental illness contribute to society while living a life of acceptable quality. The main obstacle to this development is the stigma attached to mental illness which is at the basis of the low priority given to mental health programs in most countries of the world and at the origin of many difficulties that arise in care for people with mental illness.

A number of programs combating stigma have been started and carried out in the recent past. They have demonstrated that it is possible to reduce or prevent stigmatization and its consequences. They have also shown that the traditional strategies of fighting stigma need to be reviewed and revised. This chapter reports on some of the insights gained in the course of these programs and presents some of the suggestions that those interested and willing to fight against stigma might wish to examine. Until the time when treatments of mental illness become so effective that mental illness becomes a banality, the fight against stigma must become and remain a priority and a routine part of health and other social service programs. The insights presented here might help in this effort.

References

1. Sartorius, N. & Schulze, H. (2005). *Reducing the stigma of mental illness. A report from a global programme of the World Psychiatric Association.* Cambridge: Cambridge University Press.
2. Pickenhagen, A. & Sartorius, N. (2002). *Annotated bibliography of selected publications and other materials related to stigma and discrimination because of mental illness and intervention programmes fighting it.* World Psychiatric Association Global Programme to Reduce the Stigma and Discrimination Because of Schizophrenia. Also on www.openthedoors.com
3. Aichberger, M. & Sartorius, N. (2006). *Annotated bibliography of selected publications and other materials related to stigma and discrimination. An update for the years 2002 to 2006.* The World Psychiatric Association Global Programme to Reduce the Stigma and Discrimination Because of Schizophrenia. Also on www.openthedoors.com

4. Sartorius, N. (2005). Stigma and discrimination because of schizophrenia: A summary of the WPA Global Programme Against Stigma and Discrimination Because of Schizophrenia. In H. Stuart, J. Arboleda-Flórez, N. Sartorius, (Eds.). *Stigma and Mental Disorders: International Perspectives. World Psychiatry Volume 4,* Supplement.
5. Thornicroft, G., Brohan, E., Rose, D., Sartorius, N., & Leese, M, for the INDIGO Study Group. (2009). Global pattern of experienced and anticipated discrimination against people with schizophrenia: A cross-sectional survey. *Lancet, 373,* 408–415.

12

The Social Determinants of Mental Health

SANDRO GALEA AND MARIA STEENLAND

Introduction

There is a long tradition of conceptual and theoretical work that has been concerned with social influences on mental disorders.[1,2,3] To name one prominent historical example, Faris and Dunham published seminal early work in 1939 using data from Chicago that suggested an inverse relationship between social organization and schizophrenia.[4] In subsequent years, empiricists[5] and theorists[6] from disciplines including medical sociology and social epidemiology, to name a few, have presented data linking social processes to mental illness. However, during the past two decades, the disciplines that are principally concerned with the origins of psychopathology—particularly psychiatry and epidemiology—have focused much of their attention on individual factors that are linked with particular mental illness. This increasing focus on individual risk factors—particularly molecular and genetic—as determinants of mental illness has yielded tremendous gains. For example, recent research has identified genetic markers associated with several forms of dementia,[7] and the biologic mechanisms that lead to depressive symptoms are becoming clearer.[8] Unfortunately, the growing sophistication of risk-factor epidemiologic research, of molecular biology and molecular genetics, has come, to some extent, at the expense of building on the seminal work that was conducted in the first half of the twentieth century that laid the groundwork for much of our current understanding of how social processes contribute to mental health in populations.

Recent shifts in several of the key relevant disciplines suggest, however, a resurgence of interest in the social determinants of health in general. Several authors have proposed frameworks that suggest how factors at multiple "levels" of influence, ranging from macrosocial processes, to individual behaviors, to molecular factors are causes of health states.[9,10,11] Methodologic developments[12,13] have allowed the introduction of factors at different levels of influence—including, for example, neighborhood levels[14]—in empiric analyses that aim to understand the factors that are associated with risk of mental illness. This work has set the stage for a resurgence of interest in the systematic study of the social factors that influence risk of psychopathology.

There are two overarching perspectives that have emerged in recent years that may usefully frame our thinking about the social determinants of mental health. The first, social epidemiology, has recently grown dramatically as a formal discipline.[15] Generally, social epidemiology is concerned with understanding how various aspects of the social environment are related to health.[16] Social epidemiology has contributed to the field a growing number of empirical studies that explore how exogenous factors are associated with health and disease, although most of these studies have been concerned with the health outcomes that have historically been the core focus of epidemiology, including cardiovascular disease,[17] cancer,[18] and infectious diseases.[19] Increasingly, social epidemiologists have also been considering the determinants of mental health and illness within a multilevel framework that incorporates social[20] and behavioral[21] factors as determinants of mental illness.

A second perspective that is instructive is the population health perspective proposed by Geoffrey Rose whose contributions were clarifying and a clarion call for subsequent work.[22] A direct consequence of Rose's work is that it may be more fruitful to consider the factors that influence *population* patterns of risks and of disease than it is to consider the factors that influence *individual* risks.[23] Rose further suggested that while traditional public health efforts have attempted to influence individual behavior, to change individual risk, more successful efforts could target the social factors that shaped the distribution of risk factors.[24] Both social epidemiology and the population health perspective provide a theoretic foundation for the importance of social determinants in our understanding of mental health.

Mental disorders account for about 14% of the global burden of disease, most of which is attributed to depression and other common mood-anxiety disorders.[25] Although we are increasingly understanding the individual and biological determinants of some mental illness, particular psychotic disorders,[26] our ability to explain patterns of common mood disorders such as depression remains limited.[27] Arguably, this limitation stems from the limited, individual, explanatory covariate set that is considered in most studies concerned with the determination of risk of psychopathology. This paper suggests, building on social epidemiologic and population health perspectives, that a full understanding of the production of mental illness also needs to take into account exogenous—or social—factors that also influence mental health and disease. Centrally, the ubiquity of social exposures suggests that intervening on the social exposures associated with mental illness may substantially reduce mental illness.

This chapter is a synthesis of the extant evidence and a call for more work in the area. To illuminate the state-of-the science about how social factors, at different levels of influence, are associated with psychopathology. Although we do not here offer our own explicit conceptual framework about how social factors influence mental illness, we build on extant frameworks[11] and review individual, inter-individual, and ecological social factors that have compelling conceptual reasons to be associated with mental disorders. At the individual level, we discuss socioeconomic position (SEP) and race/ethnicity, at the inter-individual level we discuss violence and social support, and at the ecologic level we discuss features of place, particularly urban places, and social capital as determinants of mental illness. Though we recognize the considerable importance of gender in shaping mental health, it is not discussed because the association between gender and mental health is likely explained by a combination of complex social and biological factors. Depression, for example has been shown to increase in women at puberty, due to changing hormone levels. While this evidence is not entirely consistent it does point to the possibility that biological factors are involved.[28] It is also possible that women are more susceptible to risk factors, such as life stressors associated with depression.[29] Other summaries of the literature would productively contribute to the field by considering the conjoint influence of social and behavioral factors and genetic variability in mental illness.

This chapter focuses on common mood, anxiety, and substance use disorders, specifically major depression, posttraumatic stress disorder (PTSD), generalized anxiety disorder, and substance use disorders. An understanding of the social determinants of these disorders can lead to interventions that aim to reduce the population morbidity associated with these common mental illnesses, effectively, "shifting the curve" of disease.

Individual Factors

Socioeconomic Position

Socioeconomic position (SEP) is the position that individuals and groups hold within the structure of society. In practice, SEP is typically quantified as the social and economic factors that determine an individual's place in society, most often income, education, and occupation.[30] It is hypothesized that different social strata experience differing levels of vulnerability to experienced stressful events, and that they also have different resources available to them to cope with these events.[31] Although overall there is a well-documented inverse relation between SEP and mental illness, this finding is not consistent across disorders and contexts. Several large community-based studies in the US have examined the effect of SEP on different mental disorders. Using data from the National Comorbidity Survey, Kessler and colleagues estimated lifetime and 12-month prevalence of 14 DSM-III-R psychiatric disorders. Disorders were classified into any affective disorder, any anxiety disorder, any substance use disorder, and antisocial personality disorder. In their full model, adjusting for other demographic factors, persons in the lowest level of income category (earning $0–$19,000 per year) had greater odds of all disorder categories as compared to the persons in the highest income category (greater than $70,000 a year). The relation of education and mental health was less consistent; lower levels of education were associated with increased anxiety and substance use disorders but not significantly associated with affective disorders.[32] These findings have not been consistent across all published research, particularly research conducted using European samples.

Laaksonen and colleagues investigated the association between SEP and common mental disorders in middle-aged Finnish and British public sector employees in the Helsinki Health and the Whitehall II Studies. They assessed mental health using Golberg's General Health Questionnaire (GHQ-12), and found that only childhood and current economic difficulties were associated with GHQ-12 score.[33] More traditional indicators such as respondent's education and occupational class were not statistically significant. Weich and colleagues found, in a prospective study of adults in England, Wales, and Scotland, that poverty and unemployment were associated with the maintenance but not the onset of common mental disorders. Financial strain, however, was associated with both the maintenance and onset of disorders even after adjusting for indices of standard of living.[34] It is plausible that the relation between SEP and mental illness is more marked in countries such as the US, where inter-individual SEP is more heterogeneous than it is in European countries where it is less so.

There has been substantial interest in the association between SEP and depression. A meta-analysis of 56 studies found that low-SEP individuals had higher odds of being depressed (OR 1.81).[35] Among the five incidence studies included, the lowest SEP group had a 1.24 times greater odds of depression than the highest SEP group. In addition, in studies of the persistence of depression, already depressed individuals from lower SEP groups had a twofold greater odds of remaining depressed (OR 2.06).[35] Lynch and colleagues measured SEP in a less traditional way through the measurement of three different time periods of economic hardship rather than a single measurement of income. The odds of depression were more than three times greater in individuals who experienced three episodes of economic hardship than those with consistently higher incomes.[36]

It is possible that the central driver of the relation between SEP and common mental illness is the experience of stressful life events.[37] Unemployment has been studied relatively frequently as a sentinel stressful life event. Dooley and colleagues used a continuum of employment to investigate whether movement from employed to unemployed or from employed to underemployed increased the likelihood of depression among 5,113 respondents from a nationally representative survey, The National Longitudinal Survey of Youth. After controlling for prior depression, both changes from employment to either unemployment or underemployment resulted in a similar increased risk of depression.[38]

The association between SEP and substance abuse and dependence has also been examined and is reviewed more exhaustively elsewhere.[39] In general, this literature suggests that substance use disorders are more prevalent among persons with lower SEP, even though substance use itself may not be. Montgomery et al. examined alcohol problems among 2,887 British men in the 1958 longitudinal British birth cohort study. When compared to men who had never been unemployed, men with over three years of unemployment had a 2.15 times greater odds of problem drinking. Men who were unemployed in the past year had a 1.73 times greater odds of heavy drinking and a 2.90 times greater odds of having a drinking problem.[40] Kadushin and colleagues examined 9,762 adults in 42 urban communities in the US and found that among binge drinkers (those who consumed more than four drinks on one occasion in the last year) mean income was associated with alcohol dependence.[41]

A meta-analysis of risk factors for PTSD found that education and general childhood adversity predicted PTSD relatively consistently but to a varying extent.[42] Other studies have found no association between income or education and PTSD. A study conducted in Detroit found that income and education levels were not associated with PTSD after adjustment for other sociodemographic factors such as sex, race, marital status, and residence.[43] Kilpatrick and colleagues explored whether SEP and crime characteristics predicted the development of crime-related PTSD among women from Charleston County, South Carolina and found that crime-related PTSD was not associated with sociodemographic characteristics including education and income.[44]

Race and Ethnicity

The difference in physical health between racial and ethnic groups is well documented; there is abundant evidence that racial/ethnic minorities have worse physical health than do members of majority racial/ethnic groups.[45] In terms of mental health, theorists have proposed several mechanisms that could explain a differential association between race/ethnicity and psychopathology. It has been suggested that "the structural location of blacks in society would lead them to have higher levels of stress than whites," and that "the experience of specific incidents of racial bias can generate psychological distress and lead to alteration in physiological processes that can adversely affect health."[46] It also has been suggested that groups who have historically been exposed to discrimination develop adaptation strategies that mitigate or reduce to some extent their vulnerability to unfair treatment.[47]

Empirical evidence suggests that the association between race and ethnicity and mental health is complex. McGuire and Miranda note that minorities, in general, have equal or better mental health than White Americans.[48] There is evidence, however, that minorities have less access to mental health services and report more severe symptoms than Whites.[48] Further increasing the complexity of these associations, SEP and race are highly correlated and adjusting for SEP in models of race and health outcomes often eliminates the association between race and mental health altogether.[45] Race/ethnicity can also modify the relation between SEP and mental health. Jones-Webb and colleagues found that lower social class was associated with drinking problems among Black men but not among White men.[49]

Evidence about the relation between race/ethnicity and depression is mixed.[50] Riolo and colleagues examined the National Health and Nutrition Examination Survey III, a representative U.S. sample of 8,449 respondents aged 15–40 years of age, and found that prevalence of major depression was significantly higher among Whites than African Americans and Mexican Americans. However, the opposite association was found for dysthymic disorder, or long-term depression.[51] Adding to Riolo's findings, Williams and colleagues used the National Institute of Mental Health's Collaborative Psychiatric Epidemiology Surveys to examine the relation between ethnicity and depression and found that lifetime prevalence of major depressive disorder (MDD) was highest among Whites, followed by Caribbean Blacks and African Americans. However, the 12-month MDD estimates were similar for the three groups.[52]

Large national surveys have shown that the relationship between race/ethnicity and anxiety disorders varies by disorder. One study used both the National Survey of American Life and the National Comorbidity Survey Replication to examine racial and ethnic variation in the prevalence of anxiety disorders.[53] The study used the Diagnostic and Statistical Manual of Mental Disorders, Fourth Edition (DSM-IV) and the World Mental Health Composite International Diagnostic Interview (WMH-CIDI) to assess GAD, social anxiety disorder (SAD), PTSD, and panic disorder (PD). Whites were at a greater risk of developing GAD, PD, and SAD compared to Caribbean Blacks and African Americans. Black respondents however, had increased odds of developing PTSD.[53]

Large national studies have not identified consistent differences in drug use between racial and ethnic groups in the US.[54] Grant and colleagues investigated trends of alcohol abuse and dependence between 1991/1992 and 2001/2002 and found that the prevalence of abuse was higher among Whites than among Latinos, Blacks, and Asians, and that the prevalence of dependence was higher in Whites, Native Americans, and Latinos than Asians. They also found that abuse had not increased among young White adults but had increased among minority young adults, specifically Black and Hispanic males and Asian women.[55] Studies also have found racial/ethnic differences in the consequences of drug use and the patterns of treatment for drug use. A study of accidental drug overdose in New York City between 1990 and 1998 found that rates of overdose were consistently higher among Blacks and Latinos compared to Whites,[56] but differences in mental health between racial and ethnic groups were related to treatment rather than differences in incidence. Using data from the national Healthcare for Communities survey, Wells and colleagues found that African Americans were less likely to have access to alcoholism, drug abuse, or mental health care than Whites. Latinos were more likely to report delayed care or less care than needed.[57]

Empirical research has begun to focus on understanding the mechanisms that may explain why there are differences in racial/ethnic group membership and common mental illness. Kessler and colleagues examined the association between perceived discrimination and major depression, generalized anxiety disorder, and psychological distress controlling for exogenous predictors of both perceived discrimination and mental health disorders. Although the authors did not confirm their hypothesis that differential exposure to discrimination plays an important role in explaining the associations between disadvantaged social status and mental health, they did find strong associations between perceived discrimination and mental health disorders.[58]

Inter-Individual Factors

Violence

The best available evidence about the relation between an inter-individual factor and mental illness is focused on interpersonal violence. Interpersonal violence is a relatively common phenomenon both in the United States as well as in the rest of the world. The US has particularly high rates of violence compared to other high-income countries. In 2000, the US violent death rate was 6.2 per 100,000—about twice as high as the rate in other high-income countries. Fatal injuries are only part of the burden of interpersonal violence; other forms of nonfatal violence produce substantial health costs,[59] such as intimate partner violence consisting of psychological, physical, and sexual violence generally directed towards women. The World Health Organization considers violence to be the principal gender-related contributor to depression among women.[60]

The WHO's multi-country study on women's health aims to document the variation in the prevalence of intimate partner violence between countries and its relation to common mental disorders. Evidence from Brazil shows that several forms of violence including physical violence, psychological violence, and sexual violence were all associated with poor mental health after adjustment for demographic and socioeconomic characteristics.[60] A study of 1,994 Ethiopian women in rural Ethiopia focused on different types of intimate partner violence and experience of a depressive episode. Women who had ever experienced physical violence had more than two times greater odds of a depressive episode than women who had never experienced physical violence. Women reporting two or more types of emotional violence were almost four times more likely to report having experienced a depressive episode in the past 12 months.[61]

Exposure to community violence may also lead to increased rates of mental disorders in populations. Clark and colleagues examined the psychopathology associated with witnessing community violence among low income women living in urban areas in the northeastern United States. After controlling for sociodemographic factors, women who witnessed violence in their community were more than twice as likely to experience depressive and anxiety symptoms than women who did not.[62] This study found that witnessing violence was associated with anxiety and depression even among women who are not direct participants in the violent acts.[62]

Using data from the South African Stress and Health Study (SAHS), a national probability sample of South Africans, Kaminer and colleagues examined the association between multiple forms of violence and PTSD. The study found that among men, political detention and torture were the forms of violence most strongly associated with a lifetime diagnosis of PTSD. Among women, rape was most strongly associated with risk of PTSD.[63]

There is substantial evidence that the population prevalence of psychopathology is higher among populations who experience mass conflict or traumatic events. Studies documenting the prevalence of mental health disorders have found high rates of depression and PTSD in veteran as well as refugee populations. A study investigating the prevalence and determinants of mental health disorders among 289,328 veterans from Iraq and Afghanistan entering Veterans Affairs health care from 2002 to 2008 found that 21.8% of this population was diagnosed with PTSD and 17.4% with depression. The authors do not describe the specific event that was associated with PTSD; however, questions about traumatic events were likely part of the diagnostic assessment. The authors also found that greater combat exposure was associated with an increased risk of PTSD.[64] Refugee populations have also been shown to have high rates of mental illness. Among Cambodian refugees in Thailand, for example, 37% reported symptoms of PTSD and 68% reported symptoms of depression.[65] Again, no specific traumatic event is reported; however, probably it is the experiences of violence, conflict, and displacement that are associated with PTSD. Slightly lower but still high rates were found among Bosnian refugees in Croatia, of which 26% reported symptoms of PTSD and 39% reported symptoms of depression.[66]

De Jong and colleagues investigated whether individuals in Algeria, Cambodia, Ethiopia, and Palestine exposed to armed-conflict-associated violence (ACAV) were more likely to experience common mental disorders. Persons with exposure to 1 of 17 assessed conflict-related events were more likely to meet criteria for PTSD (RR = 10.03 in Palestinians and RR = 3.14 in Algerians) and mood disorders (RR = 6.06 in Ethiopians and RR = 4.53 in Palestinians). The risk ratio for anxiety disorders ranged from 2.10 to 3.16, but was not significant in Cambodia.[67] Steel and colleagues examined the mental health of Vietnamese refugees resettled in Australia. Using the International Classification of Disease version 10 (ICD-10), the authors examined mental disorders and exposure to traumatic events in a community sample of 1,413 refugees. The mean time that refugees had been in Australia was 11.2 years with a mean of 14.8 years since the time of the last traumatic event. The authors found that risk of mental illness decreased with time, and that more traumatic events increased the risk of mental illness.[68]

Social Support

Several types of social support have been operationalized. Perceived social support is considered to be the cognitive appraisal of being reliably connected to others. Enacted support is the actions others perform when they render assistance to focal personal contacts.[69] There is also a distinction between structural social support, that is, the number of existing relationships, and the function of these relationships that more appropriately represents received support.[70] Two dominant models aim to explain how social support could affect health—the stress-buffering model and the main effects model. The stress-buffering model hypothesizes that social networks affect well-being only for those individuals under stress. The main effects model contends that social capital has a salutary effect regardless of whether an individual is experiencing stress.[70]

Social support is operationalized inconsistently across studies making generalizable inference difficult. Most studies in the area have examined the relation between social support and depression and anxiety. One study examined the effect of social support and depression among 422 households in a southern Black community and measured social support through extended kin support, non-kin support, and kin interaction. Those who perceived their kin to be more supportive reported fewer symptoms of depression, though the number of extended kin and perceived support from non-kin were not associated with depression.[71] Aneshensel and Frerichs measured stress, social support, and depression in the Los Angeles Area Sample, a three-stage cluster sample based on the 1970 census. Social support, as defined by the number of close friends or relatives, and a measure of perceived support, were negatively associated with depression.[72]

The relationship between social support and substance abuse has also been studied. One study in Göteborg, Sweden analyzed alcohol dependence and abuse in relation to social variables including social network, leisure time, social class, and education and found that women with only one or no friends had a 2.6 times greater odds of alcohol dependence and abuse than women with more than one friend.[73] In addition, women who seldom had contact with friends, relatives, and neighbors had a 2.7 times increased odds of alcohol dependence and abuse than women who had daily contact with friends. All of the author's models were adjusted for age.

There has been a great deal of interest in the relationship between social support and PTSD. Kawachi and Subramanian suggest that differences in the level of social support between communities accounts for variation in the success of community recovery following a traumatic event.[74] A meta-analysis of predictors of PTSD found that in 11 studies the weighted average correlation between perceived social support and PTSD was -.28 which was statistically significant. The authors describe the effect size as small to medium in relation to the other factors in the review (e.g. history of prior trauma, family history of psychopathology).[75] Social support has also been examined extensively as a mitigating factor in the association between other social determinants and PTSD. Coker and colleagues showed that social support is a protective factor in the association between intimate partner violence (IPV) and mental health. In their study, IPV was associated with substance abuse, PTSD symptoms, current depression, and anxiety. Among women who were experiencing IPV, greater social support was associated with a decreased risk of anxiety, current depression, and PTSD symptoms.[76]

Ecologic Factors

Urban and Neighborhood Environment

The urban environment broadly has been the subject of mental health research for more than a century. In early work in the field, cities have typically been the relevant ecologic unit of interest and empiric work has aimed to understand how living in urban areas may be associated with mental illness, often in contrast to living in nonurban areas. The work of Faris and Dunham, introduced earlier, noted differences in mental disorders across particular areas of cities.[3] Other landmark work, much of it focused on the etiology of psychotic disorders, sought to understand why these disorders were more prevalent in urban versus nonurban areas.[4] Aspects of the urban environment including social disorganization, social strain, social resources, and spatial segregation have all been defined as possible mechanisms for the relation between urban life and mental health.[78] One study using data from the U.S. Epidemiologic Catchment Area study found a two-fold greater prevalence of major depression in urban areas as compared to rural areas but found no difference between small metropolitan areas and rural areas.[79] Similar results were found in a study from England that examined the prevalence of nonpsychotic mental disorders in urban and rural areas using the National Morbidity Survey in Great Britain. Using data from 9,777 participants, the authors found that urban participants had higher rates of psychiatric morbidity as assessed by the Revised Clinical Interview Schedule (CIS-R) as well as greater drug and alcohol dependence. These differences, however, were no longer significant after adjustment for life stress, deprivation, and living conditions.[80] Other studies using similarly large samples and classification systems have not found differences in prevalence between urban and rural areas. For example, Kessler and colleagues found no difference in major depression between rural, small, and large metropolitan areas in the United States.[32]

In the past couple of decades there has been a growing interest in the effects of neighborhood-level characteristics on public health.[81] This interest has generated research investigating the role of the neighborhood environment in the mental health of its residents. Schulz and colleagues propose that mental and emotional well-being is affected by the social environment such as experiences of unfair treatment and living in areas with a high concentration of households below the poverty level.[82] In a prospective population-based cohort study in New York, 1,570 adult residents were contacted 6 and 18 months after an initial interview and a greater incidence of depression was found in "poor" neighborhoods compared to "rich" neighborhoods. After adjusting for sociodemographic characteristics including individual SEP, the odds of depression were 2.19 times greater in low SEP neighborhoods than in high SEP neighborhoods.[83] In a similar study of Illinois residents, neighborhood disadvantage was associated with depression and remained significant after adjusting for individual socioeconomic factors. Interestingly, this study did not find that there were differences in depression between Chicago residents and suburb, city, and town residents.[84] Other studies have measured neighborhood quality to assess the relationship between neighborhood characteristics and mental health. Echeverría and colleagues, for example, found that individuals living in neighborhoods with the fewest problems related to income/wealth, education, and occupation were significantly less likely to report depressive symptoms than those living in the neighborhoods with the highest number of problems.[85]

A review by Mair and colleagues concerned with neighborhood-level factors and depression found that 37 out of 45 papers reviewed found an association between at least one aspect of the neighborhood environment and depression. Of the ten longitudinal studies, seven reported associations between at least one neighborhood factor and depression. The review found that structural features such as socioeconomic and racial composition and built environment were less consistently associated with depression than social processes such as disorder, social interactions, and violence.[86] A unique experimental study examined the effect of a program called "Moving to Opportunity," a program that places residents of public housing in more affluent neighborhoods, on participants' mental health. This randomized controlled trial found that parents who moved to low-poverty neighborhoods reported significantly less distress than control parents. The models were adjusted for sex, race, ethnicity, age, education, and employment status.[87]

Although most studies of neighborhood characteristics have focused on neighborhood income, there is a limited but growing body of work that has been concerned with the relation between the built environment and mental health. Residential crowding and loud exterior noise have been shown to be associated with nonspecific psychological distress.[88] Galea and colleagues investigated the relationship between neighborhood built environment and both six-month and lifetime depression among a sample of New Yorkers and found that residents of neighborhoods characterized by poor quality built environment were 29%–58% more likely to report past-six-month depression and 36%–64% more likely to report lifetime depression than respondents in neighborhoods with higher quality built environments.[89] These estimates are adjusted for neighborhood income and individual income, age, sex, and race/ethnicity.

The relationship between the neighborhood environment and substance use has also been explored, although in relatively few studies. Boardman et al. examined the relationship between neighborhood disadvantage and drug use using data from the 1995 Detroit area study in conjunction with tract-level data from the 1990 census. This study defined neighborhood disadvantage in terms of area level income as well as percent of female-headed households, male unemployment rate, and public assistance and found a positive relationship between neighborhood disadvantage and drug use, even after adjusting for individual-level SEP.[90]

Social Capital

There is a growing body of work focusing on social capital as an ecologic or group-level factor that may be associated with mental health. Putnam, one of the key theorists in the area, defines social capital as community and personal networks, civic engagement, local civic identity, reciprocity and norms of cooperation, and trust in the community.[91] Most of this work has suggested that living in areas characterized by more social capital is associated with better mental health.[92]

Fujiwara and Kawachi examined the association between measures of social capital and depression in a nationally representative prospective study of 724 U.S. adults and found that persons who trusted their neighbors (a typical measure of social capital) had lower odds of developing major depression in a model adjusted for major depression at baseline, age, gender, race, education, working status, marital status, physical health, and extroversion.[93] Another study conceptualized social capital as the amount of trust between individuals and societal institutions, measured by mean voting participation. This study monitored hospital visits for depression or psychosis among the entire Swedish population aged 25–64 from 1997 to 1999. Mean voting participation in neighborhood units was categorized into tertiles. Adjusting for both individual and neighborhood level factors, the authors found that lower levels of neighborhood social capital increased an individual's odds of hospital admission for depression or psychosis. The association between depression and social capital however, was nonsignificant after adjusting for neighborhood deprivation.[94] Another study that focused on institutional level social capital investigated whether trust in the national parliament of Sweden was associated with psychological health, taking into account "horizontal trust," that is, trust in other people. After adjusting for age, country of origin, economic stress, and horizontal trust, having no trust at all in the parliament was associated with an increased odds of reporting poor psychological health as opposed to very high trust.[95] Other studies have included different aspects of social capital. A study by Silove and colleagues measured social capital through feelings of trust and safety, community participation, and neighborhood connections and reciprocity, and found that higher levels of trust and feeling safe were associated with lower levels of psychological distress after adjusting for demographics.[96]

Social capital may function differently within different racial groups. A study of African American and White adults living in Baltimore, Maryland found that community cohesion and the perception that people generally work together was associated with better mental health among Whites only.[97] This difference in association has been noted in the past by researchers cautioning that social connections may increase levels of psychopathology in low-income women if these connections mean that they must provide support for an increased number of people.[92]

Methodologic Challenges

In summarizing the extant evidence about the relationship between features of the social environment and mental health, it is worth noting that challenges are pervasive in this area of research. Perhaps the most central of these challenges is the difficulty in determining selection versus causality. The directionality of causation challenges many of the studies in the field, particularly cross-sectional studies. Authors have commented on the challenges of distinguishing between social causation—where social causes influence the production of mental illness—and social selection—where mental illness results in a drift toward poorer social conditions—for more than 30 years.[6] For example, the association between SEP and depression could result from the effect of adversity and stress in lower social strata leading to psychopathology or from the effect of depression leading to downward economic mobility.[98] A similar question of causation exists between the relation of social support and mental health. Are people with poorer health less likely to make social connections or does a lack of social relations produce poorer health? Complicating matters, both social selection and social causation may play a role in explaining the relation between social factors and mental illness and may be combined over the life course. Longitudinal research methods have been used to help clarify this issue. These methods allow for the adjustment of baseline mental health disorders and the follow-up reporting of incident cases. Such studies, although still quite limited in number, have been able to move the field forward substantially. For example, studies that collect baseline mental health data and follow-up mental health data allow investigators to adjust for baseline mental health. Other studies follow participants for a long follow-up period and measure incidence of new disease. For example, a longitudinal study of 756 participants interviewed up to four times over 17 years found that low parental education was associated with subsequent increased risk of child depression after controlling for parental depression, child's age, and gender. However, neither parent nor child depression predicted the level of child education or income later in life.[99] There is still much ongoing discussion with respect to selection and causation and much we do not yet understand. The use of longitudinal methods can help clarify some of the inconsistent findings in the field. The adoption of methods that take into account bidirectional and nonlinear relations may also be promising in this regard.[100]

A central challenge to the research concerned with ecologic social factors as determinants of mental health is unmeasured individual-level confounding. Putman originally conceived of social capital as a group level or ecologic variable. Individual-level processes, however, must mediate the relation between group-level social capital and individual mental health. It is possible then that the observed relations between ecologic characteristics and individual mental illness reflect simply unmeasured individual-level factors that are ultimately causal. We refer the reader to several reviews and commentaries in the area that have considered this issue.[101,12,13]

Another persistent challenge to the way that we study mental health is the comorbidity of many common mental disorders. The National Comorbidity Survey found that most incident cases of major depressive disorders occur in individuals who have previously been diagnosed with another mental disorder with anxiety disorders being the most common of such disorders.[102] Comorbidity challenges the notion that a given social exposure is associated with a specific mental health indicator and might even suggest that social determinants are associated with pathophysiologic pathways that lead to overall mental illness. Complicating matters, social factors are also seldom independent. For example, racial segregation and low socioeconomic status are often associated phenomenon. Evidence from the Detroit area studies has shown that Whites moving out of the city between 1970 and 1990 decreased the tax base, property values, and employment opportunities in Detroit. As a result of this migration between 1970 and 1980, the number of census tracks in which 40% of the residents were below the poverty line significantly increased from 24 to 51.[82] Schulz and colleagues explained that "racial integration of Detroit's neighborhoods was undermined by stereotypes that fueled White residents' fears, contributing to their attempts to prevent African Americans from moving into their neighborhoods."[82] (p. 684). Thus, while differences in mental health between Whites and Blacks may be explained statistically by SEP, it is possible that race was a driving factor in initiating and perpetuating differences in SEP. These interrelations abound, and challenge efforts at isolating a single "causal" factor. Similarly, a given social factor may decrease the adverse effect of another. For example, an earlier study showed that social support mitigates the deleterious effect of intimate partner violence on women's mental health.[76]

Conclusions

In general, economic and social vulnerability are associated with an increased risk of mental illness. These relationships, however, are not consistent across social factors and across mental disorders. Low income, economic hardship, and unemployment appear to be more associated with depression than PTSD for example. Other social factors, such as race, have a more complex relation with mental illness that is inconsistent with the general trend of social vulnerability increasing mental disorder. Minorities often have lower rates of mental illness; however, they tend to have more persistent disease which is likely due to less access to treatment. Factors such as community- and conflict-related violence have consistent and sometimes strong associations with PTSD, as well as other mental health disorders such as depression. Other features of the social environment such as social connections and community engagement or trust are also associated with better mental health. Interestingly, some studies have shown that group level factors such as neighborhood income are associated with mental health disorders such as depression, independently of individual risk.

As we have discussed, there are complex theoretical questions and methodological issues when considering the relationship between social factors and mental health. Despite these issues, it is likely that social factors do affect the risk of mental disorders. Some of these associations are relatively weak; however, it is possible that even the weak associations may have a large public health importance. Many of these social factors such as low income, unemployment, and low social support are common exposures and therefore a change in one of these factors would result in a large change in population level of disease.

It then follows from our earlier discussion of the population health perspective that interventions that aim to influence social environmental factors that "shift the curve" have a greater potential to reduce the population burden of mental illness than do interventions that target only individual risk factors.

Although the trend in recent years has been to focus on individual, and increasingly molecular, determinants of psychopathology, an emerging body of work is building on earlier traditions in psychiatry and public health to document associations between social factors and mental illness. We intend this summary of extant work both to provide a perspective on the state-of-the-science, and also to motivate new research in the area. However, as we summarize the evidence about the relation between social factors and mental illness, we note that some of the most exciting work in the field aims to study not only the role of social factors but rather how social and biologic factors *jointly* shape common mental illness. For example, the children of alcohol dependent parents have a 4- to 10-fold increased probability of alcohol use and subsequent abuse and dependence compared to children of nonalcoholics.[103] This suggests that our summary of the literature in the field is not so much a call for more work that focuses exclusively on how social factors produce mental illness as it is a call for the integration of social factors in multilevel causal frameworks that consider the contribution of social, individual, and biologic factors in the production of mental illness.

References

1. Odegard, O. (1932). Emigration and insanity. *Acta psychiat.scand, Suppl. 4*, 1–206.
2. Hollingshead, A. B. & Redlich, F. C. (1958). *Social class and mental illness.* New York, NY: Wiley.
3. Faris, R. E. L. & Dunham, H. W. (1939). *Mental disorders in urban areas.* Chicago, IL: The University of Chicago Press.
4. March, D., Hatch, S., Morgan, C., et al. (2008). Psychosis and place. *Epidemiol Rev, 30,* 84–100.
5. Strole, L., Langer, T. S., Michael, S. T., Opler, M. K., & Rennie, T. A. C. (1962). *Mental health in the metropolis: The Midtown Manhattan Study.* New York, NY: McGraw-Hill.
6. Dohrenwend, B. P. (1966). Social status and psychological disorder: An issue of substance and an issue of method. *Am Sociol Rev, 31,* 14–34.
7. Kim, J., Basak, J., & Holtzman, D. (2009). The role of apolipoprotein E in Alzheimer's disease. *Neuron, 63,* 287–303.
8. aan het Rot, M., Mathew, S., & Charney, D. (2009). Neurobiological mechanisms in major depressive disorder. *CMAJ, 180,* 305–313.
9. Susser, M. & Susser, E. (1996). Choosing a future for epidemiology: II. from black box to Chinese boxes and eco-epidemiology. *Am J Public Health, 86,* 674–675.
10. Krieger, N. (2008). Proximal, distal, and the politics of causation: What's level got to do with it? *Am J Public Health, 98,* 221–230.

11. Kaplan, G. A., Everson, S. A., & Lynch, J. W. (2000). The contribution of social and behavioral research to an understanding of the distribution of disease: A multilevel approach. In: *Promoting health: Intervention strategies from social and behavioral research* (pp. 37–80). Washington, DC: National Academy Press.
12. Subramanian, S. V., Glymour, M. M., & Kawachi, I. (2007). Identifying causal ecologic effects on health: A methodological assessment. In *Macrosocial determinants of population health* (pp. 301–332). New York, NY: Springer.
13. Curtis, S. & Cummins, S. (2007). Ecologic studies. In *Macrosocial determinants of population health* (pp. 333–354). New York, NY: Springer.
14. Diez Roux, A. V. (2001). Investigating neighborhood and area effects on health. *Am J Public Health, 91,* 1783–1789.
15. Kaplan, G. A. (2004). What's wrong with social epidemiology, and how can we make it better? *Epidemiol Rev, 26,* 124–125.
16. Berkman, L. F. & Kawachi, I. (2000). *Social epidemiology*. New York, NY: Oxford Univ Press.
17. Diez-Roux, A. V., Nieto, F. J., Muntaner, C., et al. (1997). Neighborhood environments and coronary heart disease: A multilevel analysis. *Am J Epidemiol, 146,* 48–63.
18. Schootman, M., Jeffe, D., Gillanders, W., & Aft, R. (2009). Racial disparities in the development of breast cancer metastases among older women: A multilevel study. *Cancer, 115,* 731–740.
19. Ramesh, B., Moses, S., Washington, R., et al. (2008). Determinants of HIV prevalence among female sex workers in four south Indian states: Analysis of cross-sectional surveys in twenty-three districts. *AIDS, 22* Suppl 5, S35.
20. Cifuentes, M., Sembajwe, G., Tak, S., Gore, R., Kriebel, D., & Punnett, L. (2008). The association of major depressive episodes with income inequality and the human development index. *Soc Sci Med, 67,* 529–539.
21. Ezoe, S. & Morimoto, K. (1994). Behavioral lifestyle and mental health status of Japanese factory workers. *Prev Med, 23,* 98–105.
22. Rose, G. (1992). *The strategy of preventive medicine.* Oxford, England: Oxford University Press.
23. Ahern, J., Jones, M. R., Bakshis, E., & Galea, S. (2008). Revisiting Rose: Comparing the benefits and costs of population-wide and targeted interventions. *Milbank Q, 86,* 581–600.
24. Rose, G. (2001). Sick individuals and sick populations. *Int J Epidemiol, 30,* 427–432.
25. Prince, M., Patel, V., Saxena, S., et al. (2007). No health without mental health. *The Lancet, 370,* 859–877.
26. Li, X., Sundquist, J., & Sundquist, K. (2007). Age-specific familial risks of psychotic disorders and schizophrenia: A nation-wide epidemiological study from Sweden. *Schizophr Res, 97,* 43–50.
27. Levinson, D. (2006). The genetics of depression: A review. *Biol Psychiatry, 60,* 84–92.
28. Silberg, J. (1999). The influence of genetic factors and life stress on depression among adolescent girls. *Arch Gen Psychiatry, 56,* 225–232.
29. Nolen-Hoeksema, S. (2002). Gender differences in depression. In I. Gotlib, C. Hammen, (Eds.). *Handbook of depression.* 2nd ed. (pp. 492–509). New York, NY: Guilford.
30. Lynch, J. & Kaplan, G. (2000). Socioeconomic position. In L. F. Berkman & I. Kawachi, (Eds.). *Social epidemiology* (pp. 13–35). New York, NY: Oxford University Press.
31. McLeod, J. D. & Kessler, R. C. (1990). Socioeconomic status differences in vulnerability to undesirable life events. *J Health Soc Behav, 31,* 162–172.

32. Kessler, R. C. (1994). Lifetime and 12-month prevalence of DSM-III-R psychiatric disorders in the United States. Results from the national comorbidity survey. *Arch Gen Psychiatry, 51,* 8–19.
33. Laaksonen, E., Martikainen, P., Lahelma, E., et al. (2007). Socioeconomic circumstances and common mental disorders among Finnish and British public sector employees: Evidence from the Helsinki health study and the Whitehall II study. *Int J Epidemiol, 36,* 776–786.
34. Weich, S. & Lewis, G. (1998). Poverty, unemployment, and common mental disorders: Population based cohort study. *Br Med J, 317,* 115–119.
35. Lorant, V., Deliège, D., Eaton, W., Robert, A., Philippot, P., & Ansseau, M. (2003). Socioeconomic inequalities in depression: A meta-analysis. *Am J Epidemiol, 157,* 98–112.
36. Lynch, J. W., Kaplan, G. A., & Shema, S. J. (1997). Cumulative impact of sustained economic hardship on physical, cognitive, psychological, and social functioning. *N Engl J Med, 337,* 1889–1895.
37. Kessler, R. C. (1997). The effects of stressful life events on depression. *Annu Rev Psychol, 48,* 191–214.
38. Dooley, D., Prause, J., & Ham-Rowbottom, K. A. (2000). Underemployment and depression: Longitudinal relationships. *J Health Soc Behav, 4,* 421–436.
39. Galea, S., Nandi, A., & Vlahov, D. (2004). The social epidemiology of substance use. *Epidemiol Rev, 26,* 36–52.
40. Montgomery, S. M., Cook, D. G., Bartley, M. E. L. J., & Wadsworth, M. E. J. (1998). Unemployment, cigarette smoking, alcohol consumption and body weight in young British men. *Eur J Public Health, 8,*21–27.
41. Kadushin, C., Reber, E., Saxe, L., & Livert, D. (1998). The substance use system: Social and neighborhood environments associated with substance use and misuse. *Subst Use Misuse, 33,* 1681–1710.
42. Brewin, C. R., Andrews, B., & Valentine, J. D. (2000). Meta-analysis of risk factors for posttraumatic stress disorder in trauma-exposed adults. *J Consult Clin Psychol, 68,* 748–766.
43. Breslau, N. (1998). Trauma and posttraumatic stress disorder in the community: The 1996 Detroit area survey of trauma. *Arch Gen Psychiatry, 55,* 626–632.
44. Kilpatrick, D. G., Saunders, B. E., Amick-McMullan, A., Best, C. L., Veronen, L. J., & Resnick, H. S. (1989). Victim and crime factors associated with the development of crime-related post-traumatic stress disorder. *Behavior Therapy, 20,* 199–214.
45. Williams, D. R. & Collins, C. (1995). US socioeconomic and racial differences in health: Patterns and explanations. *Annu Rev Sociol, 21,* 349–386.
46. Williams, D. R., Yu, Y., Jackson, J. S., & Anderson, N. B. (1997). Racial differences in physical and mental health: Socio-economic status, stress and discrimination. *J Health Psychol, 2,* 335–351.
47. Brown, T. N., Williams, D. R., Jackson, J. S., et al. (2000). "Being black and feeling blue": The mental health consequences of racial discrimination. *Race and Society, 2,* 117–131.
48. Miranda, J. & McGuire, T. (2008). New evidence regarding racial and ethnic disparities in mental health: Policy implications. *Health Aff, 27,* 393–403.
49. Jones-Webb, R. J., Hsiao, C. Y., & Hannan, P. (1995). Relationships between socioeconomic status and drinking problems among black and white men. *Alcohol Clin Exp Res, 19,* 623–627.
50. Breslau, J., Aquilar-Gaxiola, S., Kendler, K. S., Maxwell, S., Williams, D., Kessler, R. D. (2006). Specifying race-ethnic differences in risk for psychiatric disorder in a US national sample. *Psychol Med, 36,* 57–68.

51. Riolo, S. A., Nguyen, T. A., Greden, J. F., & King, C. A. (2005). Prevalence of depression by race/ethnicity: Findings from the national health and nutrition examination survey III. *Am J Public Health, 95*, 998–1000.
52. Williams, D. R., Gonzalez, H. M., Neighbors, H., et al. (2007). Prevalence and distribution of major depressive disorder in African Americans, Caribbean blacks, and non-Hispanic whites: Results from the national survey of American life. *Arch Gen Psychiatry, 64*, 305–315.
53. Himle, J. A., Baser, R. E., Taylor, R. J., Campbell, R. D., & Jackson, J. S. (2009). Anxiety disorders among African Americans, blacks of Caribbean descent, and non-Hispanic whites in the United States. *J Anxiety Disord, 23*, 578–590.
54. Ompad, D. & Fuller, C. (2005). The urban environment, drug use and health. In S. Galea & D. Vlahov, (Eds.). *Handbook of urban health populations, methods, and practice* (pp. 127–154). New York, NY: Springer.
55. Grant, B. F., Dawson, D. A., Stinson, F. S., Chou, S. P., Dufour, M. C., & Pickering, R. P. (2004). The 12-month prevalence and trends in DSM-IV alcohol abuse and dependence: United States, 1991–1992 and 2001–2002. *Drug Alcohol Depend, 74*, 223–234.
56. Galea, S., Ahern, J., Tardiff, K., et al. (2003). Racial/ethnic disparities in overdose mortality trends in New York City, 1990–1998. *J Urban Health, 80*, 201–211.
57. Wells, K., Klap, R., Koike, A., & Sherbourne, C. (2001). Ethnic disparities in unmet need for alcoholism, drug abuse, and mental health care. *Am J Psychiatry, 158*, 2027–2032.
58. Kessler, R. C., Mickelson, K. D., & Williams, D. R. (1999). The prevalence, distribution, and mental health correlates of perceived discrimination in the United States. *J Health Soc Behav, 40*, 208–230.
59. Mercy, J. A., Krug, E. G., Dahlberg, L. L., & Zwi, A. B. (2003). Violence and health: The United States in a global perspective. *Am J Public Health, 93*, 256–261.
60. Ludermir, A. B., Schraiber, L. B., D'Oliveira, A. F., França-Junior, I., & Jansen, H. A. (2008). Violence against women by their intimate partner and common mental disorders. *Soc Sci Med, 66*, 1008–1018.
61. Deyessa, N., Berhane, Y., Alem, A., et al. (2009). Intimate partner violence and depression among women in rural Ethiopia: A cross-sectional study. *Clin Pract Epidemol Ment Health, 5*, 8.
62. Wright, R., Berkman, L., Canner, M., Kawachi, I., Ryan, L., & Clark, C. (2008). Witnessing community violence in residential neighborhoods: A mental health hazard for urban women. *J Urban Health, 85*, 22–38.
63. Kaminer, D., Grimsrud, A., Myer, L., Stein, D. J., & Williams, D. R. (2008). Risk for post-traumatic stress disorder associated with different forms of interpersonal violence in South Africa. *Soc Sci Med, 67*, 1589–1595.
64. Seal, K., Metzler, T., Gima, K., Bertenthal, D., Maguen, S., & Marmar, C. (2009). Trends and risk factors for mental health diagnoses among Iraq and Afghanistan veterans using Department of Veterans' Affairs health care, 2002–2008. *Am J Public Health, 99*, 1651–1658.
65. Cardozo, B. L., Vergara, A., Agani, F., & Gotway, C. A. (2000). Mental health, social functioning, and attitudes of Kosovo Albanians following the war in Kosovo. *JAMA, 284*, 569–577.
66. Mollica, R. F., McInnes, K., Sarajlic, N., Lavelle, J., Sarajlic, I., & Massagli, M. P. (1999). Disability associated with psychiatric comorbidity and health status in Bosnian refugees living in Croatia. *JAMA, 282*, 433–439.
67. de Jong, J. T., Komproe, I. H., & Van Ommeren, M. (2003). Common mental disorders in postconflict settings. *Lancet, 361*, 2128–2130.

68. Steel, Z., Silove, D., Phan, T., & Bauman, A. (2002). Long-term effect of psychological trauma on the mental health of Vietnamese refugees resettled in Australia: A population-based study. *The Lancet, 360,* 1056–1062.
69. Barrera, M. (1986). Distinctions between social support concepts, measures, and models. *Am J Community Psychol, 14,* 413–445.
70. Cohen, S. & Wills, T. A. (1985). Stress, social support, and the buffering hypothesis. *Psychol Bull, 98,* 310–357.
71. Dressler, W. W. (1985). Extended family relationships, social support, and mental health in a southern black community. *J Health Soc Behav, 26,* 39–48.
72. Aneshensel, C. S. & Frerichs, R. R. (1982). Stress, support, and depression: A longitudinal causal model. *J Community Psychol, 10,* 363–376.
73. Thundal, K. L., Granbom, S., & Allebeck, P. (1999). Women's alcohol dependence and abuse: The relation to social network and leisure time. *Scand J Public Health, 27,* 30–37.
74. Kawachi, I. & Subramanian, S. V. (2006). Measuring and modeling the social and geographic context of trauma: A multilevel modeling approach. *J Trauma Stress, 19,* 195–203.
75. Ozer, E. J., Best, S. R., Lipsey, T. L., & Weiss, D. S. (2003). Predictors of posttraumatic stress disorder and symptoms in adults: A meta-analysis. *Psychol Bull, 129,* 52–73.
76. Coker, A. L., Smith, P. H., Thompson, M. P., McKeown, R. E., Bethea, L., & Davis, K. E. (2002). Social support protects against the negative effects of partner violence on mental health. *J Womens Health Gend Based, 11,* 465–476.
77. Morgenstern, H. (1982). Uses of ecologic analysis in epidemiologic research. *Am J Public Health, 72,* 1336–1344.
78. Galea, S., Goldmann, E., & Maxwell, A. (2009). City living and mental health in history. In S. Loue & M. Sajatovic, (Eds.). *Determinants of minority mental health and wellness* (pp. 15–37). New York, NY: Springer.
79. Blazer, D., George, L. K., Landerman, R., et al. (1985). Psychiatric disorders. A rural/urban comparison. *Arch Gen Psychiatry, 42,* 651–656.
80. Paykel, E. S., Abbott, R., Jenkins, R., Brugha, T. S., & Meltzer, H. (2000). Urban–rural mental health differences in great Britain: Findings from the national morbidity survey. *Psychol Med, 30,* 269–280.
81. Diez Roux, A. V. (2001). Investigating neighborhood and area effects on health. *Am J Public Health, 91,* 1783–1789.
82. Schulz, A. J., Williams, D. R., Israel, B. A., & Lempert, L. B. (2002). Racial and spatial relations as fundamental determinants of health in Detroit. *Milbank Q, 80,* 677–707.
83. Galea, S., Ahern, J., Nandi, A., Tracy, M., Beard, J., & Vlahov, D. (2007). Urban neighborhood poverty and the incidence of depression in a population-based cohort study. *Ann Epidemiol, 17,* 171–179.
84. Ross, C. E. (2000). Neighborhood disadvantage and adult depression. *J Health Soc Behav, 41,* 177–187.
85. Echeverría, S., Diez-Roux, A. V., Shea, S., Borrell, L. N., & Jackson, S. (2008). Associations of neighborhood problems and neighborhood social cohesion with mental health and health behaviors: The multi-ethnic study of atherosclerosis. *Health Place, 14,* 853–865.
86. Mair, C., Roux, A. V., & Galea, S. (2008). Are neighbourhood characteristics associated with depressive symptoms? A review of evidence. *Br Med J, 62,* 940–946.
87. Leventhal, T. & Brooks-Gunn, J. (2003). Moving to opportunity: An experimental study of neighborhood effects on mental health. *Am J Public Health, 93,* 1576–1582.

88. Evans, G. W. (2003). The built environment and mental health. *J Urban Health, 80,* 536–555.
89. Galea, S., Ahern, J., Rudenstine, S., Wallace, Z., & Vlahov, D. (2005). Urban built environment and depression: A multilevel analysis. *Br Med J, 59,* 822–827.
90. Boardman, J. D., Finch, B. K., Ellison, C. G., Williams, D. R., & Jackson, J. S. (2001). Neighborhood disadvantage, stress, and drug use among adults. *J Health Soc Behav,* 42, 151–165.
91. Whitley, R. & McKenzie, K. (2005). Social capital and psychiatry: Review of the literature. *Harv Rev Psychiatry, 13,* 71–84.
92. Kawachi, I. & Berkman, L. F. (2001). Social ties and mental health. *J Urban Health, 78,* 458–467.
93. Fujiwara, T. & Kawachi, I. (2008). A prospective study of individual-level social capital and major depression in the United States. *J Epidemiol Community Health,62,* 627–633.
94. Lofors, J. & Sundquist, K. (2007). Low-linking social capital as a predictor of mental disorders: A cohort study of 4.5 million Swedes. *Soc Sci Med, 64,* 21–34.
95. Mohseni, M. & Lindstrom, M. (2009). Social capital, political trust and self-reported psychological health: A population-based study. *Soc Sci Med, 68,* 436–443.
96. Silove, D., Brooks, R., Bauman, A., Chey, T., & Phongsavan, P. (2006). Social capital, socio-economic status and psychological distress among Australian adults. *Socl Sci Med, 63,* 2546–2561.
97. Gary, T. L., Stark, S. A., & LaVeist, T. A. (2007). Neighborhood characteristics and mental health among African Americans and whites living in a racially integrated urban community. *Health and Place, 13,* 569–575.
98. Muntaner, C., Eaton, W. W., Miech, R., & O'Campo, P. (2004). Socioeconomic position and major mental disorders. *Epidemiol Rev, 26,* 53–62.
99. Ritsher, J. E. B., Warner, V., Johnson, J. G., & Dohrenwend, B. P. (2001). Intergenerational longitudinal study of social class and depression: A test of social causation and social selection models. *Br J Psychiatry Suppl, 178,* 84–90.
100. Galea, S., Hall, C., & Kaplan, G. (2009). Social epidemiology and complex system dynamic modelling as applied to health behaviour and drug use research. *Int J Drug Policy, 20,* 209–216.
101. Galea, S. & Ahern, J. (2006). Invited commentary: Considerations about specificity of associations, causal pathways, and heterogeneity in multilevel thinking. *Am J Epidemiol, 163,* 1079–1082.
102. Kessler, R. C., Nelson, C. B., McGonagle, K. A., Liu, J., Swartz, M., & Blazer, D. G. (1996). Comorbidity of DSM-III-R major depressive disorder in the general population: Results from the US national comorbidity survey. *Br J Psychiatry Suppl, 168,* 17–30.
103. Spanagel, R. (2009). Alcoholism: A systems approach from molecular physiology to addictive behavior. *Physiol Rev, 89,* 649–705.

PART V

New Approaches to Include Mental Health in Public Health

13

HealthStreet

A Community-Based Approach to Include Mental Health in Public Health Research

LINDA B. COTTLER, CATINA CALLAHAN O'LEARY, AND CATHERINE W. STRILEY

Introduction

The focus of this 100th APPA meeting, mental health in public health, catalyzed creative thinking about mental health disparities and populations at risk for illness, shifting demographics, changes in mental health from youth to older age, issues that shape the debate about public mental health parity, and new approaches to including mental health in public health. Topics addressed disorders conditional upon exposure; intersections of criminal behaviors, mental illness, and addiction; perceived stigma and discrimination; economic predictors of mental health; and others. In sharing our vision for the next 100 years, we all focused our discussions on reducing mental health and addiction disparities. The conference presentations culminated with a focus on developing new strategies to increase the numbers of people from all walks of life, and with all medical and psychiatric histories and risk factors, into clinical trials and to link people, in real time, to health services. This paper reports on one of those strategies.

There is an ever-increasing literature on how to link people, as well as how to engage the community, in research; in summary, the field believes that the process must begin by allowing potential participants to have genuine input as to how they want to be recruited, what the protocol should look like, and how to retain them in studies. Although there have been innovative practices for recruitment and retention developed recently, they have not been widely disseminated.[1] However, even if every clinical trial were enrolling and retaining an adequate sample of people, or using innovative practices, if the samples recruited are not representative of diverse populations, the results of the trials will not be generalizable to diverse populations, making it difficult to translate the findings to routine clinical practice.[2]

Comparative effectiveness research is a new paradigm for clinical trials and requires that studies are conducted in real world settings. In its report to the President and Congress, the Federal Coordinating Council for Comparative Effectiveness Research documented its insistence that there be inclusion in research of racial and ethnic minorities, persons with disabilities, the elderly, children, and persons with co-occurring disorders, including mental illness.[3]

The rate of participation of U.S. citizens in about 80,000 clinical trials is less than 1%,[4] suggesting that research is conducted without authentic community involvement.[5,6] This leads to findings that do not account for a range of genetic, cultural, racial, gender, age, and linguistic factors, which in turn impacts how well new drugs and treatments perform in the real world. Women, elderly, racial and ethnic minorities, and rural populations are particularly underrepresented in research. Thus, there is a discrepancy between participants enrolled in research studies and the general U.S. population to whom the findings relate.

Past studies that evaluated barriers to research participation indicated that minority group members favored research but have concerns regarding inconvenience, burden, risk, and fear that they will be treated as "guinea pigs."[7,8,9] Additionally, other identified barriers included mistrust of the research community and medical profession, skepticism of the consent process, and inappropriate incentives.[10] The climate may be changing with new community-based participatory research efforts that take into account new approaches intended to foster sustainable participation.[11] A continued focus on these new approaches is necessary to understand the complex needs of research volunteers.

Prevention research trials suggest that efforts tailored to the needs of the community are necessary, and that one-size-fits-all efforts are no longer viable.[12,13,14] Participation in research may be improved by surmounting key barriers such as lack of knowledge about what a study entails, transportation to the research site, meeting other needs to reduce burdens of participation, and proper remuneration for a participant's time and inconvenience.[15,16] A focus on these key areas that are important to community members could alleviate potential fears.[17,18,19]

Protocols and strategies to recruit out-of-care community volunteers are being developed sporadically across the country. Top-down approaches such as practice-based networks (PBRNs) are creative ways to help bring clinical trials to the community. PBRNs do not solve all of the problems because the participants from those networks are only as diverse as the practice; further, since the data come from a myriad of practitioners' offices the databases are fragmented.[3] Additionally, since the people in those settings are already connected to health care, one downstream advantage of the PBRN—linkage to research opportunities—is unrealized. Other creative approaches for linking community volunteers to research include patient registries, powered by search engines. This approach requires individuals to log on to a Web site where their lifetime medical history is taken without any human contact. This passive strategy may be ideal for highly motivated patients with a specific research interest; the burden of updating both individual records and a fresh sample pool is shifted away from trained research staff to motivated volunteers. Because of these issues, registries have been associated with demographically skewed samples.

There is a "paucity of translational results,"[20] and a real need to bring findings from the bench to the bedside and now curbside. One major challenge has been a lack of integrated and comprehensive programs, also called "one-stop shops" or "front-door services" that connect people to resources. To truly transform the research enterprise, another tool must be added to the toolbox—community-based entry portals. Such a portal would assess concerns and health priorities; facilitate matching people to services relevant to their needs; put investigators in touch with the people who are suffering from the disorder and who need intervention; and lead to sustainable strategies for partnerships. Finally, such a portal would be the missing link in helping to retain research participants in longitudinal follow-up studies, where dropout rates are high, hovering near 30% to 40%.[1] Such high attrition rates at follow-up affect the generalizability of study findings and their implications.[14] The requirement to achieve high follow-up rates has been used by investigators as the rational for hand-picking samples to obtain the cream of the crop; this may happen to minimize attrition some associate with community populations, often perceived to be incapable of adhering to a research protocol.

One of the most exciting outcomes of engaging underrepresented populations in conversations about their health is the resultant ability to link them to services, based on their needs, concerns, and priorities. The one-stop approach, just described, allows real-time referrals that reduce barriers to access and disparities in health care, which ultimately improves the health of the community. Barriers to care are similar to those for engaging in research and include irrelevance of services being delivered, lack of awareness of the benefits of care, mistrust in the provider or staff, lack of transportation, inconvenient hours, and cultural insensitivity on the part of the staff. Better methods to reduce these barriers, to track success with these methods, and to increase the inclusion of underrepresented populations are needed as we strive to link people to medical and psychiatric care and to social services.

People with two of the most prevalent conditions in the world—addiction and depression—are especially underrepresented in research.[21] For example, persons who use illicit drugs or who abuse licit drugs may be especially likely to either exclude themselves from research or be excluded from research. Blanco and colleagues conducted two analyses using the National Epidemiologic Survey for Alcohol Related Conditions (NESARC) data. In one, they found that the exclusion criteria commonly used in clinical trials, when applied to NESARC participants, would result in the inclusion of "pure" rather than "typical" or "representative" participants.[22] They found that 51% of individuals with a DSM-IV alcohol dependence disorder and 79% of those who endorsed having sought alcohol treatment would have been excluded from participation. One or more of the standardized study criteria would result in excluding 0.9% to 48% of the overall sample and 0.8% to 44% of the treatment-seeking sample.[22]

Depression commonly excludes one from research studies. Blanco and colleagues also assessed the proportion of community-dwelling adults with major depressive disorder (MDD) who would meet eligibility criteria for an MDE treatment trial and found that 76% of those with MDE would have been excluded by one or more study eligibility criteria. Two-thirds (67%) of the subsample of those who previously sought treatment would have been excluded; exclusions ranged from 2% to 47% in the overall sample and 0% to 38% in the treatment-seeking sample.[23] These findings corroborate those of other studies.[24–27] In their meta-analysis, Westen and Morrison[28] showed that exclusions are primarily due to disorders that are commonly comorbid with those under study, explaining why depressed people might be commonly excluded from studies on diabetes, for example, leading to findings not being generalizable.

Additionally, people with drug or alcohol dependence also have comorbid medical or psychiatric conditions.[29,30] This is another example of how exclusion of one condition also excludes the other. Concerns have emerged about whether the findings from these studies can be generalized to nonpatient community members.[31,32,33] Humphreys and Weisner[34] found that significant proportions of potential research subjects in clinical trials of alcohol dependence were excluded under most protocols. Compared to enrolled participants, those excluded were more likely to be African American, to report low incomes and more severe alcohol, drug, and other psychiatric problems. Extending this study, Humphreys et al.[35] noted that patients were often excluded on the basis of their alcohol problems (39%), comorbid psychiatric problems (38%), past or concurrent utilization of alcohol treatment (32%), comorbid medical conditions (32%), and perceived noncompliance and poor motivation (32%). These exclusions result in samples that are more heavily White, economically stable, and higher-functioning when compared to the general population; this leads to a significant bias in estimates of outcomes.[36]

Excluding a substantial proportion of the sample from participating in clinical research has ethical, as well as scientific, ramifications.[37] FDA and pharmaceutical study protocols generally have a long list of exclusion criteria, generally resulting in samples being unrepresentative. Unfortunately, this exclusion occurs in the context of high treatment need. Drug users are commonly untreated, despite their significantly impairing comorbidities,[38] and we should do all we can to consider only evidence-based, medically necessary, exclusions.[14]

With health care reform in our immediate future and a significant need for real-time data from the community, new models must be launched to meet this challenge immediately and into the future. This final chapter describes one research group's response to scale up efforts at collecting real-time data from all, including underrepresented populations. The effort includes an entry portal that links people to medical, psychiatric, and social services, as well as one that recruits, navigates, and enrolls people into research studies and sustains their participation. The attractiveness of this model is that it is based on an established community effort that relies on community health workers (CHWs) to fulfill its mission. The model is transdisciplinary in a truly participatory way, involving partners in federally qualified health centers, the health department, HIV/AIDS community-based organizations, Department of Human Services, criminal justice, drug treatment programs, and others. This blending of community-based participatory research science with bioinformatics is at the cutting edge of a new frontier in community-engaged research. Our success with this model is shown, as well as the methodology used to initiate the model.

The Model

As the Institute of Medicine stated in their report,[39] there is a quality chasm between the promise of evidence-based medicine and the reality of community practice. This could be alleviated through more access to care and increased trust in the health care system for all, not just the tip of the iceberg, which is the population usually reached. One model that operationalizes this is facilitated by the Washington University Clinical and Translational Science Award (CTSA), funded by the National Center for Research Resources (NCRR) of the National Institutes of Health (NIH). This award creates a definable academic home for translating science from the bench to the bedside; community engagement is a required component of the CTSA and with 55 sites participating across the United States, with a cap of 60 sites to be funded by 2012, there is significant momentum to contribute to the science of community-engaged research. The CTSA has five strategic goals: to build national clinical and translational research capacity, to provide training for such careers, to advance bench science discoveries and knowledge, and to improve the health of the nation. Community engagement fits under this last goal. At Washington University, the Community Engagement core is headed by the first author of this chapter. The Center for Community Based Research has three arms; one of the arms is the Community Engagement arm, which functions through a site called HealthStreet, which actually began in 1989.

From 1989 through 2005, with funding from the National Institute on Drug Abuse (NIDA) and the National Institute on Alcohol Abuse and Alcoholism

(NIAAA) of the NIH, the Cottler team partnered with the St. Louis City Department of Health to conduct street outreach to recruit persons for studies to reduce high-risk behaviors putting them at risk for HIV/AIDS and sexually transmitted diseases (STDs). The team achieved a 96.6% 18-month follow-up rate of 479 drug abusers enrolled in a NIDA-funded project aimed at reducing HIV transmission among St. Louis injection drug users. Gender, race, age, education, and psychiatric status did not predict recruitment difficulty. A comprehensive tracking strategy as well as persistence and creative team work were more important determinants of successful retention than participant characteristics.[12] For these studies, two storefront satellite offices of the Health Department were established, called HealthStreet, to "pave the way to good health"; community health workers (CHWs) engaged individuals in conversation about our studies and invited them to HealthStreet to participate. To reduce skepticism and unwillingness of neighbors to allow such a storefront in their area, the team attended town hall meetings and met with aldermen and neighbors to explain the purpose of the office. Over the years, members of the team have been involved with the Public Safety Task Force, AIDS Task Force, the HCV Task Force, the Syphilis Elimination Task Force, and the Re-Entry Effort, all of which have responded to the needs of the community by maintaining continuity and by bringing in needed services to the communities.

Partnering with committee leaders and neighbors increased acceptance; residents gained trust in the research team and accepted the presence of researchers in their community. We, as researchers, learned to rely on the members of the community we worked in to guide us in all next steps. In addition to signing up for research studies, community members also took advantage of other needed services, such as food pantry referrals, blood pressure checks, flu shots, and housing referrals, all offered free of charge in direct response to need.[40,41,14]

Our innovative and successful methods for enrolling and retaining vulnerable research participants with mental illness, drug abuse, and high risk behaviors were sought by the Washington University School of Medicine when they were writing the Clinical and Translational Science Award grant, and the Cottler team scaled up the effort for the treatment, early detection, and prevention of medical conditions such as diabetes, hypertension, heart disease, cancer, other physical and mental disorders, and their risk factors.

The model underwent a transformation for this new effort to coincide with its increased responsibilities and focus. HealthStreet's goals are to assess medical problems and health concerns from community residents, share findings with the community and investigators, educate researchers about the importance of diversity in research, contribute to the science of community-engaged research, and improve the public health through referrals to social and medical services and through increasing participation of underrepresented populations into research. Two specific theoretical frameworks have relevance to our community engagement efforts—positive deviance, and diffusion of innovation. Sternin's positive deviance theory posits that solutions to community problems exist within the community.[42] A second theory, diffusion of innovations theory, is based on three insights relevant to social change: the factors that spread an idea, peer-to-peer conversations and networks, and the needs of potential implementers.[43,44]

Recruitment Strategy

The recruitment strategy begins with CHWs reaching people where they are: at barbershops and beauty shops, parks, shelters, bus stops, community agencies, churches, neighborhood associations, health care facilities, sports venues, grocery stores, laundromats, nail salons, fitness centers, YMCAs, colleges, gas stations, check cashing venues, and many others, including the street. CHWs, indigenous to the city, engage potential volunteers in a brief explanation of what they are trying to accomplish and describe the community engagement process, a particular study or project, and their interest in linking them to services. Data are then collected on first name and last initial, age, gender, ethnicity, primary health concerns, level of education, zip code area and place of contact, whether the individual has participated in a research study before, and their perceptions about research. These anonymous data allow us to calculate both numerators and denominators of ratio measurements to evaluate the impact of our efforts in the community and characteristics of people who participate further compared to those who don't. People are then asked to sign a consent form to allow us to ask them protected health information about their medical history and other information.

CHWs rely on a two-prong approach to reach people all over the city: a study van and HealthStreet. The van is equipped with GPS navigation system for the safety of our CHWs and for geocoding the areas we visit. All areas of the city are identified with a unique code which allows us to track areas that are visited each day, at a level that is smaller than a zip code. This allows the team to determine reach and effectiveness of the outreach efforts.

CHWs are lay members of the community who either volunteer or work for pay and share a common language with the people they serve. They have been called the "PhDs of the sidewalk."[45] The CHWs are dedicated to the philosophy of community-engaged research and to the actual nitty-gritty of such engagement.

Recruitment, Navigation, and Enrollment of the Community

Since opening HealthStreet in January 2009, through July 2010, there have been 3,230 people contacted by HealthStreet staff and CHWs or who walked into the HealthStreet site (see Figure 13.1). A contact is a meaningful connection with someone where at the minimum, an introduction to the effort and some of the elements of consent have been provided to the community member. Over time, 156 persons have begun this meaningful contact but then refused to continue (mostly at bus stops). Persons who refuse any contact with a CHW are not counted.

Recruitment of community participants is exceedingly high; the recruitment yield is 95.2%. This is the percent of the population contacted (3074/3230) out of all those who completed a HealthStreet informed consent. The consent invites potential participants to answer questions with the health intake form after the initial data are collected, yielding data on demographic characteristics of the respondent, age and gender of all children, number of persons in household, best times of day to reach the potential participant, and phone numbers for future contact. Such locating information boosts enrollment rates as well as recruitment; these detailed tracking and locating data resulted in the superb follow-up rates, repeatedly topping 95%, among the hardest-to-reach populations.[12] Other data collected includes the participant's top health concerns, medical history (including allergies [5 items]; arthritis [4 items]; autoimmune diseases [3 items]; disorders of the blood [5 items]; brain, spinal, or nervous system [20]; lungs [9]; cancer [1]; dental health [7]; diabetes or thyroid disorder [7]; digestive problems [18]; hearing loss [4]; heart or circulatory problems [11]; kidney, urinary [5] or infectious diseases [19]; mental health problems [13]; muscle and bone problems [7]; reproductive health problems; skin [10], sleep [5] and vision problems [6]; gynecological/obstetric problems [11]; male health [2]; alcohol [2] and drug use [18]; smoking [2]; and gambling [2]; and all current medications). Access to health care, insurance, and doctor visits are also assessed. Recently, questions were added concerning participants' perceptions about research participation. Finally, CHWs obtain the GPS coordinates of the location where they met the respondent for geographic analyses.

As shown, health intake forms were completed with 2,854 people out of the 3,074 who started the process (92.8%). The 220 people who did not complete the intake form, also known as breakoffs, did not have time to finish the assessment or decided against participating after beginning the intake process.

After the health intake is completed, the CHWs use the data to individually link participants to medical and social referrals based on their history and their health concerns, invite them to participate in educational classes, or navigate them to a research opportunity at Washington University. This can be done

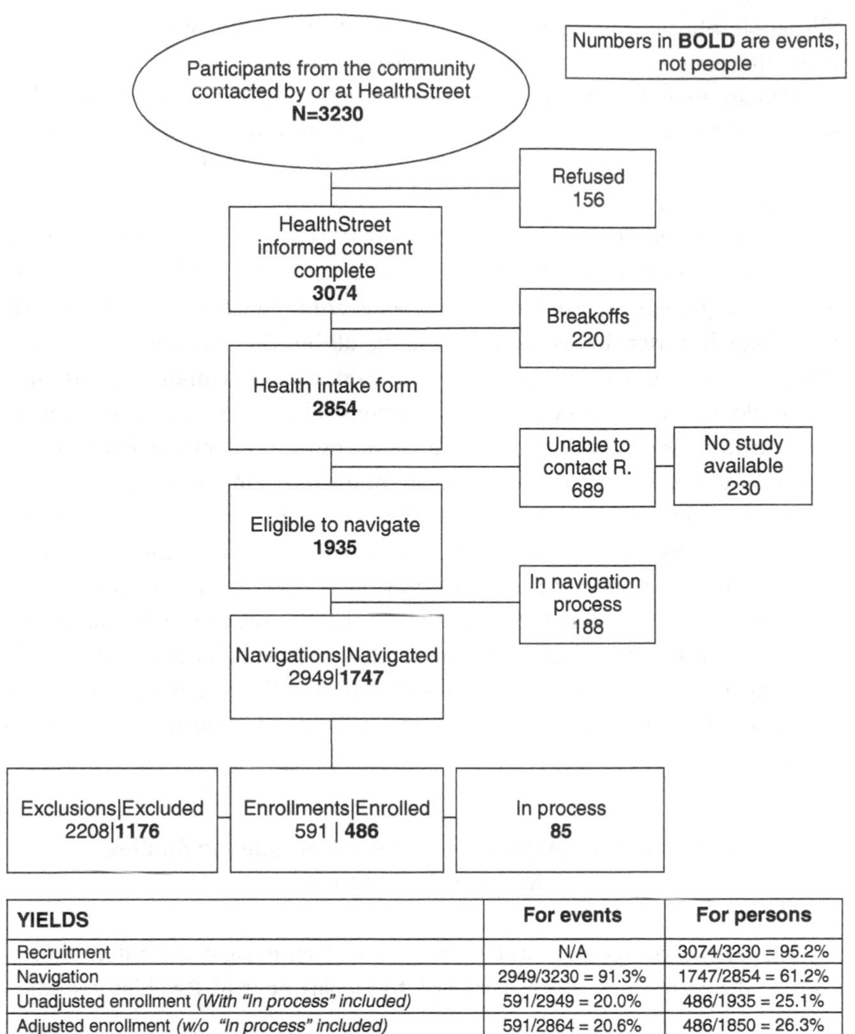

YIELDS	**For events**	**For persons**
Recruitment	N/A	3074/3230 = 95.2%
Navigation	2949/3230 = 91.3%	1747/2854 = 61.2%
Unadjusted enrollment *(With "In process" included)*	591/2949 = 20.0%	486/1935 = 25.1%
Adjusted enrollment *(w/o "In process" included)*	591/2864 = 20.6%	486/1850 = 26.3%

Figure 13.1 HealthStreet flow chart from HealthStreet opening (mid-January 2009) through July 31, 2010.

either in the field or later via phone contact. As shown, among those who completed the intake form (n=2,854), 1,935 people were eligible to navigate—that is, the CHW was able to contact the person, and a study was available for him/her (67.8%). The HealthStreet staff successfully navigated 90% (1,747) of the 1,935 eligible persons to a study coordinator for further research screening.

One of the most important functions of the HealthStreet model is its ability to link people to research opportunities to give everyone a voice in the research enterprise. HealthStreet has a high record of success in this effort. As shown,

486 people who were navigated have been enrolled a total of 591 times, yielding an enrollment rate of 26.3%, if the 85 people who are still in the process of being enrolled are excluded. When no adjustment is made for those who are still in process, that is, when they are included in the denominator, the yield is 25.1%. The yields for all events, which allows for more than one effort per person, are also shown in Figure 13.1.

The top five health concerns of those who completed this section of the survey and who reported at least one concern are shown in Table 13.1, by age, in decades. Hypertension, asthma, and diabetes are top health concerns, regardless of age; hypertension is ranked 1 among all but the younger respondents. Mental health was ranked among the top health concerns among all but those 60 and older. Diabetes is ranked second among all of the respondents. A mention of arthritis is reported as a top health concern by those 50 and older. Among those 60 and older, heart problems was mentioned as a top health concern.

As shown in Figure 13.2, residents have been recruited from all city zip codes; some outlying areas to the west of the city have been recruited more heavily than others (63136, 63121, 63130), but on the whole, nearly all zip codes contiguous to the city have been reached. In the city, the area with the highest recruitment is 63110 (the zip code where HealthStreet is located), followed by 63118 and 63115. Mapping our recruitment sample allows us to plan where the CHWs should go next, and to evaluate where the greatest needs and successes are for recruitment.

Characteristics of Persons Who Are Navigated to Studies through HealthStreet

Among persons navigated to studies, 32% have been navigated to internal medicine studies, 24% have been navigated to Department of Psychiatry studies,

Table 13.1 Top 5 Health Concerns of Community Recruited Persons from HealthStreet by Age, in Decades (among those who mentioned at least one concern)

Less than 30 Years of Age (n = 501)	*30 to 39 Years of Age (n = 352)*	*40 to 49 Years of Age (n = 490)*	*50 to 59 Years of Age (n = 444)*	*60+ Years of Age (n = 125)*
Asthma	Hypertension	Hypertension	Hypertension	Hypertension
Diabetes	Diabetes	Diabetes	Diabetes	Diabetes
Hypertension	Mental Health	Mental Health	Arthritis	Arthritis
Weight	Weight	Asthma	Cancer	Heart Problems
Mental Health	Asthma	Weight/Cancer (tie)	Mental Health	Cancer

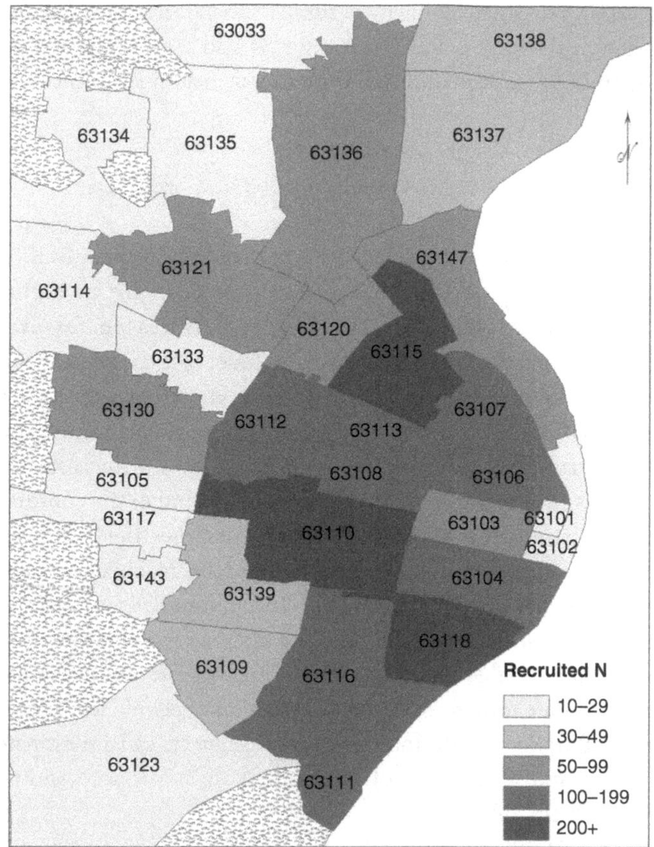

Figure 13.2 Zip codes of residents recruited by community health workers.

12% to psychology, 10% to neurology, and 8% to the Institute for Public Health. Other participants have been navigated to the Physical Therapy and Occupational Therapy departments (4% each). Pathology and Immunology, Otolaryngology, Ophthalmology, and Radiation Oncology departments have each received 2% of the navigations.

The sample of persons who are navigated to studies is diverse: 61% are females; the mean age is approximately 40 years of age, skewed due to the fact that we have recruited people 6 to 91 years of age. Minorities represent 85.2% of the sample, with 82% African American. Most participants have never been married (67%) or are high school graduates (77%). Over one-third (39%) are employed either full time or part time. Most of the participants are from St. Louis City proper (84%), and are recruited from all city zip codes. The need for this effort is acute, as there are few health care facilities in the north city. Over three-quarters of the sample (78%) had never been in a study before being recruited by our staff. Most of the participants were recruited by CHWs in our study van (76%). The participants have some connection to health care: 60% had seen a doctor in the past 6 months, 66% had had a checkup in the previous 12 months, and 52% reported that they had some health insurance.

Differences Between Enrolled and Excluded

A number of persons were excluded from participating in research (n = 1176). There are many reasons that potential respondents might be excluded from research studies and HealthStreet staff code every reason for exclusion as reported by the study coordinator. Reasons include: 1) the respondent might not meet the eligibility criteria of a selected study after they are navigated (age, gender, threshold of the particular criterion of interest, etc.); 2) the study might be closed to recruitment after the respondent shows up for screening; 3) the respondent feels that the study is not a good match; and 4) the coordinator feels the potential respondent is not a good match. At times the coordinators have told us that "the people we send them cannot be reached" or "community respondents are not compliant and do not return phone calls" or the "community respondents have a lot of needs." There are also perceptions that underserved individuals are not capable of participating in or adhering to research protocols. These views translate into the systematic exclusion of people from research. The HealthStreet effort is helping to educate coordinators and investigators about the enthusiasm and willingness of respondents to participate and the importance of research equality.

Because the HealthStreet model assesses demographic, medical, and psychiatric history and other characteristics of community members, it is able to contribute to our understanding of the differences between those who enroll or are excluded from research studies. Our hypothesis is that individualized recruitment efforts will increase enrollment as well as study retention and that these efforts will minimize exclusions that occur due to stereotyping.

Demographic Characteristics

Shown in Table 13.2 are the differences between the 1,662 persons navigated to a study who were either enrolled (29%) or excluded from the study (71%). Demographic characteristics differed statistically in several areas: people enrolled compared to excluded were older; more likely to be widowed, separated, or divorced; more educated; and less likely to be employed. They were also more likely to have been involved in research previously and to have been seen by a doctor in the past 6 months. Surprisingly, they were also less likely to have been recruited through the van; walk-ins were more likely to be enrolled. This could

Table 13.2 Characteristics of Enrolled vs. Excluded Community Recruited Persons from HealthStreet Through 7/31/10

Demographics	*Enrolled* *N = 486*	*Excluded* *N = 1176*	*P-Value*
Female	57.24%	62.24%	.06
Mean Age	43.35 years (6–77)	37.82 years (6–91)	<0.0001
Ethnicity/Race Reported			
Asian	0.43%	0.26%	NS
African American	82.17%	81.74%	
Caucasian	15.22%	15.27%	
Other	2.17%	2.73%	
Minority	84.78%	84.73%	NS
Hispanic/Latino	1.00%	2.24%	NS
Marital Status			
Never Married	61.59%	68.77%	.007
Married	13.69%	13.20%	
Separated/divorced/widowed	24.72%	18.03%	
Education			
<High School	21.4%	24.5%	
High School	40%	44.7%	
> High School	40.6%	30.8%	.0009
Employed	33.69%	40.72%	.04
Geographic Location			
North City	40.8%	40.6%	NS
North County	14.3%	13.2%	
South City	42.4%	42.8%	
South County	2.5%	3.4%	
Been in Research Before	25.69%	18.04%	.005
Referral Source			
Van	63%	81%	<0.0001
Walk-In	26%	12%	
Friend or Relative	7%	2%	
Health Fair	2%	3%	
Seen a Doctor in Past 6 Months	64%	57%	.03
Had Check-up in Past 12 Months	65%	67%	NS
Any Insurance	50%	54%	NS
STDs	*Enrolled* *N = 486*	*Excluded* *N = 1176*	*P-Value*
Chlamydia	6.5%	3.9%	.05
Gonorrhea	2.3%	2.8%	NS
Hepatitis	4.3%	3.0%	NS
Herpes	1.4%	0.84%	NS
HIV/AIDS	2.7%	0.95%	.01
Syphilis	0.85%	0.48%	NS
Any STD Above	11.97%	7.0%	.001

(Continued)

Table 13.2 (*Contd.*)

Mental Health Disorders	*Enrolled N = 486*	*Excluded N = 1176*	*P-Value*
Affective Disorder	22.9%	23.5%	NS
Anxiety	10.6%	10.7%	NS
ADD/ADHD	2.3%	1.7%	NS
Autism	0.28%	0.36%	NS
Eating Disorder	0.88%	1.4%	NS
Personality Disorder	1.7%	0.96%	NS
Schizophrenia	4.6%	3.7%	NS
Gambling Problem	4.2%	6.2%	NS
Any Mental Health Disorder Above	29.8%	30.9%	NS
Medical Disorders	*Enrolled N = 486*	*Excluded N = 1176*	*P-Value*
Hypertension	32.8%	25.9%	.006
Diabetes*	9.3%	8.2%	NS
Asthma*	17.4%	18.3%	NS
Any Cancer*	2.7%	3.7%	NS
Weight Problem/Obesity	14.3%	15.7%	NS
Heart Problem*	2.9%	1.6%	NS
Arthritis	20.8%	19.1%	NS
Digestive Problem	13.9%	19.3%	NS
Neurological Problems*	6.4%	6.0	NS
Any Medical Disorder Above with *	31.3%	29.3%	NS
Recent (past 30 day) Substance Use	*Enrolled N = 486*	*Excluded N = 1176*	*P-Value*
Tobacco	55.3%	51.45%	NS
Marijuana*	15.3%	21.1%	.04
Cocaine*	3.1%	1.7%	NS
Heroin*	0.85%	0.72%	NS
Opioids	7.9%	5.9%	NS
Any Drugs Above with *	15.2%	18.9%	.13

be attributed to the fact that many people came to HealthStreet after they had been contacted on the street by a CHW and thus were primed for study enrollment. Males tended to be more likely to be enrolled than females.

STDs

The rate of STDs in this sample ranged from 0.85% for syphilis to 6.5% for chlamydia among enrolled. Among the excluded, the range was 0.48% for syphilis to 3.85% for chlamydia; nearly 12% of the enrolled versus 7% among excluded had at least one STD. Only a few differences between enrolled and excluded persons were noted regarding their sexually transmitted disease history; those with a history of chlamydia or HIV/AIDS were more likely to be enrolled compared to those without that history. A history of at least one STD also was associated with being more likely to be enrolled than excluded.

Mental Disorders

The rates of mental disorders were not unlike the rates published in general population studies.[46–49] Approximately 23% reported being told by a health professional that they had depression, nearly 11% were told they had anxiety; the rate was about 2% for ADD/ADHD. Rates of gambling and schizophrenia were slightly higher than the general population rates. Surprisingly though, reporting a mental disorder, in and of itself, was not associated with being excluded from a research study.

Medical Disorders

The rates of common medical conditions and disorders are shown in Table 13.2. Approximately 30% of the sample had at least one of the more significant medical disorders such as diabetes, asthma, cancer, or heart or neurological problem. The only condition that distinguished enrolled participants from the excluded was hypertension. It also was the most prevalent condition reported by the sample regardless of enrollment status. Arthritis was the next most common condition, followed by asthma.

Substance Use

As shown in Table 13.2, the reported rates of substance use in the last 30 days were higher than rates from other studies.[38] The 2008 National Survey on Drug Use and Health reported past-month use of 8% among persons 12 and older; the inclusion of a larger number of pre-teens and teenagers may have decreased this rate of use.[50] A fairly high proportion of respondents reported having used a drug, not including tobacco. Persons who used marijuana were less likely to get enrolled in a study; no other differences were found. However, there was a trend towards people who were enrolled to have reported cocaine or heroin use at higher rates.

Use of and Referrals to Health Care and Social Services

As one satellite office for community-based efforts for Washington University, HealthStreet also links people to services. As shown in Figure 13.3, there were

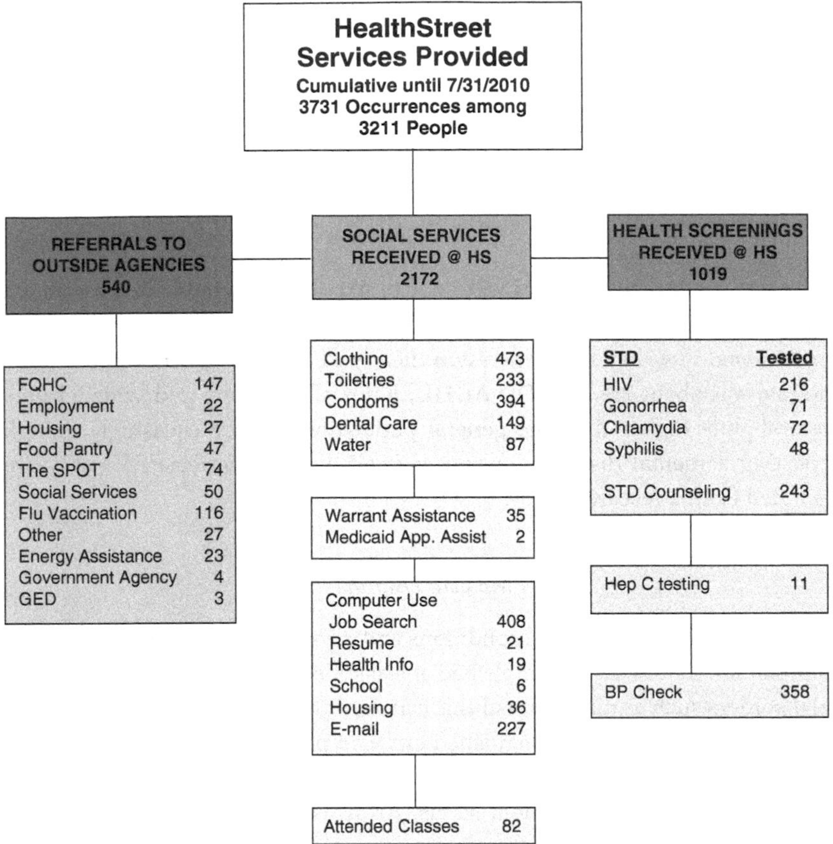

Figure 13.3 Medical and Social Services Provided through HealthStreet.

3,731 occurrences of services provided to 3,211 people through HealthStreet. Most received social services (n = 2172) ranging from visits to the clothing closet and toiletry giveaways, to condom, toothbrush, and toothpaste giveaways. HealthStreet recently became an official cooling station for the City of St. Louis, which necessitates distributing bottled water. People also received assistance with a warrant and were able to re-schedule their hearing with the Municipal Court. A fair number of residents came to HealthStreet to use the computers to obtain help with a job search (n=408), to learn how to use the computer for their resume, to get health or housing information, or to get their email. In fact, several people have been hired as a result of the efforts of our staff. HealthStreet is also a conduit for delivering educational messages; 82 residents took advantage of the classes taught by staff, investigators, Occupational Therapy Department and College of Pharmacy students, and others.

Health screenings were provided at HealthStreet for over 1,000 residents; many received HIV testing and counseling at no cost, provided by the City of St. Louis Department of Health and a local HIV-testing agency. STD counseling was also provided. Because the staff has been taught to do blood pressure checks, this is offered daily. In several instances, participants found to have high pressure were taken to the emergency department for further screening. Body-mass indices (BMIs) are also calculated daily by the staff.

Finally, at HealthStreet and in the van, CHWs use the data collected in the intake form to make referrals to federally qualified health centers, social service agencies, and employment and housing agencies. Residents are referred to food pantries, government agencies, places for flu shots, and other medical and social needs based on their history or request.

Neighborhood of Residence and Prevalence of Disorders

The needs assessment has been useful for indicating the health and health needs of our community—necessary for responding appropriately with referrals for services, prevention, and treatment. Figure 13.4, with six maps, shows the zip codes where people live who self-reported affective disorders, schizophrenia, illicit drug use, cigarette use, and mental and medical problems—two composite variables. Although these maps are descriptive in nature, they allow for a comparison of areas of concern. The shades of salmon go from low rates to highest rates. It must be remembered that although all of the zip codes were visited, the base rate of population assessed,differs by zip code, making some of the rates unstable, given that the total population to analyze is about 2,900.

The demographic distribution of our city shows significant racial imbalance[51]; zip codes that are predominantly African American are those in the north city (63115, 113, 106, 120, 101, 147, 107, and 112). Those that are mixed race are predominantly 63118, 104, 110 103, 102, and 108. The area in the south city tends to be racially isolated with non-African Americans predominating (63116, 111, 139, and 109).

Because the map legends are equivalent for all conditions, comparisons can be made between them. As shown, a higher prevalence of drug use, tobacco use, and medical and mental disorders (specifically affective and schizophrenia disorders) seems to be concentrated in certain zip codes primarily in the south city. With data such as these, we can begin to address the needs of the people in our city, and target where to begin implementing evidence-based practices. The zip code maps are especially important for mental disorders and drug use because the city's needs assessment does not assess or track mental illness or drug use.

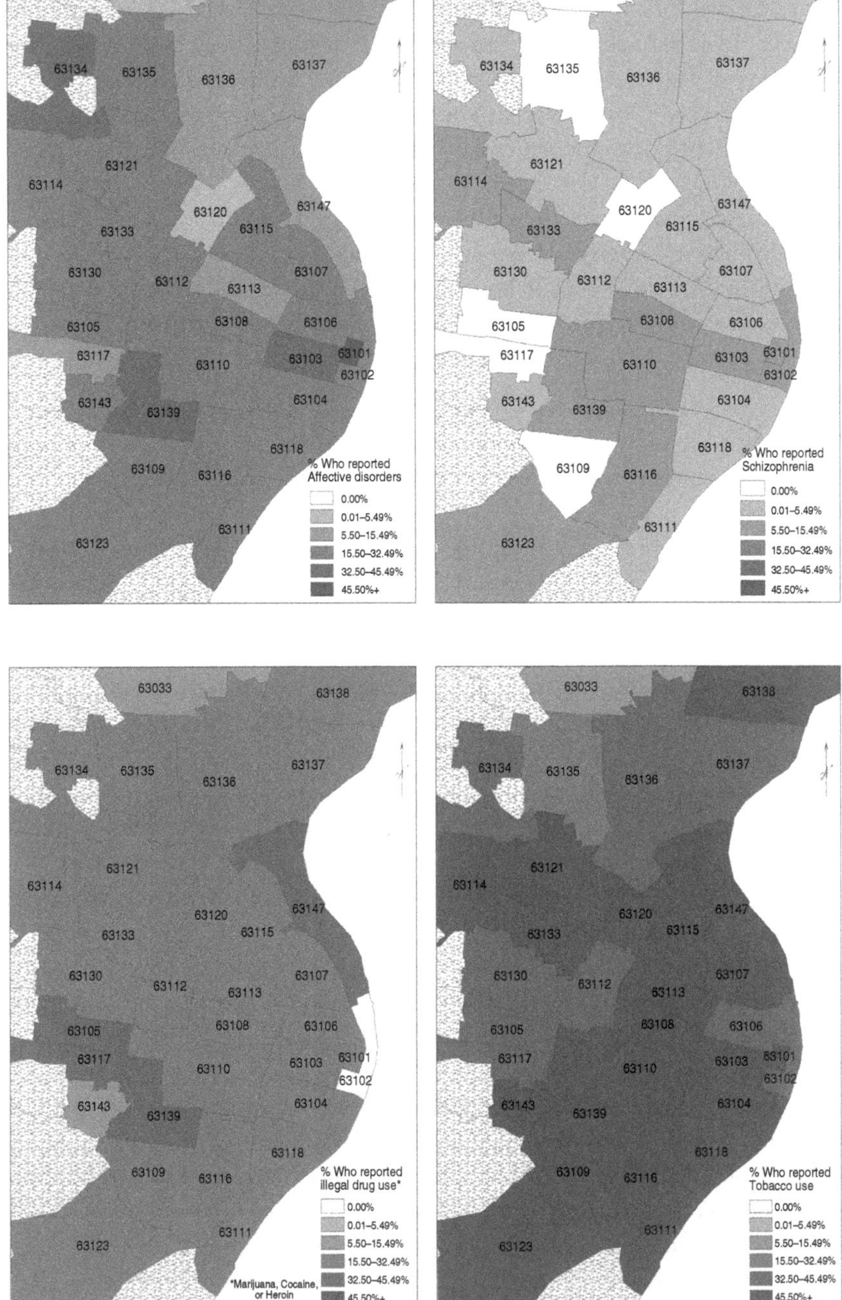

Figure 13.4 Medical and mental problems and drug use by zip code.

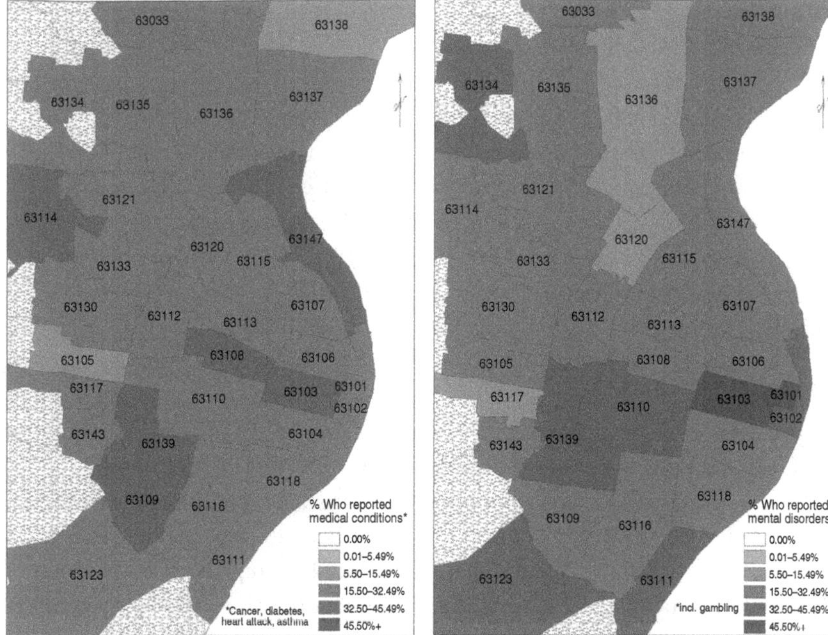

Figure 13.4 (Contd.)

Discussion

The data presented in this chapter bring us closer to understanding the needs of our community. We have contributed to the science of community-engaged research with the development of a robust health intake form that assesses medical history and important risk factors for conditions; by task-shifting the collection of the data from public health professionals to trained CHWs; by developing a human resource job description for the CHW that has been shared with other investigators; and by enriching a previously used model for contacting and linking populations in need to medical, psychiatric, and social services and recruiting, navigating, and enrolling underrepresented populations into research.

We had hypothesized that concierge recruitment efforts would increase enrollment; this was accepted, using the field's enrollment rates as a comparison. Our most conservative rate of enrollment, out of everyone we had intake data on, is 17% compared to the rate in a doctor's office where patients with one illness only (cancer) are asked to participate in a cancer trial (14%).[52] When we use only the people who were eligible to participate in the denominator, as most doctor's offices would, our rate increases to 25%. Additionally, with the exception of a few characteristics and conditions, we found few differences between persons who had been enrolled and excluded. As the model matures, these differences will likely be further reduced.

Our success is being accomplished, one community at a time, using community-based efforts that are robust, unique, creative, and relatively inexpensive. (Cost accounting data are not presented in this chapter, though the CTSA has been tracking cost per person enrolled. The cost began high, but was quickly halved. More analyses are needed in this area.) The new HealthStreet model has done this by task-shifting with the hiring of CHWs, indigenous to the area, who can get more people linked to services, get health education messages to the community, give more people opportunities to get involved in health research, and ultimately give all communities a voice.[53] It has done this effectively through diffusion of innovation techniques using CHWs as innovators, and also through the positive deviance model, which is internally fueled with a grassroots effort that focuses on solutions rather than problems.

Though the model has many strengths, it does suffer from some weaknesses. For example, the CHWs go to areas of the city according to planned activities, health fairs, and where people congregate, thus limiting the sample to those who are able to be reached through community outreach methods. They target all areas of the city, but oftentimes the CHWs tend to feel more comfortable going to places they are familiar with. Scheduling their outreach activities in advance spurs them to include all areas. While other recruitment strategies may be less efficient at reaching minorities, the HealthStreet model may be less efficient at reaching majority populations, populations that are affluent, and populations that are less likely to use public transportation in St. Louis, less frequently leave their homes, or feel uncomfortable speaking to "strangers." Health problem data rely on self-report and are only in response to a question about diagnosed conditions; thus, if people are seeking less care and not being diagnosed with a condition, that condition is not reported. A needs assessment that identifies mortality statistics or an epidemiological study could overcome this weakness; however, such an epidemiological study would be more costly and would likely suffer from low response.[54] While there are limitations, the HealthStreet model does reach the elderly, persons from all over the city (and parts of the county), minorities, persons who use drugs, persons with mental illness, persons who have never been in a research study and persons with health concerns who might not be linked to services. Further, through the mapping and geocoding, the model allows for a better understanding of how conditions cluster, where they cluster, and what areas could be targeted for risk reduction.

CTSAs have been discussing the benefits of a national recruitment registry—a database for people interested in research studies, who guide themselves through a web registry. As discussed, these strategies are cost effective but do not focus on reaching out to persons with lower health literacy and those without access to computer resources. Furthermore, the people who are able to sign up with a registry tend to be those with access to health care, predominantly female (69%), Caucasian (83%), and considered themselves to be healthy (75%). The respondents were allowed to select three diseases they were concerned about, and the top three choices were weight control, mental health, and women's health (reflecting the predominance of female respondents).[55]

The blending of all of these approaches is most likely to build trust in the community, identify and match underrepresented populations (URPs) to services, and ensure retention of people in research. With respect and trust dominating the model, the hope is that URPs will experience more positive outcomes, will be more likely to follow through on the referrals given, and will report more satisfaction with their decision to participate. Additionally, persons who come to a one-stop shop will be more satisfied with their physicians, and have a better understanding and perceived control over their illness, leading to improvements in their medical conditions. They might also be more likely to report more trust in and more adherence to care, and to receive optimal preventive care. The early linkages to care might also have a positive effect on better health outcomes in general. An unintended consequence of our model, however, would be high demand from URPs to participate in studies which might not be available.

The HealthStreet model is being recognized nationally as an important and robust model for clinical and translational research. Additional opportunities have arisen since we began the effort: an NCRR CTSA American Recovery and Reinvestment Act (ARRA) Supplement; a GO! ARRA grant from the National Heart, Lung, and Blood Institute (NHLBI), a NIDA CTSA R01, and a National Institute of Mental Health (NIMH) Small Business Innovation Research (SBIR) subcontract from TerraNova Incorporated.

The CTSA supplement, called the Sentinel Network, is modeled after the NIDA Community Epidemiological Work Group. It is a partnership with four other universities and two national community partnerships to detect emerging community issues regarding participation of underrepresented populations in health research through CHWs. At each site, CHWs are collecting identical data to report back to communities and NCRR about top health and neighborhood concerns, common disorders, and perceptions about research participation. Even though funding is limited, CHWs provide referrals to community participants for health and social services as needs arise. To date, we have collected over 4,000 surveys from the five sites and have established guidelines for the CHW role.

The GO! Grant is funded to automate the workflow of the CHW to facilitate linkages and navigations in the field and at HealthStreet. With the use of a comprehensive web system and portal that mimics human decision making, along with sensitive and persistent recruiters who build sustainable relationships with participants, high recruitment and follow-up rates will be achievable.[12] Further, this model should be utilizable nationally to translate the HealthStreet model to other locations.

The NIDA CTSA grant was funded to understand the attitudes of primary investigators (PIs), study coordinators, Institutional Review Board (IRB) members and Human Studies staff towards persons with mental illness and drug use histories and to increase their numbers into clinical trials. This is being done through a stepped up HealthStreet model where persons are randomized to either the HealthStreet model or a "study ambassador" who helps navigate research milestones. The idea for the ambassador model originated with the patient navigation medical model which improved screening rates from 11% to 17%, increased adherence to follow-up visits from 21% to 29%, and dropped days from diagnosis to follow-up to 25 days from 42.[56] An Institute of Medicine report[2] "Engaging the Public in the Clinical Research Enterprise" noted that spending time with a knowledgeable person can nearly double one's likelihood of ending up in a trial.[57] Our data to date support this: persons who are enrolled versus those excluded are more likely to be "walk ins" to HealthStreet or be referred through a relative or a friend. Nationally, experts are recommending clinical trial support and processing centers[1] with trained, culturally competent engagement specialists or ambassadors to increase enrollment in clinical studies. Ensuring the participation of minority members and drug users is a necessary element of clinical and translational research and is one of the "pillars" of community engagement.[58] This cannot be achieved without addressing the very real biases and prejudices of research scientists, research coordinators, and the involvement of IRB members. This grant will help with clearer guidelines for educating IRBs and strategies for increasing and sustaining participation in research.

Finally, the TerraNova SBIR is a partnership between HealthStreet and a private company in Wisconsin to increase the number of people with depression into research using a randomized trial to compare a psychoeducational model conducted with a facilitator and a family member to an arm that allows the family pair to self-guide through the materials. CHWs recruit participants through HealthStreet and follow up the participants to determine the effectiveness of the paradigms.

In summary, HealthStreet has received the attention of multiple NIH institutes and partners, and has grown since its early days as a satellite site to recruit for one study. The value added of HealthStreet is substantial: we are task-shifting through the use of the CHW to give voice to all of the community, to improve mental health and addiction parity in research, to understand the risk factors of our local population, to provide needed referrals and services to people who might otherwise not have gotten them, to disseminate research findings to young and old, to help shape local and national policy, to contribute to the science of community-engaged work, to teach our professional community, to build research and community capacity, and to ultimately transform the culture. This transformation will be needed for the new health care reform act that will require more real-time data from individuals and communities to improve the quality of the care given.[59]

The future of HealthStreet is boundless. The model can be a research incubator for investigators to test their protocols, it can be a hub for telemedicine, for mHealth initiatives, for bringing research to the people where they live, whether in rural areas, or cities. CHWs have become an integral part of this model, and their role in the research enterprise and as navigators to care and services is significant.

All across the US, researchers at medical centers and public health institutes are combining efforts towards improving the health of communities. In an effort to make the largest impact, there is a focus on reducing the prevalence of two or three outcomes at most. The disorders and conditions that are being selected usually include heart disease, cancer, asthma and obesity. Though these are important and prevalent, mental health conditions which are often more prevalent, co-morbid with many medical conditions, and among the top health concerns reported by the community, are being overlooked. NIH has invested millions of dollars into translating findings to the public through clinical trials. If persons with mental illness or persons with addiction are being excluded from these studies, they are being excluded from participation in making research relevant to them. This translates to poorer outcomes and ultimately poorer health. As discussed at the 100th conference, there can be no health without mental health. The next 100 years of medicine will need to address and represent the needs of all. Until mental health is part of the public health, we cannot rest.

Acknowledgments

The authors would like to thank the participants, the CHWs who have worked on this project over the years, the Commissioners of Health throughout the funded periods and current Commissioner Melba Moore, Center for Community Based Research Co-Investigators Drs. Jane Garbutt, Katherine Mathews, and Consuelo Wilkins, Arbi Ben Abdallah and Susan Bradford at EPRG for their statistical help, Amy Hepler and Dan Martin (HealthStreet coordinators), Ann Schwartz for data entry, Tamara Millay for editorial assistance, and student and community volunteers. The authors gratefully acknowledge funding of NIDA (DA06163, DA05585, DA08324, DA11622), NIAAA (AA12111) and NCRR (RR024992), and Dean Larry Shapiro, Drs. Kenneth Polonsky and Brad Evanoff, PI and Co-PI of the CTSA, for vision and support.

References

1. Faster Cures, The Center for Accelerating Medical Solutions. (2006). *Clinical trials recruitment and retention: Best practices and promising approaches.* Meeting Report.
2. Institute of Medicine. (2003). *Exploring challenges, progress and new models for engaging the public in the clinical research enterprise.* Washington DC: The National Academies Press.
3. Federal Coordinating Council for Comparative Effectiveness Research. (2009). *Report to the President and the Congress.* Department of Health and Human Services.
4. US News. (2008). Report claims clinical trials miss many populations-Women, elderly, minorities among those routinely excluded or under-represented, researchers say. http://health.usnews.com/usnews/health/healthday/080401/report-claims-clinical-trials-miss-many-populations.htm
5. Killien, M., Bigby, J. A., Champion, V., et al. (2000). Involving minority and under-represented women in clinical trials: The National Centers of Excellence in Women's Health. *J Womens Health Gend Based Med, 9,* 1061–1070.
6. Merton, V. (1993). The exclusion of pregnant, pregnable, and once-pregnable people (a.k.a. women) from biomedical research. *Am J Law Med, 19,* 369–451.
7. Corbie-Smith, G., Thomas, S. B., Williams, M. V., & Moody-Ayers, S. (1999). Attitudes and beliefs of African Americans toward participation in medical research. *J Gen Intern Med, 14,* 537–546.
8. Giuliano, A. R., Mokuau, N., Hughes, C., et al. (2000). Participation of minorities in cancer research: The influence of structural, cultural, and linguistic factors. *Ann Epidemiol, 10,* S22–34.
9. Comis, R. L., Aldige, C. R., Stovall, E. L., Krebs, L. U., Risher, P. J., & Taylor, H. J. Coalition of National Cancer Cooperative Groups, Cancer Research Foundation of America. Cancer Leadership Council, and Oncology Nursing Society. (2000). *A quantitative survey of public attitudes towards cancer clinical trials.*
10. Fouad, M. N., Partridge, E., Green, B. L., et al. (2000). Minority recruitment in clinical trials: A conference at Tuskegee, researchers and the community. *Ann Epidemiol, 10,* S35–40.
11. Horowitz, C., Robinson, M., & Seifer, S. (2001). Community based participatory research from the margin to the mainstream? Are researchers prepared? *Circulation, 119,* 2633–2642.
12. Cottler, L. B., Compton, W. M., Ben-Abdallah, A., Horne, M., & Claverie, D. (1996). Achieving a 96.6 percent follow-up rate in a longitudinal study of drug abusers. *Drug Alcohol Depend, 41,* 209–217.
13. Fitzgibbon, M. L., Prewitt, T. E., Blackman, L. R., et al. (1998). Quantitative assessment of recruitment efforts for prevention trials in two diverse black populations. *Prev Med, 27,* 838–845.
14. Striley, C. W., Callahan, C., & Cottler, L. B. (2008). Enrolling, retaining and benefitting out-of-treatment drug users in intervention research. *J Empir Res Hum Res Ethics, 3,* 19–25.
15. Brown, D. R., Fouad, M. N., Basen-Engquist, K., & Tortolero-Luna, G. (2000). Recruitment and retention of minority women in cancer screening, prevention, and treatment trials. *Ann Epidemiol, 10,* S13–21.
16. Shavers-Hornaday, V. L., Lynch, C. F., Burrmeister, L. F., & Torner, J. C. (1997). Why are African Americans under-represented in medical research studies? Impediments to participation. *Ethn Health, 2,* 31–45.

17. Robinson, J. M. & Trochim, W. M. (2007). An examination of community members,' researchers' and health professionals' perceptions of barriers to minority participation in medical research: An application of concept mapping. *Ethn Health, 12,* 521–539.
18. Wendler, D., Kington, R., Madans, J., et al. (2006). Are racial and ethnic minorities less willing to participate in health research? *PLoS Med, 3,* e19. Epub 2005 Dec 6.
19. Wendler, D., Krohmal, B., Emanuel, E. J., & Grady, C.; ESPRIT Group. (2008). Why patients continue to participate in clinical research. *Arch Intern Med, 168,* 1294–1299.
20. Heller, C. & Melo-Martin, I. (2009). Clinical and Translational Science Awards: Can they increase the efficiency and speed of clinical and translational research? *Acad Med, 84,* 424–432.
21. World Health Organization. (2009). *Global health risks: Mortality and burden of disease attributable to selected major risks.* Geneva, Switzerland.
22. Blanco, C., Olfson, M., Okuda, M., Nunes, E. V., Liu, S. M., & Hasin, D. S. (2008). Generalizability of clinical trials for alcohol dependence to community samples. *Drug Alcohol Depend, 98,* 123–128.
23. Blanco, C., Olfson, M., Goodwin, R. D., et al. (2008). Generalizability of clinical trial results for major depression to community samples: Results from the National Epidemiologic Survey on Alcohol and Related Conditions. *J Clin Psychiatry, 69,* 1276–1280.
24. Haberfellner, E. M. (2000). Recruitment of depressive patients for a controlled clinical trial in a psychiatric practice. *Pharmacopsychiatry, 33,* 142–144.
25. Zetin, M. & Hoepner, C. T. (2007). Relevance of exclusion criteria in antidepressant clinical trials: A replication study. *J Clin Psychopharmacol, 27,* 295–301.
26. Zimmerman, M., Mattia, J. I., & Posternak, M. A. (2002). Are subjects in pharmacological treatment trials of depression representative of patients in routine clinical practice? *Am J Psychiatry, 159,* 469–473.
27. Zimmerman, M., Chelminski, I., & Posternak, M. A. (2004). Exclusion criteria used in antidepressant efficacy trials: Consistency across studies and representativeness of samples included. *J Nerv Ment Dis, 192,* 87–94.
28. Westen, D. & Morrison, K. (2001). A multidimensional meta-analysis of treatments for depression, panic and generalized anxiety disorder: An empirical examination of the status of empirically supported therapies. *J Consult Clin Psychol, 69,* 875–899.
29. Hasin, D. S., Stinson, F. S., Ogburn, E., & Grant, B. F. (2007). Prevalence, correlates, disability, and comorbidity of DSM-IV alcohol abuse and dependence in the United States: Results from the National Epidemiologic Survey on Alcohol and Related Conditions. *Arch Gen Psychiatry, 64,* 830–842.
30. Mannelli, P. & Pae, C. U. (2007). Medical comorbidity and alcohol dependence. *Curr Psychiatry Rep, 9,* 217–224.
31. Institute of Medicine. (1998). *Bridging the gap between practice and research.* Washington DC: The National Academies Press.
32. Velasquez, M. M., DiClemente, C. C., & Addy, R. C. (2000). Generalizability of project MATCH: A comparison of clients enrolled to those not enrolled in the study at one aftercare site. *Drug Alcohol Depend, 59,* 177–182.
33. Rothwell, P. M. (2005). External validity of randomized controlled trials: "To whom do the results of this trial apply?" *Lancet, 365,* 82–93.
34. Humphreys, K. & Weisner, C. (2000). Use of exclusion criteria in selecting research subjects and its effect on the generalizability of alcohol treatment outcome studies. *Am J Psychiatry, 157,* 588–594.

35. Humphreys, K., Weingardt, K. R., Horst, D., Joshi, A. A., & Finney, J. W. (2005). Prevalence and predictors of research participant eligibility criteria in alcohol treatment outcome studies, 1970–98. *Addiction, 100,* 1249–1257
36. Humphreys, K., Harris, A. H., & Weingardt, K. R. (2008). Subject eligibility criteria can substantially influence the results of alcohol-treatment outcome research. *J Stud Alcohol Drugs, 69,* 757–764.
37. DuBois, J., Callahan, C., & Cottler, L. B. (2009). The attitudes of females in Drug Court toward additional safeguards in HIV prevention research. *Prev Sci, 10,* 345–352.
38. Compton, W. M., Thomas, Y. F., Stinson, F. S., & Grant, B. F. (2007). Prevalence, correlates, disability, and comorbidity of DSM-IV drug abuse and dependence in the United States: Results from the National Epidemiologic Survey on Alcohol and Related Conditions. *Arch Gen Psychiatry, 64,* 566–576.
39. Institute of Medicine. (2001). *Crossing the quality chasm: A new health system for the 21st century.* Washington, DC: National Academies Press.
40. Cottler, L. B., Compton, W. M., Price, R., et al. (1993). St. Louis' efforts to reduce the spread of AIDS. In J. A. Inciardi, F. Tims, & B. Fletcher, (Eds.). *Innovative approaches to the treatment of drug abuse: Program models and strategies* (pp. 205–218). Westport, CT: Greenwood Press.
41. Cunningham-Williams, R. M., Cottler, L. B., Compton, W. M., Desmond, D. P., Wechsberg, W., Zule, W. A., et al. (1999). Reaching and enrolling drug users for HIV prevention: A multi-site analysis. *Drug Alcohol Depend, 54,* 1–10.
42. Walker, L. O., Sterling, B. S., Hoke, M. M., & Dearden, K. A. (2007). Applying the concept of positive deviance to public health data: A tool for reducing health disparities. *Public Health Nurs, 24,* 571–576. Erratum in: *Public Health Nurs.* 2008; 25(3):292.
43. Berwick, D. M. (2003). Disseminating innovations in health care. *JAMA, 289,* 1969–1975.
44. Rogers, E. M. (1995). *Diffusion of innovations.* New York, NY: The Free Press.
45. Personal communication, Loretta Jones, CEO of Healthy African American Families, Los Angeles, CA. See Jones, L., Wells, K. (2007). Strategies for academic and clinician engagement in community-participatory partnered research. *JAMA, 297,* 407–410.
46. Hasin, D. S., Goodwin, R. D., Stinson, F. S., & Grant, B. F. (2005). Epidemiology of major depressive disorder: Results from the National Epidemiologic Survey on Alcoholism and Related Conditions. *Arch Gen Psychiatry, 62,* 1097–1106.
47. Grant, B. F., Hasin, D. S., Stinson, F. S., et al. (2005). Prevalence, correlates, comorbidity, and comparative disability of DSM-IV generalized anxiety disorder in the USA: Results from the National Epidemiologic Survey on Alcohol and Related Conditions. *Psychol Med, 35,* 1747–1759.
48. Kessler, R. C., Berglund, P. A., Demler, O., Jin, R., & Walters, E. E. (2005). Lifetime prevalence and age-of-onset distributions of DSM-IV disorders in the National Comorbidity Survey Replication. *Arch Gen Psychiatry, 62,* 593–602.
49. Kessler, R. C., Chiu, W. T., Demler, O., & Walters, E. E. (2005). Prevalence, severity, and comorbidy of 12-month DSM-IV disorders in the National Comorbidity Survey Replication. *Arch Gen Psychiatry, 62,* 617–627.
50. Substance Abuse and Mental Health Services Administration. (2009). *Results from the 2008 National Survey on Drug Use and Health: National findings* (Office of Applied Studies, NSDUH Series H-36, HHS Publication No. SMA 09–4434). Rockville, MD.
51. The City of St. Louis Department of Health. (2007). Understanding our needs, update, 2007. http://stlouis.missouri.org/citygov/health/pdf/UON_2007_Web.pdf.

52. Lara, P. N., Jr. Higdon, R., Lim, N., Kwan, K., & Tanaka, M. (2001). Prospective evaluation of cancer clinical trial accrual patterns: Identifying potential barriers to enrollment. *J Clin Oncol, 19,* 1728–1733.
53. Patel, V., Koschorke, M., & Prince, M. (in press). Closing the treatment gap: A global health perspective. In L. B. Cottler, (Ed.). *Mental health in public health: The next 100 years.* New York, NY: Oxford University Press.
54. Galea, S. & Tracy, M. (2007). Participation rates in epidemiologic studies. *Ann Epidemiol, 17,* 643–653.
55. Harris, P., Lane, L., & Biaggioni, I. (2005). Application of information technology: Clinical research subject recruitment: The Volunteer for Vanderbilt Research Program. *J Am Med Inform Association,* 12, 608–613.
56. Wells, K., Battaglia, T., Dudley, D., et al. (2008). Patient navigation: state of the art or is it science? *Cancer, 113,* 1999–2010.
57. Fallowfield, L. J., Jenkins, V., Brennan, C., Sawtell, M., Moynihan, C., & Souhami, R. L. (1998). Attitudes of patients to randomized clinical trials of cancer therapy. *Eur J Cancer, 34,* 1554–1559.
58. Michener, L., Scutchfield, F. D., Aguilar-Gaxiola, S., Cook, J., Strelnick, A. H., Ziegahn, L., et al. (2009). Clinical and Translational Science Awards and Community Engagement: Now is the time to mainstream prevention into the nation's health research agenda. *Am J Prev Med, 37,* 464–467.
59. Orszag, P. & Emanuel, E. (2010). Health care reform and cost control. *NEJM, 363,* 601–603.

14

Presidential Perspectives

For the 100th anniversary meeting, the past APPA presidents were invited to give their perspectives on the future of psychiatry. Living presidents Bob Cloninger, Myrna Weissman, Alfred Freedman, and Jim Barrett were not able to attend.

The forum remarks made at the meeting were written up for this publication. Members at the 200th meeting will see which predictions were most accurate.

ALFRED M. FREEDMAN, MD
PRESIDENT 1972
NEW YORK MEDICAL COLLEGE
NEW YORK, NEW YORK
ALFREDM@PIPELINE.COM

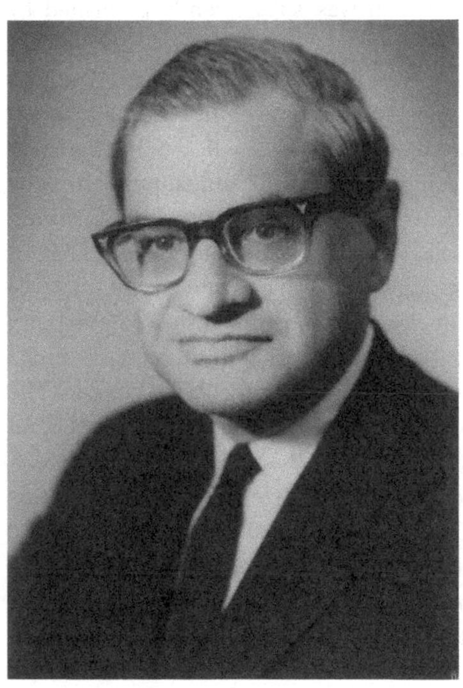

For an organization to celebrate its Centennial Anniversary is always a joyous occasion. This is particularly true for the APPA, and congratulations are in order for the current officers and members as well as those who worked for the success and continuation of the APPA for the past hundred years. Unfortunately, I deeply regret my inability to be present at this happy occasion.

This celebration is particularly evocative for me since it brings to mind memories of the APPA forty or more years ago. I joined the APPA in 1960 and after having served on committees was elected Treasurer and President-Elect and was President in 1972. During that period the APPA was a smaller organization but had a successful and well-attended annual meeting that was guided by Paul Hoch and Joseph Zubin, both professors at the Psychiatric Institute of the College of Physicians and Surgeons of Columbia University. Both made major contributions to the continuation of the APPA as well as played a principal role in the organization of the program at the annual meeting. At that time, the papers delivered at the meeting were collected quickly and edited mostly by Joseph Zubin and published in a very short time in a volume put out by Gruen and Stratton. Mr. Stratton was a good friend of Paul Hoch and was very cooperative in the rapid publication of the meeting. There is a whole series of annual volumes consisting of the papers presented at the annual meeting of the APPA. The early ones are edited by Hoch and Zubin but later the

President of the APPA participated in developing the program and in the editing of the annual volume. Thus, while President-Elect, I was able to choose the topic for our annual meeting, namely "The Psychopathology of Adolescence." At that time I had great interest in child and adolescent psychiatry, the area of my psychiatric training. Further, when I became Chairman of the Department of Psychiatry of the New York Medical College I became very aware of the heroin epidemic of adolescents in New York City. Heroin abuse was prevalent throughout the city but particularly in East Harlem where our services were located. There was widespread concern in regard to the involvement of adolescents. Dr. Zubin and I developed the program which was subsequently published by Gruen and Stratton with the title "The Psychopathology of Adolescence," edited by Zubin and Freedman. Not long after this, Dr. Hoch moved up to Albany as Commissioner of Mental Health, and Dr. Zubin retired from Columbia to join the faculty of Psychiatry at the University of Pittsburg Medical School. Also at that time Mr. Stratton died and the arrangement for our annual publication by Gruen and Stratton came to an end. The organization of the program was taken over by the membership and no annual volume was produced. An affiliation with Comprehensive Psychiatry was set up which still exists today.

My memory of that period is one of close relationships with a membership both before and after my Presidency. During that period of time the meetings were held at the Park Central Hotel, which later became the Park Sheraton. The hotel was famous because a notorious gangster, Albert Anastasia, was shot and killed while sitting in a chair in the barber shop in the hotel. During the meeting, in the years following this episode, participants who knew or heard of this event would go down and peek into the famous barber shop.

The accepted wisdom at that time was that the APPA had been formed in 1910 as a group opposed to the American Psychiatric Association (APA) of that period. Whether this was true or not, there certainly was no such antagonism, and most of the psychiatrists in the APPA had been or were active in the APA and often achieved high office in that organization.

But what of the future of psychiatry? Although hazardous, prediction is necessary for sensible progress for psychiatry. I believe the future compels us to strive for the key to new developments, integration. Because of the multitude of variables essential for comprehending normal and abnormal behavior, a complex, all-encompassing model takes on increased importance. Dualism and reductionism have had a chilling effect on progress in developing psychiatric models. Biopsychosocial models, as elaborated by Dr. George Engel, would appear to be a major step in moving toward an adequate, workable model. Dr. Engel rejected the biomedical, or Newtonian model, in favor of the biopsychosocial model, basing his conception in part on developments in the past century in modern physics, particularly the contributions of Einstein,

Heisenberg, and Planck. The implications and relevance of these advances, including the work of Niels Bohr and many others, have added to these conceptions. All of these concepts and the new thinking that arises from them reinforces notions of wholism leading to a new integration and a more humanitarian psychiatry and medicine.[1] My emphasis on the future of psychiatry is the integration of variables that might contribute to the further delineation of normal and abnormal behavior.

I wish to thank Professors Cottler and Fink for encouraging me to make this presentation which I hope you find interesting. The first part brought back memories of stimulating and rewarding meetings. I hope you find my abbreviated predictions worth consideration.

Congratulations to all of you as well as your predecessors for making this Centennial Anniversary possible.

Reference

1. Freedman, A. M. (1995). The biopsychosocial paradigm and the future of psychiatry. *Compr Psychiatry, 36*, 397–406.

MAX FINK, MD
PRESIDENT 1974
STONY BROOK UNIVERSITY
LONG ISLAND, NEW YORK
MAX.FINK@SUNYSB.EDU

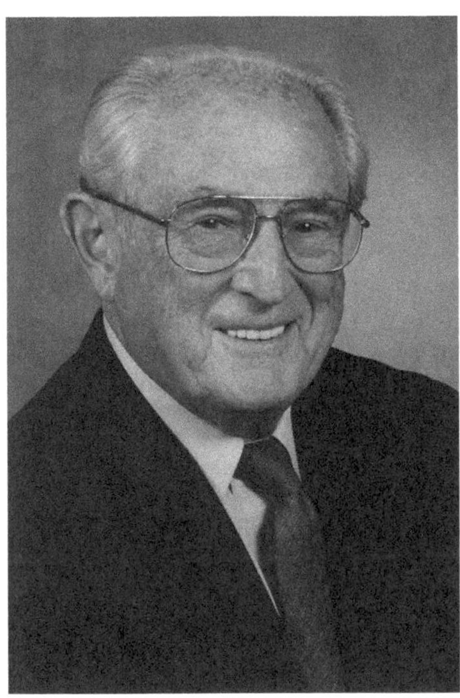

In the 17th and 18th centuries, the diagnosis of physical illnesses moved from mythology and religious beliefs to studies of the physiology of internal organs, laying the foundation for modern medical practice. Bacteriology next gave medicine a special spurt in diagnosis with effective treatments for infectious diseases. Twentieth century psychiatry, enthralled with the "mind," eschewed connections to body and brain physiology. Psychiatrists rejected the physical examination, laboratory tests, and responses to psychoactive agent in identifying psychiatric conditions, making psychiatric diagnosis a descriptive art and not a medical science.[1]

In the 1970s, clinicians at Washington University, notably Sam Guze, Eli Robins, George Winokur, Paula Clayton, George Murphy and their colleagues—all well-known members of the American Psychopathological Association—applied the Sydenham medical model of diagnosis to the identification of psychiatric disorders.[2] Clinically observed symptoms and signs and the course of the illness suggest etiologies. Examination and laboratory tests verify a syndrome that is validated by the response to specific interventions. Family history and course of illness are additional validating criteria.

DSM-III was meant to follow this model, but when the initial descriptions were presented to the Trustees of the American Psychiatric Association, their investment in the office practice of psychodynamic psychiatry and their rejection of connections to medical practice negated attempts to use verifying or validating medical criteria.[3] The resulting classification was descriptive, based on the presence of a limited number of clinical symptoms. Check-off rating scales became the principal tool in classification.

The DSM-IV iteration continued the descriptive nosology, resulting in the present muddle of ill-defined conditions rendering clinical research ineffective. The failures of the present classification are sadly demonstrated by the increasing recognition of "therapy-resistant disorders," the inability to establish "remission" as a clinical goal, and acceptance of symptom relief in treating psychiatric illnesses. The limited findings of the STAR*D[4], STEP-BD[5], and CATIE[6] studies are reflections of the diagnostic inadequacies.

Specific diagnostic progress is possible, however, by applying the medical model. Two psychiatric syndromes, *catatonia* and *melancholia*, have been effectively delineated by this method, offering clinicians guidelines for effective remission of these disorders.

Catatonia. In the 20th century catatonia was incorporated within schizophrenia only. First described as a syndrome by Karl Kahlbaum, adopted by Emil Kraepelin in his concept of dementia praecox, re-enforced by Eugen Bleuler in his image of schizophrenia, catatonia was endorsed as a principal sign of schizophrenia and is so designated in the DSM classification.[7] In the 1970s, however, clinicians commonly found catatonia among patients who otherwise met criteria for depressive and manic mood disorders and toxic medical states.[8] The neuroleptic malignant syndrome was soon delineated as a form of malignant catatonia, offering effective identification and effective treatment algorithms.[9]

In 1930, William Bleckwenn described the relief of catatonia by boluses of intravenous amobarbital.[10] In 1934, Ladislas Meduna relieved catatonia by inducing grand mal seizures chemically.[11] A few years later, electric inductions of seizures became popular, and electroconvulsive therapy (ECT) is the definitive treatment of catatonia today.

By the 1980s, a lorazepam test was developed, and effective treatments of high dose benzodiazepines and ECT were documented with full remission occurring in more than 90% of patients treated. Arguments for the separation of catatonia from schizophrenia appeared[12,13] and the DSM-V psychosis work group has the opportunity to establish catatonia as a definable syndrome in a home of its own in the classification, akin to delirium and dementia.

Melancholia. For centuries, clinicians, artists, and poets have described a syndrome of melancholic madness. Nineteenth century psychopathologists recognized melancholia as circular insanity, as manic-depressive illness, and in the past few decades as endogenous, endogenomorphic, autonomous, or psychotic depression.[14] In the 1970s, effective doses of tricyclic antidepressants failed to relieve psychotic depressed patients, although were very effective in the nonpsychotic depressed.[15] Simultaneously, hypercortisolemia was shown to be a characteristic finding in melancholia and the dexamethasone suppression test (DST) was its effective marker.[16] Other markers such as the CORE motor test[17] and sleep EEG abnormalities[18] were documented. These findings encouraged the separation of melancholia from the amorphous class of major depressive disorder, to assure more homogeneous populations for better treatment outcomes and research study.

The syndrome of melancholia is readily separated from the present criteria of major depression and bipolar disorder by "characteristic" or "prototypic" signs across multiple domains: (1) *a disturbance in affect*, disproportionate to any stressor, marked by unremitting apprehension, morbid thoughts, and blunted emotional response; (2) *psychomotor retardation* that may be expressed in reduced facial and vocal reactivity, as well as by anergia or torpor; (3) *psychomotor agitation* evinced as profound apprehension, anguish, bewilderment, perplexity, and motor agitation, or, in severe instances, by pathological guilt, importuning themes, and stereotypic movements; (4) *cognitive impairment* with distinctly impaired concentration; and (5) *vegetative dysfunction* displayed by loss of sleep (most commonly early morning wakening), loss of appetite and weight, as well as diurnal variation (with mood and energy generally worse in the morning); and (6) in the psychotic expression of melancholia, *delusions and/or hallucinations*, with nihilistic convictions of hopelessness, guilt, sin, ruin, or disease being common preoccupations.[19] This syndrome effectively identifies a population of depressed patients who remit when treated with tricyclic antidepressants and with ECT, two treatments already available.

A similar effort to identify a syndrome of hebephrenia within the present heterogeneous group of schizophrenias is in progress.[20]

The medical model of diagnosis, espoused by the clinicians at Washington University in the 1970s, is a more effective diagnostic model than the present hodgepodge of "diagnoses" based on committee agreement, response to the calls of political claques, offering no biological underpinnings, and resisting systematic procedures of verification and validation. Its efficacy in defining the syndromes of catatonia and melancholia is sufficient to recommend its broader application. The future of psychiatry hinges on the application of medical science principles to psychiatry, recognizing it as a medical discipline, and not a discipline focused on disturbance of the mind.

References

1. Fink, M. (2009). Catatonia: A syndrome appears, disappears, and is rediscovered. *Can J Psychiatry, 54*, 23–31.
2. Robins, E. & Guze, S. B. (1970). Establishment of diagnostic validity in psychiatric illness, its application to schizophrenia. *Am J Psychiatry, 126*, 983–987.

3. Shorter, E. (2009). *Before Prozac: The troubled history of mood disorders in psychiatry.* New York, NY: Oxford University Press.
4. McGrath, P. J., Khan, A. Y., Trivedi, M., et al. (2008). Response to a selective serotonin reuptake inhibitor (Citalopram) in major depressive disorder with melancholic features: A STAR*D report. *J Clin Psychiatry, 69,* 1847–1855.
5. Goldberg, J. F., Perlis, R. H., Bowden, C. L., et al. (2009). Manic symptoms during depressive episodes in 1,380 patients with bipolar disorder: findings from the STEP-BD. *Am J Psychiatry, 166,* 173–181.
6. Lieberman, J. A., Stroup, T. S., McEvoy, J. P., et al. (2005). Effectiveness of antipsychotic drugs in patients with chronic schizophrenia. *N Engl J Med, 353,* 1209–1223.
7. Fink, M., Shorter, E., & Taylor, M. A. (2009). Catatonia is not schizophrenia: Kraepelin's error and the need to recognize catatonia as an independent syndrome in medical nomenclature. *Schizophrenia Bulletin,* doi: 10.1093/schbul/sbp059.
8. Fink, M. & Taylor, M. A. (2003). *Catatonia: A clinician's guide to diagnosis and treatment.* New York, NY: Cambridge University Press.
9. Fink, M. & Taylor, M. A. (2009). The catatonia syndrome: Forgotten but not gone. *Arch Gen Psychiatry, 66,* 1173–1177.
10. Bleckwenn, W. J. *Catatonia cases after IV sodium amytal injection.* Videotape 1930. Washington, DC: National Library of Medicine. NLMID:8501040A (visual material).
11. Gazdag, G. G., Bitter, I., Ungvari, G. S., et al. (2009). Laszlo Meduna's pilot studies with camphor induction of seizures: The first 11 patients. *J ECT, 25,* 3–11.
12. Taylor, M. A. & Fink, M. (2003). Catatonia in psychiatric classification: A home of its own. *Am J Psychiatry, 160,* 1233–1241.
13. Fink, M. & Taylor, M. A. (2006). Catatonia: Subtype or syndrome in DSM? *Am J Psychiatry, 163*(11), 1875–1876.
14. Taylor, M. A. & Fink, M. (2006). *Melancholia: The diagnosis, pathophysiology, and treatment of depressive disorders.* Cambridge, UK: Cambridge University Press.
15. Glassman, A., Kantor, S. J., & Shostak, M. (1975). Depression, delusions and drug response. *Am J Psychiatry, 132,* 716–719.
16. Carroll, B. J. (1982a). The dexamethasone suppression test for melancholia. *Br J Psychiatry, 140,* 292–304.
17. Parker, G. & Hadzi-Pavlovic, D. (1996). *Melancholia: A disorder of movement and mood.* Cambridge, UK: Cambridge University Press.
18. Armitage, R. (2007). Sleep and circadian rhythms in mood disorders. *Acta Psychiatr Scand,* Suppl. *115*(433), 104–115.
19. Bolwig, T. G. & Shorter, E. (2007). Melancholia: Beyond DSM, beyond neurotransmitters. *Acta Psychiatr Scand,* Suppl. *115*(433), 1–183.
20. Taylor, M. A., Shorter, E., Vaidya, N. A., & Fink, M. (2010). The failure of the schizophrenia concept and the argument for its replacement by hebephrenia: Applying the medical model for disease recognition. *Acta Psychiatr Scand. 122,* 178–183.

DONALD F. KLEIN, MD, DSC
PRESIDENT 1980
NEW YORK UNIVERSITY LANGONE MEDICAL CENTER
NEW YORK CITY, NEW YORK
DONALDK737@AOL.COM

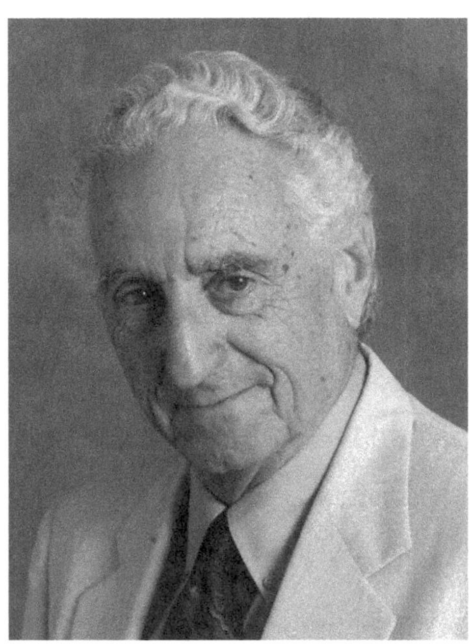

Clearly, where the field should go depends on your estimate of the fruitfulness of current trends and conceptions of possible alternatives. The most critical, fruitful, generative psychiatric events were the serendipitous discoveries that lithium, the antipsychotics (including clozapine), the antidepressants (TCAs and MAOIs), and the anticonvulsants, were uniquely powerful psychotropic agents. These powerful clinical observations took psychiatry out of the psychoanalytic cul de sac during the period bracketed by the early 1950s thru 1975. In the early 1960s, clinical scientists hoped to transcend serendipity by rational drug design. This effort, now labeled "translational research," assumed that basic genomic and synaptic biology would inform rational diagnosis as well as therapeutic agents. However, around 1975 these discoveries stopped despite enormous increases in investment by industry and NIMH in translational research. The proof of the pudding is in the eating. So far these efforts (over 35 years) have produced much wonderful biology but no useful novel therapeutics. My inference is that conventional, "translational research" vastly underestimates our ignorance of brain functions, their disorders, and the difficulty with remediation. Novel psychoactive substances regularly proved toxic or useless. This should not be surprising since most bioactive agents interfere with a finely tuned homeostasis. However, therapeutic agents either normalize or compensate for deranged adaptive functions. Since our knowledge remains primitive of just what functions became maladaptive, it is not surprising that bioactive agents, developed in ignorance of their goal, miss their target.

Unfortunately, serendipity has not been transcended. Indeed, the changes in our clinical system towards short hospitalizations and short patient contacts have been anti-serendipity, by preventing fortuitous observation of benefit. The setting for serendipity (long-term clinical observation) has been demolished. What substitute can be found? One inflaming public health issue has been the frightening perception of rare, late toxicities during long-term treatment. Since randomized controlled trials address acute effects, are of relatively short duration, and insufficient size to reliably discern rare toxicities, it is clear that another approach is required to deal with these issues. Further, it goes relatively unremarked that current trials are inadequate to affirm long-term benefit.

One safety directed possibility is the development of reliable, interlinked, computerized, longitudinal medical (prescription, practice, hospital, laboratory, autopsy, etc.) records. These could form the database for serendipitous observations of unsuspected toxicities from already marketed agents. Such a plan goes far beyond the current FDA Sentinel plan which is restricted to occasional inquiries regarding the conclusions already found from each, of multiple, databases. Further, these are not systematically monitored regarding data entry or analysis. Perhaps of equivalent, or more, importance is that such a well-developed network allows for prospective computerized serendipitous discoveries of unanticipated benefit. Clearly, this will not happen without educated public demand and legislative action.

Modifying the usual clinical trial by randomized, double-blind placebo substitution in putative responders (intensive design) isolates a clinically meaningful, experimentally defined, subsyndrome which requires specific medication for both remission and relapse prevention. This affirms specific therapeutic activity occurs by normalizing a dysfunction. Including objective baseline measures allows isolation of objective diagnostic criteria for subsyndromes. Heuristically, if such measures normalize during the course of syndrome remission, they must be an integral part of the causation of dysfunction rather than simply a correlate. Therefore, embedding objective measures within intensive clinical trials of already *known* specific therapeutic agents allows the discovery of objective, clinically relevant psychiatric diagnostic criteria. Even better, this experimental approach can define both dysfunction and the cause of specific medication benefit. However, this requires a long-term programmatic approach that substantially differs from, and exceeds, current NIH roadmaps or DSM-V discussions.

Finally, where will psychiatry be in the next 100 years? To quote Yogi Berra, "Prediction is very hard, especially about the future."

MURRAY ALPERT, PhD
PRESIDENT 1984
NEW YORK UNIVERSITY SCHOOL OF MEDICINE
NEW YORK CITY, NEW YORK
MURRAY.ALPERT@NYU.EDU

The leadership of APPA played an important role in demonstrating the inadequacy of DSM-II, and made the case for vital investment in an infrastructure for a science of psychopathology. DSM-III was to be an empirical system for establishing an experimental methodology for nosology. The evaluation of the nosology would start with demonstrations of assessment reliability: Validity can't exceed reliability. DSM-III included "field trials" which were published with the manual. In comparison with DSM-II, the results were encouraging. But the improvement in reliability was insufficient to support optimism that our field had a solid infrastructure. Improvement in the reliability of assessment remains a critical focus for progress in psychopathology.

With the explosive growth in psychopharmacology at mid-century, psychopathology evolved from a speculative to an empirical science. The pharmacologists were lucky, the drugs were relatively blunt instruments and their efficacy could be demonstrated across poorly defined diagnostic boundaries. If the drugs were effective for a range of psychotic conditions, or a range of mood disorders, precision of diagnosis was less necessary. NIMH led a program to develop a series of rating instruments to operationalize assessment of pathological behaviors.

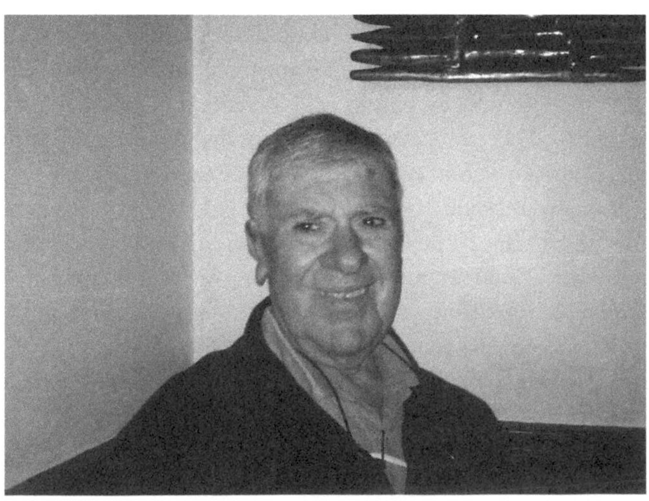

The rating scales are convenient and can be administered by technicians or, even, self administered by patients (for conditions where motivation or cognitive impairment are not an issue). The scales aren't, however, "bottom up" instruments and are less useful in forming a diagnosis. Also, they seem to have an upper limit of reliability of about 0.8 and are vulnerable to halo effects. They are most useful in clinical treatment trials aimed at capturing change over time.

When the genome was sequenced, a number of labs implicated specific genes for various psychiatric disorders. Studies were mounted where genes, assessed with reliabilities greater than 0.99 were examined among patients categorized with reliabilities of about 0.7 or 0.8. How many false positives could such an experiment tolerate? There was ample evidence of familial transmission for a number of disorders. Kety's adopted-away strategy for dissociating the effects of genes from the effects of familial context (in schizophrenia) strongly implicated genetic mechanisms. But the candidate genes could not be shown to segregate among the identified patients.

These observations raise concern for diagnostic precision. The DSM committee mechanism may not be the best agency to address these concerns. DSM is subject to many stakeholder pressures and has few investigative resources. For example, in schizophrenia there are no obligatory signs or symptoms for a diagnosis. An either-or approach is likely to increase heterogeneity in the category and lower reliability. With wide interest in flat affect in schizophrenia and strong interest in evaluating the possible advantage of atypical antipsychotics, DSM added flat affect as a cardinal diagnostic sign of the disorder. This action increased the numbers of patients available for clinical trials while increasing the perceived density of flat affect in the study population. In our clinic we found that other psychotic signs were rated as less severe. The profile of schizophrenic psychopathology was shifted by the DSM change, enhancing the role of atypical drugs in treatment. It was not announced why DSM made this change, nor was the effect of the change on diagnostic reliability reported.

DSM is an important profit center for the American Psychiatric Association and makes socially useful contributions to the smooth functioning of the medical insurance aspects of clinical practice. Other medical specialties don't have a DSM and must depend on other methods. However, other specialties have access to objective and quantitative lab measures which enhance the reliability of clinical impressions. It may be timely to investigate the development of a clinical laboratory infrastructure in psychiatry. It appears that rating scales have reached their maximal ability to improve assessment reliability. We have found good success with measures of voice acoustics to improve the reliability of assessment of affects, moods, and language function. There are a number of useful laboratory measures of dementia. It might be timely to encourage a systematic effort to develop a clinical laboratory for assessment of psychopathology.

JAMES E. BARRETT, MD
PRESIDENT 1985
DARTMOUTH MEDICAL SCHOOL
HANOVER, NEW HAMPSHIRE
JAMES.E.BARRETT.JR@DARTMOUTH.EDU

Shortly after my APPA Presidency, my career took a 90 degree turn, thanks to MacArthur Foundation funding, to a principal focus on psychiatric disorders as they present in primary care (general medicine). That focus had a theoretical side—utility and validity of psychiatric diagnoses suggested for primary care use—and a distinctly practical side— improving the recognition and management of the most common disorders, depressions. Thus, in recent years my direct involvement with psychiatry in general has been much more limited than previously. I feel I have little of significance to say about where the field should be going, or where psychiatry will be in the next 100 years, tempting as it is to hold forth anyway.

However, drawing on my experience in primary care, it is my belief that this sector is, and should be, one of the critical areas of focus for the field. From epidemiologic data, 80% of psychiatric disorders present first to a primary care provider (family physician or general internist), and 70% are seen only in primary care. Two-thirds of these disorders are depressions. Primary care thus has been, and remains, where the majority of depressive disorders are treated. The following are important areas for focus.

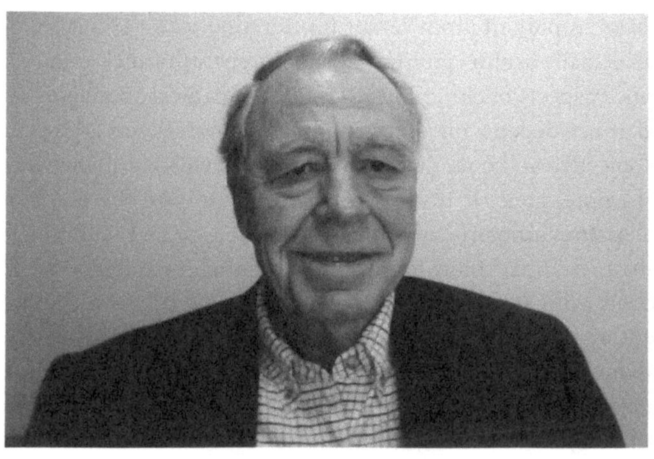

1. Diagnosis. Current psychiatric nosology has limited utility for primary care providers (PCPs). Dysthymia and major depression are relevant and useful in guiding management. But two of the most common depressions, minor depression (sometimes called sub-threshold major depression, or the RDC category episodic minor depression) and mixed anxiety depression are essentially ignored in the official DSM nosology. Effective communication between the two disciplines, thus, has been severely limited.

2. Management. The management of these disorders in primary care needs attention. What is the optimal management for minor depression, or for mixed anxiety depression, the two most common disorders? There is little established knowledge, and virtually no randomized controlled trials, to guide management, a sequellae of, as noted, these disorders being only minimally acknowledged by the field of psychiatry. There is established knowledge for management of major depression, and, to a lesser degree, for dysthymia, but further clinical trials for these disorders as well, as they present in the primary care setting itself, would have great utility.

3. The relationship between primary care and psychiatry. This is a critical area. Sadly, based on my recent 15 years of working with primary care providers (PCPs), this relationship is severely limited and often ineffective. The tendency of many psychiatrists to view PCPs as incompetent to treat depression, in spite of evidence to the contrary, and their relative inaccessibility when a consultation is sought, highlights the problem. From the PCP's perspective, psychiatrists are seen as aloof, unfamiliar with, and uninterested in the depressive disorders which are part of a PCP's daily practice, and have an inaccurate view of a PCP's effectiveness and success in managing those depressed patients.

This interface between psychiatry and primary care, where the majority of patients with psychiatric disorders, and especially depressions, are seen and treated, is a critical area deserving of attention. Well-designed and clinically relevant treatment outcome studies for presentations in primary care are needed. This knowledge, coupled with a collaboration with PCPs based on mutual respect, would lead to improved care for this large group of patients.

DAVID L. DUNNER, MD, FACPSYCH
PRESIDENT 1987
CENTER FOR ANXIETY & DEPRESSION
MERCER ISLAND, WASHINGTON
DLDUNNER@COMCAST.NET

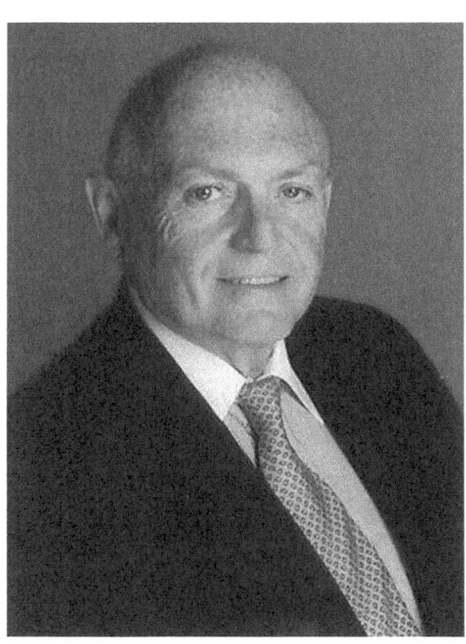

Psychiatry has been a clinically based medical specialty for the past 100 years. Our diagnoses are research based but derived by committee decisions, and our treatments are designed to alleviate the symptoms of our patients but do not address the primary pathogenesis of their disorders. It is my view that the future of psychiatry will in large part be shaped by genetic contributions—the identification of genes that define our disorders, determining the pathogenesis of these disorders by understanding how abnormal gene structure impacts cellular function, and development of treatments that might prevent the clinical manifestations of these disorders in subjects who can be identified through genetic testing. The initial phases of this process will likely be to identify genetic factors that correlate with treatment response, making it possible for clinicians to select a treatment with a higher likelihood of success than we currently experience. The second step will be to identify markers that define ill populations. The next step will be to determine the pathogenesis of these disorders, and the final step will involve appropriate treatment for individuals at high risk for the development of these disorders. The above was the theme of the meeting conducted during my presidency of APPA.

KATHERINE A. HALMI, MD
PRESIDENT 1991
WEILL CORNELL MEDICAL COLLEGE
NEW YORK CITY, NEW YORK
KAH29@CORNELL.EDU

In the next decades, a profound understanding of psychopathology should come from two areas: genetics and brain function. The rapid advance of genetic technology including epigenetic influence should provide information on the effects of various combinations of specific gene profiles for the development of traits such as perfectionism and impulsivity, behaviors such as addictions, and affective and psychotic states.

The continuing development of creative neuroimaging techniques needs to be complemented with other new imaginative assessments of brain function in various states of psychopathology.

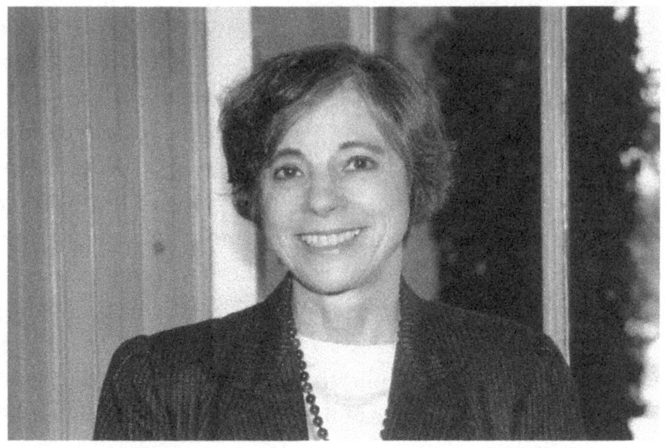

ELLIOT S. GERSHON, MD
PRESIDENT 1992
UNIVERSITY OF CHICAGO
CHICAGO, ILLINOIS
EGERSHON@YODA.BSD.UCHICAGO.EDU

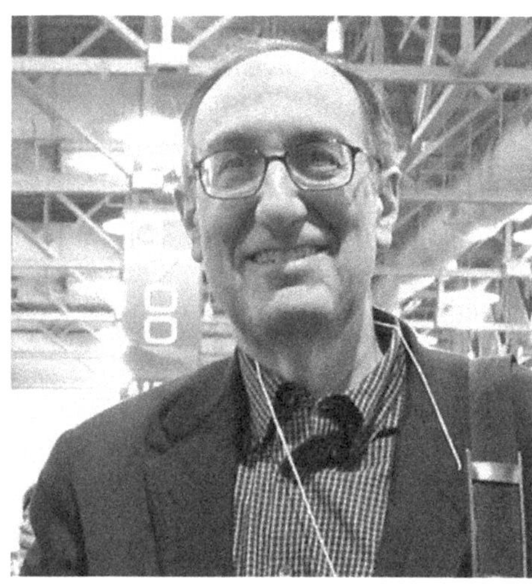

The genetics of the mood disorders and psychoses has been a most challenging problem for the past century, and has produced fewer and less satisfying solid results than genetics in multiple other common diseases. Nonetheless, progress has been made, and the field can take pride in its work.

The 1992 meeting of the APPA, when I was President and Bob Cloninger was President-Elect, was devoted to this topic. Most of the meeting was devoted to familial linkage analyses, and some very interesting results were presented. Brian Suarez presented the first coherent explanation of the "winner's curse" phenomenon, a simulation showing how replication of true linkage results can be elusive. But the retrospective truth is that the problem in the early linkage results was not true positives but false positives. The linkages to Xq28 and 11p15 in bipolar disorder, and to chromosome 5 in schizophrenia, which seemed real for a time, were not consistently replicated. The common single-locus model of these disorders, which was the basis of linkage analyses in pedigree series, now does not appear to exist.

At the time of this writing, there are several significant association results in these disorders, loci with very modest odds ratios (ORs), based on meta-analyses of very large case-control genome-wide association studies (GWAS). It remains to be seen which of them will prove replicable. One of the positive results, association of schizophrenia with a locus in the major histocompatibility region on chromosome 6, may actually relate to the earliest association findings in that disorder. The HLA type A2 was the most robust association in schizophrenia prior to the introduction of DNA marker maps, and may have been an association with the same locus.

There is also evidence for the polygenic hypothesis, genes that cannot be uniquely specified by current-size GWAS, but which in aggregate are producing a significant proportion of disease risk. Other important current leads are found in rare variants that behave somewhat like single-gene disorders, in that each of the these variants has a very potent effect on risk, with ORs between 4 and 20, as opposed to ORs less than 1.5 for all the known GWAS associations.

The rare-variant associations are all structural disorders of the genome, nearly all of them 100 kb or longer segments of microduplication or microdeletion (copy number variants, CNVs) detected through analysis of GWAS data. Based on single-gene disorders produced by large CNVs, we can expect smaller CNVs and point mutations to be detectable that produce the same syndromes. In such a case, there would be clear specification of the disease gene and of the functional changes in that gene.

So, one can look forward to further molecular progress, and to advances in phenotyping that will iterate with molecular findings. I have every confidence that the APPA, in its second century, will be the venue for many of these findings, and serve its goal of supporting the unraveling of the biology and the phenomenology of the psychiatric disorders.

C. ROBERT CLONINGER, MD
PRESIDENT 1993
WASHINGTON UNIVERSITY SCHOOL OF MEDICINE
SAINT LOUIS, MISSOURI
CLON@WUSTL.EDU

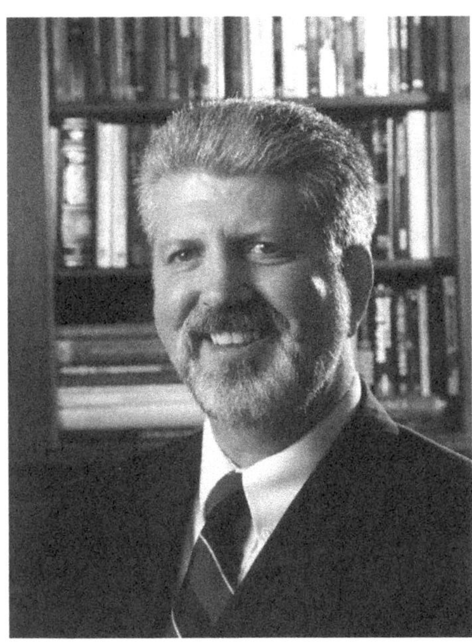

Psychiatry is at a turning point from which it can only progress if it faces the dynamic complexity of human nature and the integrative nature of health and well-being. Our clinical classification using categories is flawed in its basic conception and provides only weak utility in treatment and research. Current treatment is overly dominated by pharmacotherapy, which does not reduce vulnerability to disease. Empirical standards for evaluating efficacy are prescriptive only for groups and not specific individuals. We need to move toward person-centered analyses of functional capacities that are predictive of health and well-being, recognizing that traditional clinical syndromes are failures to achieve the integrated states of physical, emotional, social, and spiritual well-being that characterize health.

Psychiatry can advance by focusing on the well-being of the whole person. Intelligent lifestyle choices will dominate long-term health outcomes in the future because of increasing success in lengthening the lifespan by the prevention and treatment of acute physical disorders. Psychiatry is the natural leader of integrative approaches to well-being, but to play this role it will need a partnership with integrative person-centered medicine. As psychobiologists, psychiatrists are in a unique position to integrate tools of brain imaging, molecular genetics, and other psychobiological methods to develop innovative ways to assess and treat mental disorders by facilitating the development of well-being.

BRUCE P. DOHRENWEND, PhD

PRESIDENT 1994

COLUMBIA UNIVERSITY/NEW YORK STATE PSYCHIATRIC INSTITUTE

NEW YORK CITY, NEW YORK

BPD1@COLUMBIA.EDU

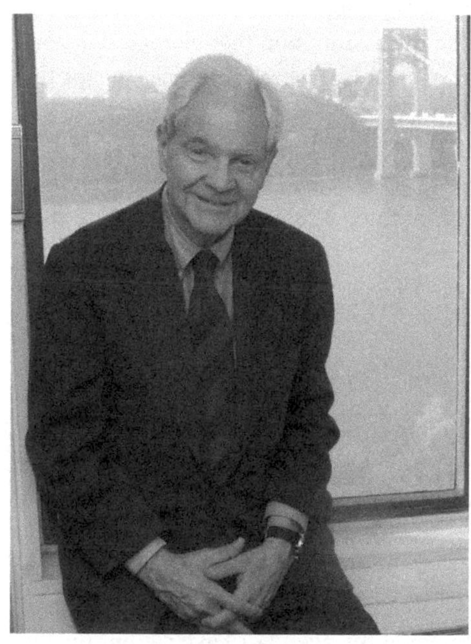

I started work in the field of psychiatric epidemiology in 1955 in my first job after getting my doctorate in psychology at Cornell. The job, still at Cornell, was on the Stirling County Study in a Canadian maritime province and directed by Alex Leighton. I have been in this field ever since.

The zeitgeist in 1955. The spirit of the times then was influenced by two major events in US history:

— The stock market crash in 1929 followed by the Great Depression when people became poor for reasons other than inherited disabilities.

— World War II, when research showed that psychiatric casualties became endemic as overall rates of killed and wounded in companies reached two-thirds. This was strong evidence that extreme environmental stress could produce serious psychopathology in previously normal persons.

In the US especially, the assumption that environmental adversity was of paramount importance in the etiology of all the major types of psychiatric disorder, including schizophrenia, became almost a given. The most sweeping statement of this position was the proposition that disorganized societies produced sick and disorganized citizens; with similar ideas about the role of low social status, especially low social class or socioeconomic status. Members of the APPA with long memories will think of the names of Lawrence K. Frank, Robert E. L. Faris, H. Warren Dunham, and Alexander H. Leighton.

This zeitgeist was compelling in focusing my interests. For over 50 years, I have been investigating the roles of adversity and stress in various types of psychiatric disorders that vary with social statuses defined by gender, ethnic/racial background, and SES. Nevertheless, it became very evident to me by the late 1960s that the pendulum had swung too far in the direction of environmental determinism. Inklings of this awareness I think are evident in Barbara Dohrenwend's and my 1969 book, *Social Status and Psychological Disorder: A Causal Inquiry.*

The zeitgeist today. Things are very different now, a half century later. The pendulum has swung—again too far in my opinion—from the assumption that environmental adversity is paramount to the assumption that biological factors, especially genetic, are paramount. There are at least three valid reasons for this momentum:

— The advances of behavior genetics, impossible to ignore with the publication in 1968 by Rosenthal and Kety of the monograph, *The Transmission of Schizophrenia.*

— New drug treatments for depression and psychosis.

— The mapping of the genome.

As Gottesman and Shields put it in their critical 1976 review, "... the burden of proof has shifted from showing that genes are important to showing that environment is important." This challenge and others like it strike home. My response has been, and continues to be, to contribute to research that will demonstrate as convincingly as the behavioral genetic studies have done for heredity, that environmental factors, especially socio-environmental factors, are important. And I have by no means finished the agenda I have set out for this purpose. This is, I think, a necessary step for me and, I hope, for others to be taking towards what we all know is ultimately needed: incisive research on interrelations between heredity and environment in the etiology of psychiatric disorders.

DAVID S. JANOWSKY, MD
PRESIDENT 1996
UNIVERSITY OF NORTH CAROLINA AT CHAPEL HILL
CHAPEL HILL, NORTH CAROLINA
DAVID_JANOWSKY@MED.UNC.EDU

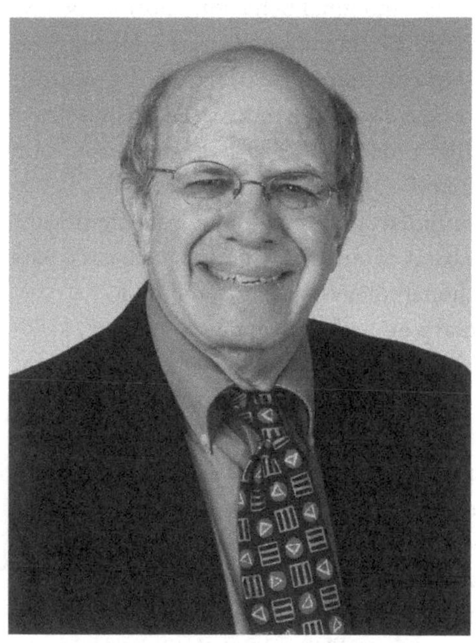

To understand the likely accuracy of predicting where psychiatry will be 100 years from now, one must look back 100 years to the year 1910 and realize how very little of what exists now was predictable then. The auto was a novelty at best, and not a common means of transportation. Air travel did not exist and airplanes barely did, nor did radio, TV, computers, antibiotics, anticancer medications, oral contraceptives, flights to the moon and beyond, weapons of mass destruction, artificial intelligence, the Internet, any idea of what genes looked like, nor the existence of megaton bombs, and this is only a tiny portion of what has developed over the past 100 years. Thus, what is most predictable is that what we consider the mental health field today will be radically changed in ways we cannot now imagine, in large part influenced by technology and equally influenced by the society to which we evolve.

That said, if there even is a field called psychiatry or psychology 100 years from now, those entities that we now call psychiatric diagnoses will almost certainly have been massively redefined and mixed to an unrecognizable level. I would guess that the categorical, rigid boundaries we now apply and call diagnoses will fall, giving way to currently unsuspected mixtures of symptoms and clusters of distress with common biologic etiologies. Major substrates underlying stress and distress and their sequelae, as well as joy, will become better known, and they will almost certainly not speak of neurotransmitters such as dopamine, serotonin, norepinephrine or glutamate, or the cherished prefrontal and limbic tracts with the reverence, focus, and respect attributed to them now.

Thus, by 2110, we will probably have learned the cascade of gene-cellular events and anatomic functions that lead to such experiences as sadness, elation, dreaming, and imagining, and how such phenomena, taken just slightly further, yield deep depression, mania, and paranoid psychosis. I would suspect that we will have learned to manipulate the above cascades at all of their levels, using psychologic and environmental influences, pharmacologic agents, and neuroanatomic perturbations, and that what is now called psychopathology will be considered an extension of normal biology, rather than a set of "illnesses."

I would suspect that inherited characteristics of personality will form a major component of the basis of understanding emotional behaviors, normal behaviors exaggerated to the point of pathology. I would not be surprised if the degree to which one is outgoing (extroverted) or shy (introverted), in need of exerting control, needing to be cherished and loved (reward dependent), being interested in new or thrilling experiences (being a novelty seeker), being chronically gloomy, irritable, depressed and anxious (i.e., having high neuroticism), being frightened of life (harm avoidant) or impulsive, to mention several significant variables, taken together, will form the basis of our understanding of a large part of human behavior, and much of psychopathology as we now define it.

I am certain that people will still crave empathy, acceptance, support, kindness, hope, and understanding from another, as they did 100 years ago, and probably since society began. However, it is not beyond the limits of feasibility that such caring and acceptance may occur as needed via computerized virtual reality scenarios as augmentors of human interactions, which make those who dial-in feel cared about, or via pharmacologic agents which selectively alter the chemistry of the brain to give the experience of being cherished.

I am quite certain that in the year 2110, very little of what we call clinical psychopharmacology will be considered relevant and probably few of our psychotherapeutic techniques as well. Our current ideas about the importance of dopamine, serotonin, norepinephrine, glutamate, and many other compounds will probably be seen as archaic and laughable, as we now consider the former use of blood letting as a valid treatment. I would suspect that the development of nanotechnology will allow very specific deliveries of chemical to behavioral target areas, thereby bypassing many of the problems and side effects our patients must now endure, and I would suspect that part of the pharmacology of the 2100s will involve alteration of specific genes and gene products to "normalize" usual biochemical pathways.

Finally, I am optimistic enough to hope that by 2110 we will have evolved as a society to the level that people can universally partake of what we have to offer as mental health professionals, and the restrictiveness of the current treatment system, being now based essentially on how well off one is economically at a given point in time, will be considered to be as archaic as the chains which bound the insane centuries ago.

ELLEN FRANK, PhD
PRESIDENT 1997
WESTERN PSYCHIATRIC INSTITUTE & CLINIC
PITTSBURGH, PENNSYLVANIA
FRANKE@UPMC.EDU

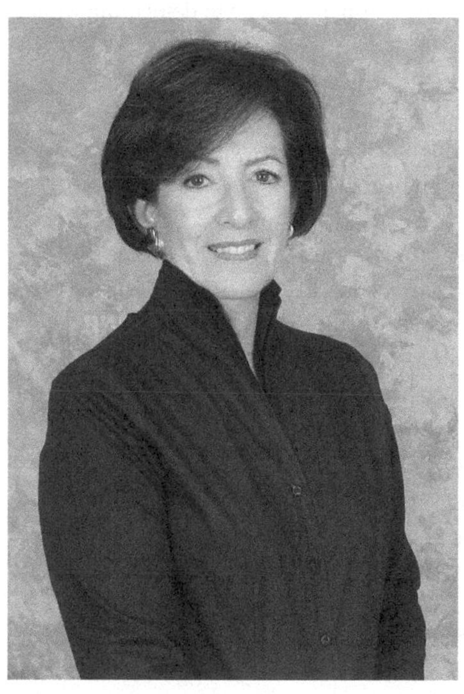

For the January, 2000 issue of the *Archives of General Psychiatry*, Jack Barchas asked my colleague, David Kupfer, and me to comment on what we thought were the questions that were ripe for answering as we entered the new millennium. We identified six such questions. A decade later, we have made some progress in each of these areas, but the questions are far from answered. I believe these remain critical areas for study—if not for the next 100 years—at least for the next several decades.

How Does Life Experience Alter Gene Expression in Vulnerable Individuals?

While some groups have published data suggesting what kinds of life experience might be important for specific polymorphisms to result in specific forms of psychopathology, consistent replication of these findings remains elusive. Additionally, these studies don't even begin to explain the *mechanisms* by which particular kinds of experience lead to, or protect from, the symptoms that constitute our current disorders.

What Are the Neurobiological Effects of Psychotherapy?

Some progress has been made particularly through the use of conventional neuroimaging, but the potential of fMRI to address the question of how so-called "nonsomatic" treatments effect change in processes that are clearly brain-based has yet to be realized. As we come to understand more about the long-term consequences of exposure to the atypical antipsychotic medications a better understanding of how behavioral and psychological interventions affect the brain seems critical.

How Does Early Trauma Lead to Such a Wide and Complex Range of Symptoms?

This is a corollary of the first question, but an area where considerably less progress has been made. Indeed, to my knowledge, no research group has attempted to address this specific, yet important, question. Certainly children exposed to early trauma, particularly chronic sexual and physical abuse, are prime candidates for indicated preventive interventions, but we probably need to know much more in this arena if we are going to be able to determine what it is we should be trying to prevent.

Can We Develop Adverse Effect-Free Pharmacotherapies?

In the mid-20th century, in the desperate search for anything that would treat severe psychopathology, we were willing to accept pharmacotherapies with substantial adverse effects. A few decades later, there were efforts to develop drugs with fewer or more benign side-effects. However, we quickly learned that often we were simply trading one set of problems for another. In some cases, the long-term consequences were actually worse for patients. Unless the contingencies that determine drug development and marketing change radically, it seems unlikely that there will be meaningful progress in this area.

What Is the Connection Between Various Physical Illnesses and Mood and Anxiety Regulation?

Substantial progress has been made, even in the last decade. Our deeper understanding of the way in which inflammatory processes may relate to both psychiatric symptoms and, for example, the metabolic syndrome, suggests that this is an area in which considerable resources should be invested in the coming decades.

How Does the Aging Process Affect Disorder Expression and Treatment?

The effect of aging on disorders is one of our greatest struggles for the DSM revision. How can we capture the diversity of expression of disorder across the lifespan without making the nomenclature so complicated as to make it unusable in conventional psychiatric practice and primary care settings? How can we convey the subtle ways in which disorders evolve over the lifespan? Even more challenging, how does lifespan development affect response to both pharmacotherapies and psychotherapies?

In the end, one thing seems certain to me: Progress will only be made if those knowledgeable about the biology of psychopathology engage in dialogue with those who are experts in the psychosocial processes associated with psychiatric disease and vice-versa. "The gene" is as much of an illusion as "the experience." Let's hope that the next 100 years is a century of such dialogue.

JUDITH L. RAPOPORT, MD
PRESIDENT 1998
NATIONAL INSTITUTE OF MENTAL HEALTH
BETHESDA, MARYLAND
RAPOPORJ@MAIL.NIH.GOV

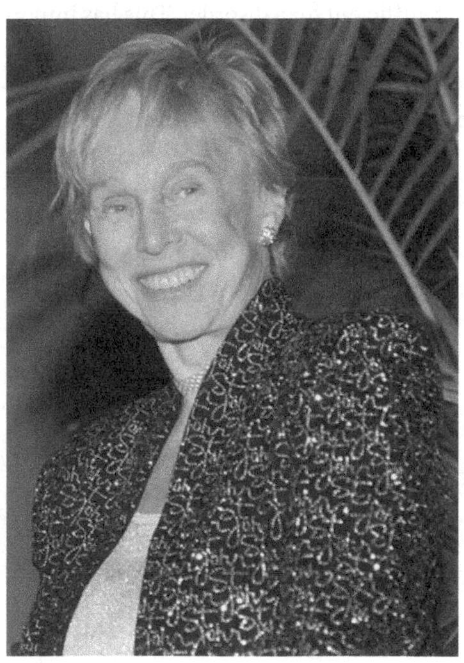

The field is undergoing remarkable intellectual change in the advances from genetics and brain imaging. In contrast, with rare exceptions, these have not translated into benefit for our patients. Almost all psychiatric medications in use today are conceptually the same as those 40 years ago. And while brain imaging is used in neurology/neurosurgery for diagnosis and treatment planning there is almost no nonresearch indication for brain imaging as part of psychiatric diagnosis and care.

The field of genetics is advancing quickly with risk gene discovery and replication for several of our most frequent psychiatric disorders. Genome-wide association studies involving very large populations provide both replications and new discoveries. Parallel studies of rare copy number variants indicate probably more penetrant individual genetic risk but with relatively few cases attributable to any individual CNV. The structural rearrangements though may lend themselves to prevention through prenatal testing as some of these subtle chromosomal abnormalities present risk for autism, retardation, or schizophrenia. Newer approaches such as genomic resequencing and epigenetic scanning will undoubtedly further contribute to clinical discovery. It is unlikely, however, that postnatal genetic testing will be clinically useful in our lifetime given the complex nature of most disorders and the elusive nature of drug discovery. To balance out the long-term promise from the translational approach to therapeutics, pharmaco-epidemiological studies should be a major focus of research for more immediate drug discovery.

Brain imaging has provided some remarkable agreement as to abnormal functional brain circuitry as that for example underlying anxiety disorders. Prospective developmental studies suggest some relatively disorder-specific anatomic and functional abnormalities, as well as possible predictive power for clinical outcome and support for plastic compensatory brain processes. Since many functional and some structural abnormalities are proving to be trait markers (i.e., present in remission in patients and seen in their well relatives) these abnormalities are neither necessary nor sufficient for a disorder. This has important research significance but makes clinical application unclear.

In summary, these are heady times for basic neuroscience but worrying for clinical psychiatry. The focus on the efficacy of focused and relatively short-term behavioral treatments has been important and reassuring.

MYRNA M. WEISSMAN, PhD
PRESIDENT 1999
COLUMBIA UNIVERSITY
NEW YORK CITY, NEW YORK
MMW3@COLUMBIA.EDU

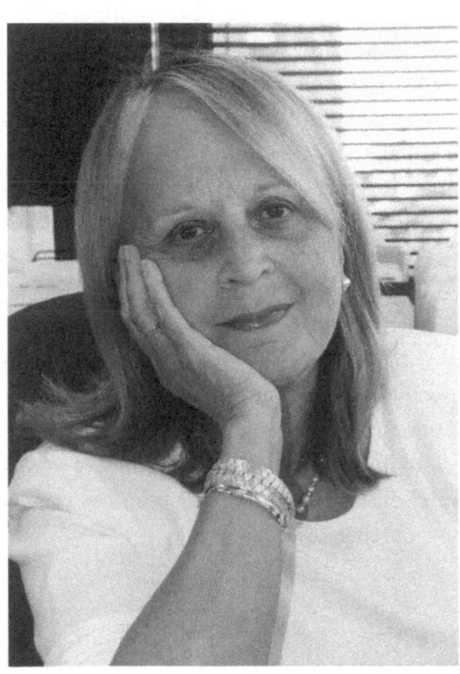

The introduction of DSM-III, with defined diagnostic criteria, and the development of assessments to collect information on signs and symptoms to make the diagnoses, facilitated the modern age of psychiatric epidemiology. In 1978, we wrote that psychiatric epidemiology was being influenced by developments in genetics, psychopharmacology, and psychopathology after the heavy influence of the social sciences during the post World War II period.[1] We called for a synthesis of these new trends in diagnosis and biology, coupled with the prior achievements in sampling and survey work for a new epidemiology of psychiatric disorders. The new epidemiology would provide information on community-based rates and risks of specific psychiatric disorders. We also noted the limitations of this approach. Knowledge of risk factors generates hypotheses within an epidemiologic framework. The testing of such hypotheses requires methods other than epidemiology, such as animal experimentation or laboratory investigation. In 1978, we did not anticipate the possibilities of imaging, or the developments in neuroscience and informatics. We did anticipate the use of genetics but nowhere near the explosion of genetic information and tools now available. Several years later, the first community-based psychiatric epidemiology study using clinical diagnostic methods was initiated, the Epidemiologic Catchment Area Study (ECA).[2]

The ECA was rapidly followed by a series of epidemiologic studies in the US by Kessler and associates, which were national samples, not just city-based as in the ECA.[3] These studies first appeared in the 1990s and were followed by more focused studies on specific ethnic groups (Asian, African American, and Hispanic American) in the 2000s. In the 2000s, the largest US survey ever (over 40,000 subjects) to determine details of alcohol abuse was launched.[4] In 2008, epidemiologic descriptive data on the rates of psychiatric disorders emerged from a landmark worldwide study by Kessler and the World Health Organization (WHO) across seven world regions in 27 countries.[5]

Research and training in psychiatric epidemiology is now ready to take the next steps suggested in 1978 and to become translational. In translational epidemiology, modifiable risk factors identified in well-designed, observational epidemiologic studies are coupled with biological studies. With these approaches, etiological mechanisms underlying the associations of risk and disorders can be identified and tested to determine how genetic and neurobiological variations can modify the associations observed. Well-known epidemiologic observations such as paternal age and schizophrenia, prenatal exposure to nicotine and offspring outcome, familial transmission of major depression, are ripe for translational approaches. Some of this research is ongoing. Training programs in epidemiology now need to strengthen their curriculum in biology. Psychiatric epidemiologists need to add to their knowledge base of sampling, design, and social risk factors, an understanding of biological risks, and of approaches to their study. With this additional perspective epidemiologists will be more likely to identify, organize, and participate as equal partners in these important collaborations. They will also be able to contribute to the design and hypothesis of biological studies. The linking of population, clinical, and basic sciences in psychiatry is what I see in the future for psychiatric research.[6]

References

1. Weissman, M. M. & Klerman, G. L. (1978). Epidemiology of mental disorders: Emerging trends. *Arch Gen Psychiatry, 35*, 705–712.
2. Robins, L. N. & Regier, D. A: (1991). *Psychiatric disorders in America: The Epidemiologic Catchment Area Study*. New York, Free Press.
3. Kessler, R. C., McGonagle, K. A., Zhao, S., Nelson, C. B., Hughes, M., Eshleman, S., et al. (1994). Lifetime and 12-month prevalence of DSM-III-R psychiatric disorders in the United States. Results from the National Comorbidity Survey. *Arch Gen Psychiatry, 51*, 8–19.
4. Grant, B. F. & Dawson, D. A. (2006). National epidemiologic survey on alcohol and related conditions: Selected findings. *Alcohol Research and Health, 29*.
5. Kessler, R. C. & Ustun, T. B (Eds.). (2008). *The WHO World Mental Health Surveys: Global perspectives on the epidemiology of mental disorders*. Cambridge University Press.
6. Weissman, M. M., Talati, A., Brown, A. (in press 2011) Translational epidemiology in psychiatry: Linking population to clinical and basic sciences. *Arch Gen Psychiatry*.

JOHN E. HELZER, MD
PRESIDENT 2000
UNIVERSITY OF VERMONT SCHOOL OF MEDICINE
BURLINGTON, VERMONT
JOHN.HELZER@VTMEDNET.ORG

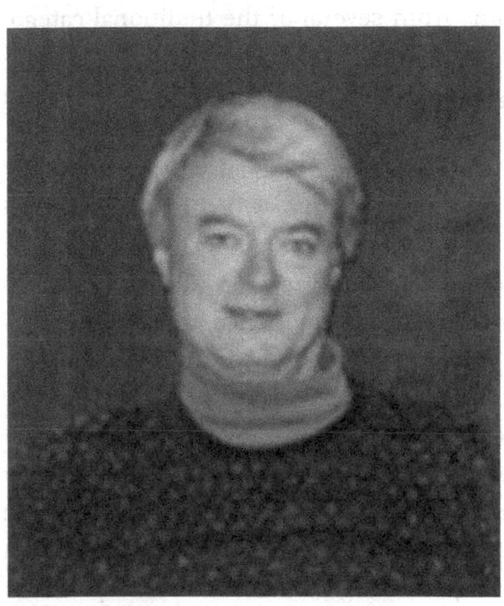

At this moment in our history, psychiatry is struggling with taxonomy—again. Thirty years ago DSM-III was a seminal advance. For the first time, the field agreed on explicit diagnostic criteria that were accepted not only in the United States but throughout much of the world. These categorical diagnoses have been revised twice since their publication. Having a well-considered, uniform set of diagnostic terms and definitions has improved clinical care, facilitated teaching, and helped to advance psychiatric research. However, in part as a consequence of the research fostered by the DSMs, we have learned a great deal about the limitations of the current taxonomy. It is now time for another seminal advance.

The most serious limitation of the current taxonomy is the strictly categorical nature of the diagnoses. This was a problem thirty years ago as well but only a few prescient experts, such as the late Robert Kendell, recognized it. Prior to DSM-III psychiatric diagnosis in the United States was in such chaos that it was difficult to fully appreciate the continuous nature of psychiatric illness. However, with the explicit definitions of the DSMs, we are now better able to see the continuous nature of illness, both within and across diagnostic groups. The Epidemiologic Catchment Area (ECA) and National Comorbidity Surveys (NCS), both based on DSM criteria, clearly demonstrated that even in the general population, single, categorically defined disorders are the exception. Someone who meets criteria for one category typically meets criteria for more than one, and often several. Furthermore, psychiatric research in many areas, particularly psychiatric genetics, has grown in sophistication to the point that a categorical system is seriously limiting. The DSM-V revision now ongoing must give this issue top priority. After two revisions since DSM-III it is not clear that the categorical definitions will benefit from further revision. Any revision to a taxonomic system is seriously disruptive in a variety of ways; therefore, revision for its own sake is not tenable.

At this point there is still debate about how best to achieve a dimensional taxonomy and there are several candidate dimensions which could form the basis for continuous definitions. Even less clear is how best to create a system that can be used to classify difficult "comorbid" cases, those which exhibit in differing degrees significant symptoms from several of the traditional categories. But there is wide recognition that a DSM-V that fails to provide for a quantitative alternative to categorical diagnoses would not begin to take us "where psychiatry needs to be going."

A second major taxonomic issue that must be addressed is whether the traditional "top-down" approach to diagnosis is optimum or whether we should be defining illness in a bottom-up manner. Top-down definitions have traditionally been used for the DSMs. A group of designated experts (a "diagnostic workgroup") is appointed to consult their own clinical experience, review the literature, analyze findings from relevant research including field trials of candidate criteria, and apply their clinical judgment to create a set of illness definitions. Conversely, a bottom-up approach begins with a broad range of symptom data from both general and ill populations and relies on statistical analysis to identify consistent symptom patterns which are then assigned appropriate diagnostic labels. Both approaches have merit, but at this point we have never tested which of these is the more valid in terms of predicting natural history, response to treatment, familial transmission, and other relevant correlates.

A third problem is how to best ascertain clinical information once agreement on illness definition has been achieved. DSM-III represented a significant advance in this regard. Just as DSM-III was being drafted, the NIMH was planning a multi-site epidemiologic survey, the ECA, and had contracted for the Diagnostic Interview Schedule (DIS) to be developed reflecting the new criteria. Since development of the criteria and the interview were occurring congruently, it was possible to compose and test questions for candidate criteria as they were being developed. The result was a diagnostic instrument usable in both clinical and general populations that closely reflected the DSM-III criteria. In the ensuing years other interview instruments, also based on the DSMs, have been developed for other clinical and research efforts. Three major problems have arisen. One is that even slight differences in question wording, choice of screening questions, symptom coding, and so forth, can result in major differences in diagnostic prevalence rates. A second problem is that the use of differing assessment instruments, although based on the same set of criteria, are typically sufficiently different that comparing results and/or pooling data across studies necessitates analytic compromises. Third, instruments designed for general population surveys are typically too extensive and complex to be useful for clinical contexts.

Designing a set of interview tools that are efficient to administer and can satisfy the needs of various users but are internally consistent and usable in both research settings and in clinical settings for diagnosis and treatment planning is challenging. But, a cumulative clinical database could significantly advance the science of psychiatry. With appropriate attention to patient confidentiality, such an assessment resource would enable the collection of a data bank for genetics and other research requiring ultra-large samples.

At this point in our history, immersed in the creation of DSM-V, where the field of psychiatry should be heading is actually DSM-VI. We should be thinking now of what the taxonomic questions will be 15 years from now and structuring DSM-V to gather the data necessary to address those questions when the time comes. For example, one delicate but important question is whether exercising our clinical judgment in creating diagnostic criteria actually improves the validity of diagnosis compared to a classification system based on a strictly empirically and statistically derived "bottom-up" classification. Or is it the case that our judgment, skewed as it is by our exposure to only those patients who come to medical attention and shaped as it is by our own proclivities, actually detracts from validity. This and the other issues raised above, the utility and added value of a quantitative classification, and the feasibility of a standard diagnostic interview, are all potentially answerable with empirical data. But they are answerable only if we begin now by structuring DSM-V in such a way as to collect the necessary data. Many, including myself, have questioned the need to revise yet again the categorical criteria of the DSM. But a DSM-V that encompasses these broader, future-oriented agendas would clearly make this massive revision effort, with all its necessary disruption, entirely worthwhile.

CHARLES F. ZORUMSKI, MD

PRESIDENT 2003

WASHINGTON UNIVERSITY SCHOOL OF MEDICINE

SAINT LOUIS, MISSOURI

ZORUMSKC@PSYCHIATRY.WUSTL.EDU

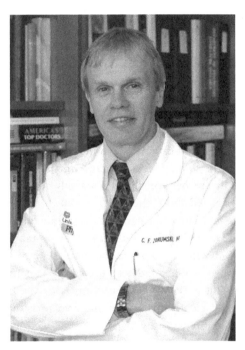

Psychiatric illnesses are disorders of the human mind. In turn, the human mind is a product of the human brain. The major problem that confronts psychiatry is how to put the brain back into diagnosis and therapeutics. Current diagnoses and treatments are not based on brain pathophysiology, and the brain has little to do with most clinical practice. Archaic concepts like "chemical imbalances" are still discussed as though they have meaning. For psychiatry to progress over the next century, it must re-establish itself as a branch of clinical neuroscience and take advantage of the explosion of information about how the brain processes information and how brain creates mind.

Advances in neuroimaging and systems biology, including the ability to image the human brain while doing complex tasks, make this a tractable problem. Functional imaging studies provide compelling evidence that the brain is organized into intrinsic connectivity networks (ICNs) that perform specific computations and interact with other ICNs to solve problems. Examples include networks for attention, decision making, language, emotion, and motivation, among others. This work has great relevance for psychiatry. Recent studies indicate that neurodegenerative illnesses such as Alzheimer's disease (AD) and frontotemporal dementia attack and percolate within specific ICNs. It is the disruption of the specific ICNs and the resulting disconnection from other ICNs that produce phenotypic expressions of illness. The underlying molecular pathology (e.g., beta-amyloid in AD) provides potential targets for pharmacological interventions while the clinical deficits more closely reflect the dysfunctional ICNs.

Of particular importance to psychiatry is the "default system," an ICN that is highly active at rest while we process information about our internal world, including emotions and autobiographical memories. When we focus on a task, we must shift out of default processing and into a mode that uses ICNs appropriate for the job at hand. Recent data indicate that subjects with several major psychiatric disorders, including depression and schizophrenia, have defects in shifting attention from default mode to external processing. Such defects in attention likely contribute to difficulties in correcting errors in thinking, emotion, and motivation that arise in psychiatric illnesses.

This work in humans is occurring in parallel to amazing advances in cellular and molecular neuroscience. Here, the field of optogenetics, in which expression of light-activated molecules in targeted brain regions allows manipulation of neuronal function in live animals, is revolutionizing how we think about brain networks and the changes that occur in illnesses. Psychiatry must embrace these advances and prepare for a future based on sophisticated brain biology—a future in which clinical psychiatry uses the science of brain networks to position itself closer to neurology and neurorehabilitative medicine.

WILLIAM W. EATON, PhD
PRESIDENT 2004
JOHNS HOPKINS BLOOMBERG SCHOOL OF PUBLIC HEALTH
BALTIMORE, MARYLAND
WEATON@JHSPH.EDU

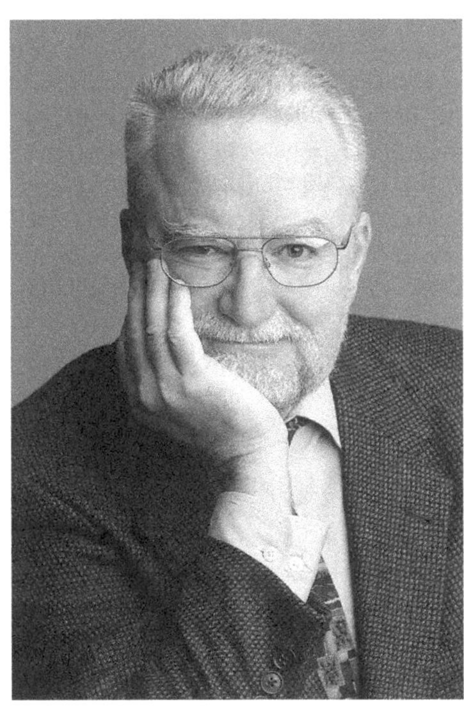

In contrast to many medical illnesses which will decline over the next century, the prevalence of mental disorders probably will increase during that time. The difference in velocities of genetic versus cultural evolution—*sociogenetic lag*—will increase. Genetic vulnerabilities for mental disorders today involve biological processes which have evolved and endured through thousands of years of evolution, and are unlikely to change much in ten decades. Social causes for mental disorders involve processes that will become more complex and challenging over the next 100 years. Adapting to social life will require higher levels of executive function as the century progresses, and the rate of social disruptions in the life course of the individual is likely to increase. The increased environmental pressure for higher levels of executive functioning, as well as the increased rate of social disruption, operating on the same set of genetic vulnerabilities, amounts to sociogenetic lag that will lead to higher prevalence of a range of disorders. Assortative mating by emotional or personality factors with continuous distributions in the population will increase. This will lead to higher levels of variability in the population for the associated emotional factors and behavioral tendencies, and push the tails of the distributions outward. The enlarged extremes of the distributions will be associated with increased rates of associated disorders, especially personality disorders. Aging and cognitive decline in the elderly—the "silver tsunami"—will change the basic structure of society, including housing, urban life, politics, and medicine.

Medications for mental disorders will continue to work on symptoms at the margin, without cure, for the most part, because the etiopathologies are too complex to respond to one or even a number of compounds. There may be dramatic breakthroughs in prevention and cure through some forms of biological management, for etiopathic subsets comprising a small percentage of the heterogeneous serious disorders such as schizophrenia, bipolar disorder, and autism. Widespread adoption of genetic screening and personalized medicine will lead to many fewer serious side effects of medications, and area-wide linkage of medical records will minimize complications from drug interactions. The result is that medications will become safer over the years, even if not much more efficacious. As treatment for other medical illnesses becomes more efficacious or automated, the specialty of psychiatry will grow compared to others. Compared to medications, talk and social therapy will maintain or even grow in their relative efficacy and efficiency. Prevention efforts will increasingly involve complex social actions of various sorts, targeting reduction of the prevalence of the common mood, anxiety, and behavioral disorders. Preventive interventions will increasingly take advantage of knowledge of individual abilities and proclivities produced by both genetic and environmental backgrounds, so that they can be tailored to individual: *personalized prevention*. But the effectiveness of preventive interventions in society as a whole will be vitiated by the increasing strength of resistant cultural localisms: that is, social groups with unique sets of beliefs, values, norms, and behaviors, different than—and possibly distrustful of—the larger society. Cultural localisms will make it hard to disseminate efficacious preventive interventions, and considerable effort will be spent re-tooling complex interventions to meet the expectations and needs of such groups.

MING T. TSUANG, MD, PhD
PRESIDENT 2005
UNIVERSITY OF CALIFORNIA, SAN DIEGO
SAN DIEGO, CALIFORNIA
MTSUANG@UCSD.EDU

Recent emphasis on the shifting paradigm in medicine from treatment to prevention calls for the restructuring of future developments and plans within psychiatry, which is a branch of medicine. Psychiatry should not be left behind while other disciplines of medicine are moving ostensibly and purposefully towards prevention and the study of wellness. Personalized medicine and the early identification of diseases, even before their onset, have become the norm in medical fields such as oncology, cardiology, and endocrinology by utilizing contemporary advances in this post-genomics era. Application of these advances should and could be made to engender positive clinical outcomes, for instance in schizophrenia. In order to develop plans for prevention of schizophrenia, early identification of the disorder before its onset is crucial. For this purpose, research in clinical, psychosocial, and biomarkers is essential for the identification of cases before their onset. The onset of schizophrenia, usually in adolescence, is difficult to differentiate from other disorders such as adolescent maladjustment or personality disorders. Before schizophrenia's onset, prodromes and premorbid personality should be studied to identify potential risk factors before its manifestation. Furthermore, it will facilitate early intervention

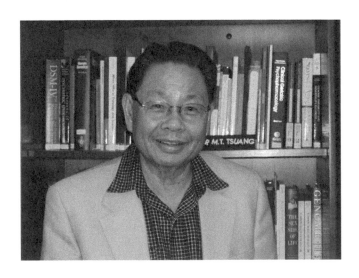

and treatment if neuroanatomical, neurophysiological, neurochemical, and genomics biomarkers can be discovered to identify the disorder before its onset. Personalized treatment for each patient could be administered, resulting eventually in prevention, by utilizing a combination of risk factors and biomarkers. In addition, determination of protective factors should be pursued to maintain wellness in physical, mental, and spiritual areas, leading to well-balanced, integrated health and well-being. Application of this line of research and its implications for promotion of psychiatry and public health in the general population should be explored and emphasized.

J. RAYMOND DEPAULO, JR., MD
PRESIDENT 2006
JOHNS HOPKINS UNIVERSITY SCHOOL OF MEDICINE
BALTIMORE, MARYLAND
JRD@JHMI.EDU

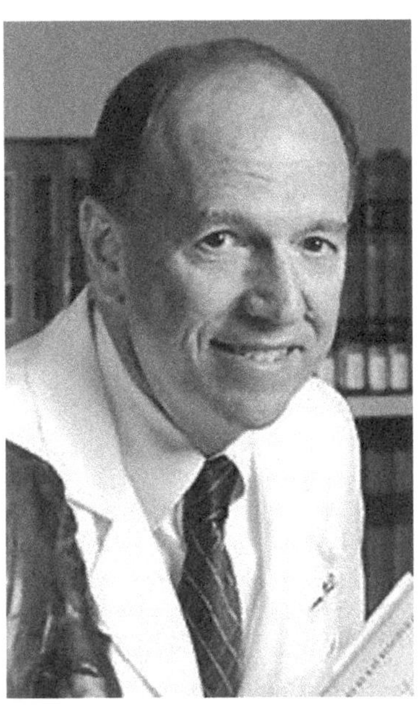

As a recent Past President of the American Psychopathological Association, I am happy to contribute some thoughts about a vision for psychiatry: where it should be going, what areas are most critical, and where we will be in 100 years. My view from the Department of Psychiatry and Behavioral Sciences at Johns Hopkins, where I have worked since I entered medical school in 1968, has been shaped by two big changes in medicine. The "war on cancer" began in 1971 when I was a junior in medical school. It was a big idea with big funding made possible by a new technology; that is, molecular biology. With this developing new method, researchers were able to interrogate tumors, but not living human brains. And even with tumors under the microscope, the initial studies were fumbling and stumbling. It took a decade before really good experiments were possible and it took until the 25th anniversary of the war before cancer death rates began to decline in the US. Psychiatry sits now somewhere in the mid 1970s (without the same presidential mandate or federal funding) if it were to be placed on the oncology calendar. We now have a mature molecular tool kit with which we can interrogate the molecules of the human brain, and we have functional brain-imaging methods, in their infancy, which have great promise. What we need now are the careers of our most ambitious medical graduates and the funding to tell the story of the brain in health and disease. Taking a long view the future of brain science and psychiatry is very bright.

The second change in medicine which has shaped my vision for psychiatry is the change in what its leaders advocate for. In particular, leaders in three medical fields that best understand the biology or pathogenesis of their respective diseases (oncology, infectious diseases, and cardiology) are now vigorous advocates for prevention. Despite the molecular advances in understanding cancers, atherosclerotic heart disease, and infections from MRSA to AIDS, prevention has proven to be surprisingly difficult work. The director of a large US cancer institute explained when asked what more he needed to ensure prevention or cures for most cancers, that the biggest obstacle was not lack of genetic or molecular knowledge but the fact that "we are no damn good at changing behavior." The message for me is that when we understand diseases from their origins we still must face the more daunting task of helping patients change their behavior.

Understanding how the brain develops and works is key to understanding the major psychiatric disorders which make up over 20% of the worldwide burden of disease according to the WHO Global Burden of Disease Studies. As the brain is our most complex organ, the scientific challenges inherent in this task cannot be underestimated. However, advances in genetics, molecular biology, systems neurobiology, and brain-imaging make radical dissection of psychiatric disorders an achievable goal.

Utilizing the knowledge already at hand from behavioral psychology and adapting it to general medical education and use is critical for the prevention of the major lethal diseases including cancer, heart disease, and AIDS. From my perspective I see psychiatry and behavioral sciences at the very center of medicine's next century.

JAMES J. HUDZIAK, MD
PRESIDENT 2007
UNIVERSITY OF VERMONT COLLEGE OF MEDICINE
BURLINGTON, VERMONT
JAMES.HUDZIAK@UVM.EDU

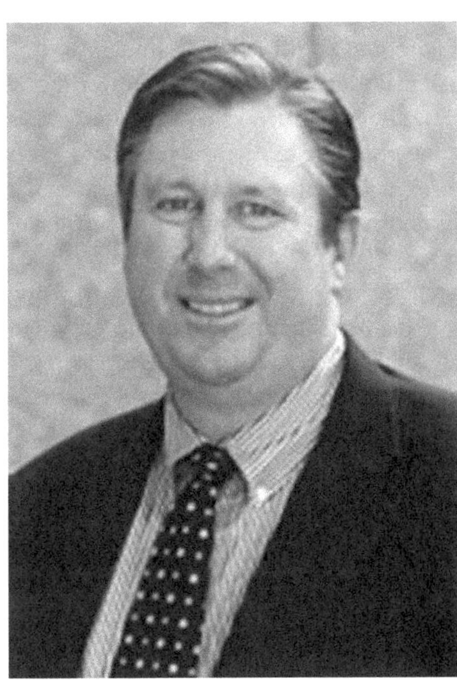

At the University of Vermont, my team and I have worked very hard at combining lessons from neuroscience and genomics to advance the assessment and treatment of the complex conditions known as psychiatric illnesses. We have developed the Vermont Family-Based Approach (VFBA), which was presented at the APPA 2007 meeting titled: *Genetic and Environmental Influences on Developmental Psychopathology and Wellness*. The principle underpinnings of the VFBA approach are that: 1. All child psychiatric illnesses (and, by extension, adult psychiatric ones) result from the influences of genes, environments, and their interplay (correlation, interaction, etc.,); 2. All psychiatric illnesses "run" in families (i.e., parents of children with psychiatric illnesses are more likely to have psychiatric illnesses, and vice versa); 3. Psychiatric illnesses in parents or children adversely affect environments that ultimately adversely affect all family members; and 4. Effective assessment and treatment of psychopathology in any member of a family requires assessment of all members of that family and treatment of those at risk or ill.

The study of environmental mediators and moderators of risk led us to build the Vermont Family-Based Environmental Treatment Formulary. We harvested data from the resilience and wellness literature and developed a rationale for health promotion, illness prevention, and intelligent family-based intervention. We developed an evidence-based approach to achieve those goals. *Well families* were defined as those in which neither children nor parents have psychopathology. For well families we recommend health promotion strategies. At our clinical research sites we have recast the job description of our social workers as "family wellness coaches." We have armed these coaches with tool kits for wellness which include lessons on sleep, nutrition, exercise, reading, music, and simple behavioral approaches to raising healthy children that all parents should, but often don't, know. *At risk families* are defined as families in which the children are currently well but where one or both parents have a psychiatric illness. We argue that research clearly tells us that children raised in homes where parents struggle with psychiatric illnesses are at both genetic and environmental risk. To these families we offer not only health promotion, but also illness prevention. In our model, our PhD- and MA-level therapists are recast as "focused family coaches." They work with evidence-based models to treat parental psychopathology (maternal depression, paternal substance abuse, etc.). In the focused family coach tool kit we include psychotherapies with demonstrated efficacy across development. Finally, *ill families* are those in which a child struggles with psychopathology. Here we provide health promotion, prevention, and intelligent family-based intervention. The family-based psychiatrist who works in this system is rewarded by being part of a multidisciplinary treatment team in which all aspects of health promotion, prevention, and intervention are being addressed.

When I present this model around the country I typically get two responses. The first is: "This makes sense." The second: "We will never be able to pay for it." While I acknowledge that our current health care system does not support such a plan, I also argue that the system is broken. In a time where health care reform is underway, I believe that psychiatry needs to be at the table to correct these problems. We currently have these VFBA programs in place in a school system, in a pediatrics office, in two federally qualified health centers via telepsychiatry, and in our Vermont Center for Children, Youth, and Families so we know that it "can be done." For psychiatrists, the work is rewarding, and the families we serve are highly invested in the approach. The critics are right to be skeptical; however, this work probably is too expensive to offer routinely in the context of our current health care culture. It certainly can not be done in 10-minute visits. However, I am of a mind that many of the bad decisions we have made in psychiatry over the past two decades are simply not good medical practice. I am certain that we should not abandon ideas rooted in our best science simply because of financial obstacles foisted upon our field by others. I am motivated that we can change our field but only if we accept the responsibility to do so.

So my first hope for the future of psychiatry is that we take back ownership of the direction of our discipline. We will need to be unified in our message that the assessment and management of psychiatric illnesses is terribly complicated and almost always requires more than writing a prescription. We need to be quite clear that 10 minutes are not enough to provide proper care to patients with the complex illnesses we treat. We offer the VFBA as one model (of what I hope will be many) that takes into account the scientific discoveries of our field. We must heed the lessons learned about genetic vulnerability and environmental mediators and moderators, and build those into new treatments for the patients and families we serve. Regardless of which specific model we ultimately embrace, we need to value our training and expertise in careful assessment, our commitment to our science, and our ability to prescribe treatment plans that include health promotion, illness prevention, and intelligent family-based intervention.

PATRICK E. SHROUT, PhD
PRESIDENT 2008
NEW YORK UNIVERSITY
NEW YORK CITY, NEW YORK
PAT.SHROUT@NYU.EDU

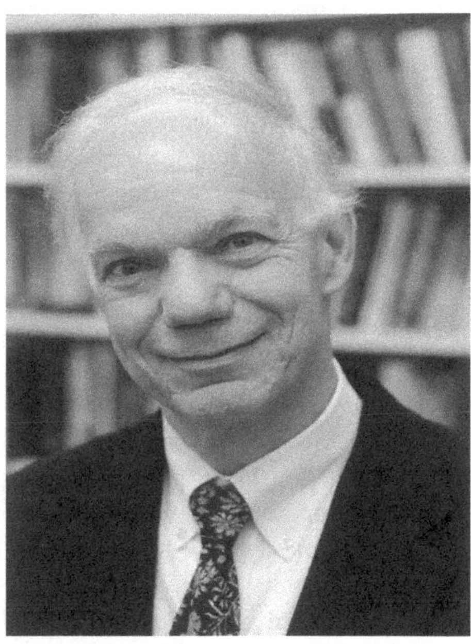

A critical question that needs to be addressed in psychiatry is the degree to which mental illness may be experienced as an acute but transient episode, much like an experience with flu, or if the concept of mental illness is going to be reserved for chronic problems that fail to remit completely.

Insofar as psychopathology researchers restrict their empirical studies to persons seeking treatment, or rely on retrospective reports of lifetime illness in cross-sectional studies, the answer will necessarily be that mental illness will be defined to be chronic and comorbid. Such restrictions make it unlikely that patterns of psychological resilience or coping will be well understood outside the therapeutic environment, and they make it likely that stigma associated with chronic mental illness will continue to discourage treatment seeking.

Modern technology will make it easier in the future to carry out prospective studies of fear, delusions, profound sadness, substance-use binges, numbing, derealization, cognitive lapses, sleep disruptions, and other problems that are often associated with mental illness. Just as cardiovascular researchers ask persons to wear ambulatory blood pressure monitors, and endocrinologists ask study subjects to provide multiple samples of saliva and other fluids over the course of a day for several days, so could psychopathology researchers devise ways to monitor behavioral, biochemical, and mental events in short time-intervals over long periods of time. Intensive data such as these can provide new insights into more subtle variations of human suffering and psychological immune responses to periods of misery.

DARREL A. REGIER, MD, MPH
PRESIDENT 2009
AMERICAN PSYCHIATRIC ASSOCIATION
ARLINGTON, VIRGINIA

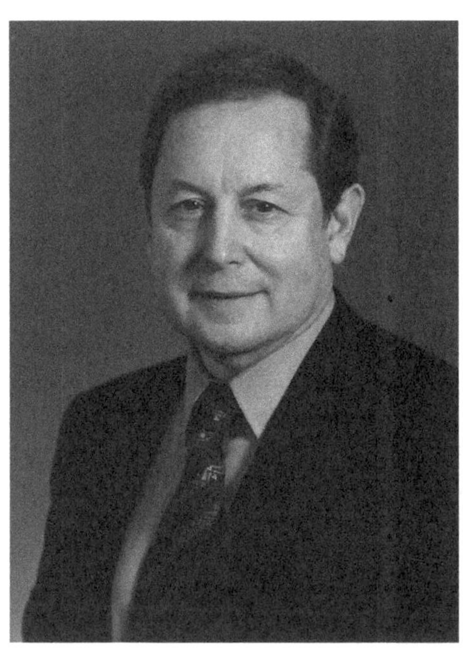

Since the mapping of the human genome was completed in 2000, our ability to understand disease on a genetic level has led to fascinating but challenging considerations about illness risk, prevention, and treatment. We are now looking beyond genetic susceptibilities and taking a broader view that encompasses the unique epigenetic mechanisms linking genes and disease to environment and behavior. Accordingly, in psychiatry, one of the most critical areas for focus is on obtaining greater understanding of the pathophysiology and the gene-environmental interactions that are the causal components of mental disorders. The methods necessary for doing this will involve a greater commitment to genetic epidemiology techniques in which environmental exposures are more carefully measured from prenatal to geriatric age groups. Family history assessments, diagnostic assessments with DSM-V type dimensional approaches, and more efficient genetic analytic techniques will evolve to support the development of longitudinal studies in which the impact of gene-environmental risks will have time to demonstrate their effects on the development of psychopathology.

In the area of pathophysiology, our ability to directly correlate the functioning of the human brain with behavioral, cognitive, and emotional expressions will depend on additional advances in structural and functional imaging techniques. Likewise, advances in molecular biology will enable additional understanding of how genetic instructions affect cellular functions that are normal or pathological. Informed by genetic studies, imaging techniques will also improve our ability to identify phenotypes between individuals with shared genetic risk for disorders, such as schizophrenia. All of these advances are critical for understanding how both pharmacologic and psychosocial interventions can effectively treat mental disorders, and in the future may play an important role in validating diagnosis.

While we are waiting for advances in the basic and applied sciences to improve our treatment capacity, we will need to focus on maximizing the effectiveness of currently available treatments and in assuring the accessibility of these treatments to the population with mental disorders. Survey data from the United States and the World Health Organization have demonstrated that, despite their high prevalence, mental disorders, both in the United States and internationally, frequently go untreated. And while a majority of these disorders may be mild in severity, as many as two-thirds of individuals with serious mental illness do not receive treatment. Mental health treatment has long been considered by insurance companies and their lobbyists less imperative than that of general medical conditions. The current focus on health reform that incorporates national parity insurance coverage for mental disorders will be critical for the mental health field to guide and study.

LINDA B. COTTLER, PhD, MPH
PRESIDENT 2010
WASHINGTON UNIVERSITY SCHOOL OF MEDICINE
SAINT LOUIS, MISSOURI
COTTLER@EPI.WUSTL.EDU

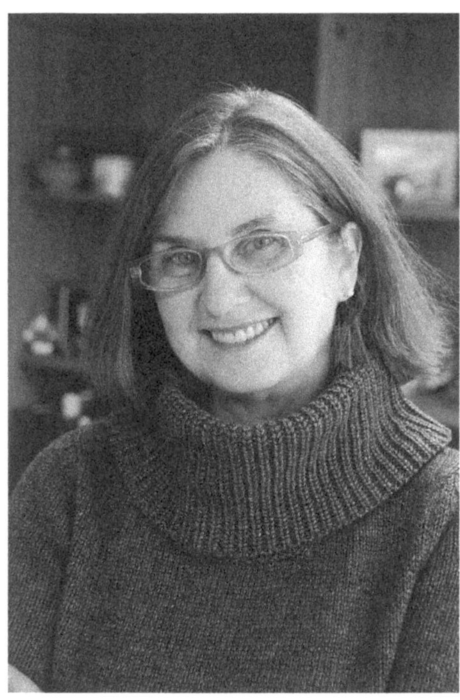

As all other Presidents have said, predicting the next 100 years is impossible. Our environment has changed dramatically in the past 100 years. Even though we are in the era of the genome, where all the functions of each gene are being identified, and where we are beginning to understand how genetic factors affect health and illness, we still don't know with certainty who will develop a mental or other illness. Given this, I believe the next 100 years will focus on preventing illness and exposures that might lead to illness.

Currently, this is an exciting time for psychiatry. It is a time when epidemiological strategies are needed more than ever to uncover risk factors related to health and disease. As an epidemiologist, this makes me happy! It is a time when disciplines are being blended together, in a meaningful way, and when our input is needed and valued. It is a time when greater emphasis is being placed on healthy lifestyles. However, the kinds of studies we conduct, in all areas of medicine, must change. We need to achieve higher response rates, recruit more underrepresented populations, collect quality data, and do these studies with the highest ethical standards. Our studies must also be culturally acceptable and globally transferrable in this age of global health. Mobile technologies will ease our recruitment problems and minimize bias.

To achieve success, our next steps require us to get back to the basics—to go farther with methods, or as people now call it, implementation science. We will need to use innovative methods to assess and uncover all environmental and behavioral modifiable factors in our world so we can link biological data to exposure variables to understand more fully what leads to health and disease.

As Rose stated so eloquently, a small reduction in risk for a large number of people could have much more impact on the public's health than a large reduction in risk for a small number of people. Thus, I believe that prevention messages—focused on small reductions in risk—will have as much or more benefits to the population than identifying the genes for individual behaviors. I also believe that holistic interventions that are adaptive in their focus will be important. There isn't a "one intervention fits all" strategy now, and there won't be one in the future either. Interventions must be tailored to a risk indicator, like is the case with cancer therapy.

I believe also that the time is overdue for community-engaged mental health research that brings our findings to the people—in the community, in vans, in storefronts –where people live. More and more community-engaged research is being conducted in the community rather than in hospitals and institutions.

Finally, I believe the future of the APPA rests with all of you reading this essay. We on the Council do our part to increase membership and plan meetings; however, the organization will survive another 100 years only if we involve more young members in a decision-making capacity in our organization. Our meeting topics must be relevant to you, and our speakers must be diverse. We urge you to come to meetings, and participate in the APPA. Only then can we move forward and make progress in the next 100 years and bring mental health into public health.

Disclosure Statements from Contributors

Sergio Aguilar-Gaxiola: S.A.-G. has no conflicts of interest to disclose. He is funded through NIH grant number UL1 RR024146 from the National Center for Research for Medical Research.

Murray Alpert: M.A. has no conflicts of interest to disclose.

James E. Barrett: J.E.B. has no conflicts of interest to disclose.

Martha L. Bruce: M.L.B. receives research funds from the NIMH and has no conflicts of interest to disclose.

O. Joseph Bienvenu: O.J.B. has no conflicts of interest to disclose. He is funded by the NIH only (NIMH and NHLBI), grants: R01 HL088045, R01 MH085016, R01 HL91760, 3R01 HL09760-02S1, and R01 MH71507.

Adrie W. Bruijnzeel: A.W.B. has no conflicts of interest to disclose. He is funded by the NIH (R01DA023575, R03DA020502), the Flight Attendant Medical Research Institute (Young Clinical Scientist Award #052312), and the James and Esther King Biomedical Research Program.

Catina Callahan O'Leary: C.C.O. has no conflicts of interest to disclose.

Redonna K. Chandler: R.K.C. is a full-time employee of the National Institute on Drug Abuse, National Institutes of Health, U.S. Department of Health and Human Services. Dr. Chandler reports no biomedical financial interests or other potential conflicts of interest.

C. Robert Cloninger: C.R.C. has no financial relationship with a commercial entity that has an interest in the subject of this manuscript.

Wilson M. Compton: W.M.C. is a full-time employee of the National Institute on Drug Abuse, National Institutes of Health, U.S. Department of Health and Human Services. He has no stock ownership positions of relevance to this chapter, but he does have stock ownership positions in Abbott Labs, General Electric, and Pfizer (between $1,000 and $15,000 each).

John N. Constantino: J.N.C. reports that to his knowledge, all of his or his coauthors' possible conflicts of interest, financial or otherwise, including direct or indirect financial or personal relationships, interests, and affiliations, whether or not directly related to the subject of the chapter, are listed as follows: He receives royalties from Western Psychological Services for commercial distribution of the Social Responsiveness Scale, a quantitative measure of autistic impairment that is unrelated to the content of this book chapter. He receives research support from the Centers for Disease Control and from the National Institute of Child Health and Human Development.

Linda B. Cottler: L.B.C. is funded by the NIH including NIDA, NIMH, NHLBI, NCRR, and NIH Fogarty International Center. She has received non-NIH funding from Pinney Associates (funded by Shire Pharmaceuticals), JMJ Technologies (funded by the U.S. Department of State), Terra Nova (funded by NIMH), and ESPN. She reports no Speakers' Bureaus. She is paid as Co-Editor of *Current Opinion in Psychiatry*, SUD.

Francine Cournos: F.C. has no conflicts of interest to disclose. Her only sources of income are derived from HRSA and PEPFAR federal funding streams and the private practice of psychiatry.

Rosa M. Crum: R.M.C. has no conflicts of interest to disclose. She is funded by the NIH only, grant support: NIAAA (AA016346 and AA014869).

J. Raymond DePaulo, Jr.: J.R.D. reports no biomedical financial interests or potential conflicts of interest.

Bruce P. Dohrenwend: B.P.D. reports no biomedical interests or potential conflicts of interest.

David L. Dunner: D.L.D. has received grant support from Neuronetics and Cyberonics. He is a consultant for Eli Lilly, Wyeth, Cyberonics, Healthcare Technology Systems, Jazz Pharma, SanofiAventis, and Medavante. He has been on the Speaker's Bureau for Eli Lilly, Wyeth, Neuronetics, Pfizer, AstraZeneca, Janssen, and BristolMyersSquibb.

William W. Eaton: W.W.E. has no conflicts of interest to disclose. His sources of research support are from the National Institute on Drug Abuse, NIH DA026652, and the National Institute of Mental Health, NIH MH53188.

Max Fink: M.F. has no conflicts of interest to disclose.

Ellen Frank: E.F. is on the Advisory Board for Servier International and receives royalties from Guilford Press.

Alfred M. Freedman: A.M.F. has no biomedical financial interests or financial conflicts of interest.

Sandro Galea: S.G. has no conflicts of interest to disclose.

Elliot S. Gershon: E.S.G. reports no biomedical financial interests or potential conflicts of interest.

Margo Genderson: M.G. has no conflicts of interest to disclose. She is currently a doctoral student at Boston University and is participating in a clinical externship at Georgetown University's Counseling and Psychiatric Services Center. She was previously funded by the NIH/NIA. Grant support: The VETSA Longitudinal Twin Study of Cognition and Aging; NIH/NIA (R01 AG018384).

Marci E.J. Gleason: M.E.J.G. has a research project that is supported by a grant from the National Institute of Mental Health (MH077840, Thomas Oltmanns, PI). With that exception, she has no biomedical financial interests or potential conflicts of interest to disclose.

Mark S. Gold: M.S.G. has no conflicts of interest to disclose.

Michael D. Grant: M.D.G. has no conflicts of interest to disclose. He is funded by the NIH/NIA only. Grant support: The VETSA Longitudinal Twin Study of Cognition and Aging, NIH/NIA (R01 AG018384); The VETSA Longitudinal MRI Twin Study of Aging, NIH/NIA (R01 AG022381).

Alden L. Gross: A.L.G. has no conflicts of interest to disclose. He is currently a postdoctoral fellow at the Aging Brain Center, Institute for Aging Research, Harvard Medical School.

Katherine A. Halmi: K.A.H. has no conflicts of interest to disclose.

John E. Helzer: J.E.H. has no conflicts of interest to disclose.

Michael Herkov: M.H. has no conflicts of interest to disclose.

James J. Hudziak: J.J.H. reports no biomedical financial interests or potential conflicts of interest.

David S. Janowsky: D.S.J. serves on the scientific board of QRxPharma.

Donald F. Klein: D.F.K. has no conflicts of interest to disclose.

Mirja Koschorke: M.K. has no conflicts of interest to disclose. She is funded by the Wellcome Trust (Clinical PhD Fellowship) through the London School of Hygiene and Tropical Medicine, London, UK.

Michael J. Lyons: M.J.L. has no conflicts of interest to disclose. He is funded by the NIH only, grant support: 1R01AG018384.

Karen McKinnon: K.M. has no conflicts of interest to disclose. She is funded by the NIMH, HRSA, and the NYS Department of Health and NYS Office of Mental Health only.

Lisa J. Merlo: L.J.M. has no conflicts of interest to disclose. She was funded by the NIDA only, grant support: National Institute on Drug Abuse training grant T32-DA-0731310 (PI: Linda B. Cottler).

Carol S. North: C.S.N. discloses research funding from the NIMH; NIAAA; NIDDK; VA; American Psychiatric Association; Tarrant County, TX; and the UT Southwestern Medical Center; employment at VA North Texas Health Care System; consulting fees from the University of Oklahoma Health Sciences Center; and speakers' fees from Washington University in St. Louis.

Vikram Patel: V.P. has no conflicts of interest to disclose. He is funded by the Wellcome Trust, the John and Catherine MacArthur Foundation, and Autism Speaks.

Thomas F. Oltmanns: T.F.O. has a research project that is supported by a grant from the National Institute of Mental Health (MH077840, Thomas Oltmanns, PI). With that exception, he has no biomedical financial interests or potential conflicts of interest to report.

Martin Prince: M.P. has no conflicts of interest to disclose. He is funded by the Wellcome Trust only, grant support: Cardiovascular Risk, Nutrition and Dementia Incidence in Admixed Populations Undergoing Rapid Health Transition–Latin America and China (080002/Z/06/Z).

Judith L. Rapoport: J.L.R. has no conflicts of interest to disclose.

Darrel A. Regier: D.A.R. reports no biomedical financial interests or potential conflicts of interest. As Executive Director of APIRE, he oversees all federal and industry-sponsored research and research training grants in APIRE but receives no external salary funding or honoraria from any government or industry sources.

Anna Roytberg: A.R. is a radiologist resident at Brown University, Rhode Island Hospital and has no conflicts of interest to disclose.

Norman Sartorius: N.S. has served as a consultant to Lundbeck and Servier, and as a member of the advisory board of Eli Lilly. He gave talks and chaired scientific symposia organized by Actelion, AstraZeneca, Janssen, and Lilly.

Patrick E. Shrout: P.A.S. has no conflicts of interest to disclose.

Maria Steenland: M.S. has no conflicts of interest to disclose.

Catherine W. Striley: C.W.S. was a paid consultant for the Robert Wood Johnson Foundation in 2009 and 2010 and has received salary support from a contract between Dr. Linda Cottler and Pinney Associates, funded by Shire Pharmaceuticals.

Ming T. Tsuang: M.T.T. has no conflicts of interest to disclose.

Milton Wainberg: M.W. has no conflicts of interest to disclose. He is funded by the NIMH, NIDA, and NIAAA as follows: 1) R01DA026775, Wainberg (PI): HIV/STI Prevention for Adolescents with Substance Use Disorder in Treatment; 2) R34MH090843, Rabkin & Wainberg (MPI): Behavioral Activation/Armodafinil to Treat Fatigue in HIV/AIDS; and 3) R01 MH65163, Wainberg (PI): RCT of a Brazilian HIV Prevention Intervention for the SMI.

Myrna M. Weissman: M.M.W. has received funding from the National Institute of Mental Health (NIMH), the National Institute on Drug Abuse (NIDA), the National Alliance for Research on Schizophrenia and Depression (NARSAD), the Sackler Foundation, the Templeton Foundation, and the Interstitial Cystitis Association; and receives royalties from Oxford University Press, Perseus Press, the American Psychiatric Association Press, and MultiHealth Systems.

Linda Ziegahn: L.Z. has no conflicts of interest to disclose. She is funded through NIH grant number UL1 RR024146 from the National Center for Research for Medical Research.

Charles F. Zorumski: C.F.Z. has no conflicts of interest to disclose.

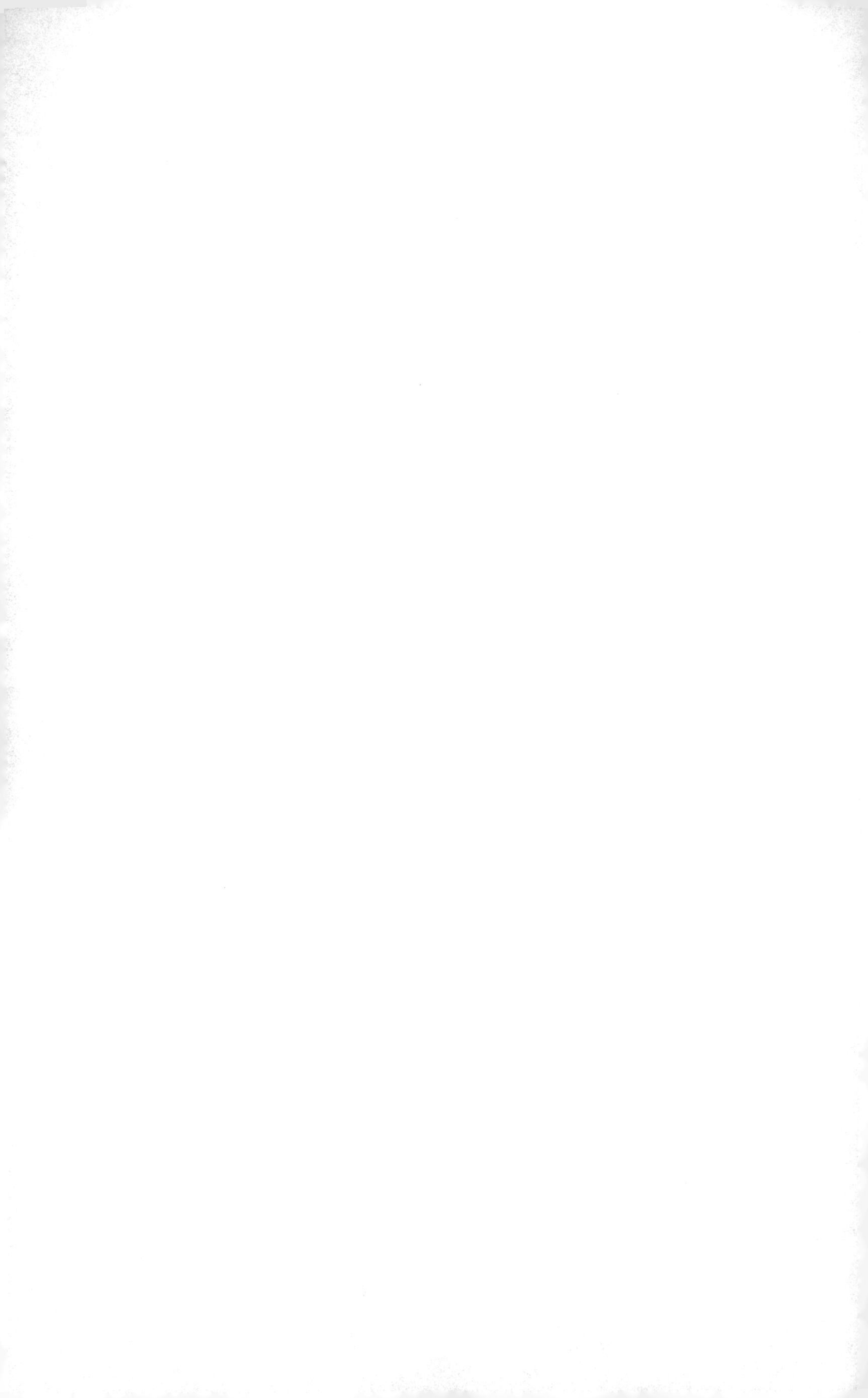

Index